COOK ONCE
Keto ALL WEEK

800
Affordable & Healthy Recipes to Speed Weight Loss, Lower Cholesterol & Reverse Diabetes for Busy People

---

4-Week
Progressive Easy Meal Prep System

NANCY TRAVIS

ISBN: 978-1-952613-11-1

TABLE OF CONTENT

Introduction..1

Chapter 1 Meal Prep for Keto Diet 101..........3
Why Choose Keto Meal Prep.................................3
The Keto Diet Principles 3
Keto Diet Food Pyramid 3
Keto Diet Macros Ratio.......................................5
How to Customizing Your Calories.....................5
The Keto Food List 5
Intermittent Fasting on Keto Diet 8

Chapter 2 Meal Prep Basics 9
Grab-and-go Containers 9
The Basic Storage Guideline..............................10
Must-have Kitchen Equipment 12

Chapter 3 Cook Once, Keto All Week.........13
Keto Meal Prep Guideline 13
4 Progressive Keto Meal Prep 14
Meal plan 1 15
Meal plan 2..19
Meal plan 3..24
Meal plan 4..29

Chapter 4 Breakfast.................................35
Pumpkin Bread And Salmon Sandwich.................36
Pancakes With Cream And Raspberries.................36
Spicy Eggs With Cheese 36
Scrambled Eggs With Salmon 37
Creamy Bagel Omelet 37
Cheesy Bacon Egg Cups 37
Buttery Eggs With Avocado Ang Spinach 37
Vinaigrette And Mushroom Frittata......................38
Goat Cheese And Asparagus Omelet......................38
Easy Sausage, Egg, And Cheese Casserole 38
Crunchy Cinnamon French Toast 39
Spicy Cheesy Eggs With Avocado And Cilantro.......39
Healthy Hemp Seed Porridge.............................39
Coffee Chia Smoothie 40
Sausage Breakfast 40
Keto Kale And Bacon With Eggs 40
Everything Bagel Seasoned Eggs 40
Walnut Granola 41
Chicken And Egg Stuffed Avocado 41

Eggs & Spinach Florentine 41
Scrambled Eggs With Cheese And Chili 41
Keto Cereal 42
Keto Cinnamon Flaxseed Bun Muffins...................42
Shrimp And Chives Omelet................................42
Waffle Sandwiches...43
Beef & Veggie Hash..43
Bacon Quiche..43
Creamy Bacon Omelet 44
Simple Scrambled Eggs 44
Basic Capicola Egg Cups 44
Stevia Chocolate Waffle 44
Bacon And Broccoli Egg Muffins..........................45
Strawberry Smoothie Bowl 45
Almond Cream Cheese Pancakes 45
Spanish Egg Frittata...45
Basic Cream Crepes 46
Low Carb Jambalaya With Chicken 46
Creamy Spanish Scrambled Eggs 46
Classic Omelet 46
Sausage And Spinach Hash Bowl 47
Lemon Allspice Muffins 47
Paleo Omelet Muffins 47
Nut-Free Granola With Clusters 48
Ham And Veggie Omelet In A Bag 48
Breadless Egg Sandwich 48

Chapter 5 Vegetable 49
Sauteed Mushroom 50
Spinach And Mushroom Italian-Style 50
Tasty Collard Greens 50
Simple Parmesan Zucchini Fries...........................50
Cauliflower Casserole 51
Spinach Casserole 51
Cheesy Cauliflower Bake 51
Syrian-Style Green Beans 51
Easy Asparagus Firy...52
Easy Baked Cabbage...52
Guacamole...52
Oven-Baked Keto Zucchini.................................52
Cauliflower, And Mushroom Casserole 53
Broccoli And Mushroom Soup Casserole 53
Ritzy Ratatouille 53
Crusted Zucchini Sticks.....................................54
Zucchini And Walnut Salad................................54

Milky Mushroom Soup..........................54
Cauliflower Hash With Poblano Peppers And Eggs..55
Asparagus And Pork Bake........................55
Easy Broccoli And Dill Salad...................55
Lemony Coleslaw 55
Spiralized Zucchini With Avocado Sauce.........56
Cheesy Cauliflower And Broccoli Bake...........56
Riced Broccoli With Almonds 56
Easy Asparagus With Walnuts 56
Vegetables Tricolor 57
Lemony Brussels Sprout Salad With Spicy Almond And Seed Mix.................57
Focaccia 57
Mushroom Pizzas With Tomato Slices 58
Stir-Fried Zucchini With Green Beans 58
Zucchini Lasagna 58
Odd Taste Vegan Pancake 59
Shichimi Collard Greens With Red Onion.........59
Zucchini Manicotti 59
Spinach, Artichoke And Cauliflower Stuffed Red Bell Peppers 60
Pecan And Veggies In Collard Wraps 60
Greedy Keto Vegetable Mix 60
Flaxseed With Olive And Tomato Focaccia 61
Seeds And Nuts Parfait 61
Riced Cauliflower And Leek Risotto 61
Zoodles With Butternut Squash And Sage 62
Luscious Vegetable Quiche 62
Sautéed Zucchini With Greens...................63
Scrumptious Briam 63

Chapter 6 Poultry 64

Creamy Chicken And Ham Meatballs...............65
Buttery Chicken And Mushrooms 65
Air-Fried Garlic-Lemon Chicken.................65
Sour Pepper Chicken 66
Italian Garlic Chicken Kebab 66
Chicken In Tomatoes And Herbs 66
Spicy Burnt-Fried Chicken 67
Crunchy Taco Chicken Wings.....................67
Spicy Cheesy Stuffed Avocados 67
Crispy Keto Wings With Rich Broccoli 67
Keto Chicken Casserole 68
Chicken Breast With Guacamole 68
Buttery Cheesy Garlic Chicken 69
Pan-Fried Creamy Chicken With Tarragon 69
Cheesy Low-Carb Chicken 69
Sour And Spicy Chicken Breast 69
Baked Chicken Thighs With Lemon Butter Caper Sauce............70
Spicy Oven-Baked Chicken 70
Grilled Spiced Chicken 70

Spicy Garlic Chicken Kebabs 71
Chicken And Herb Butter With Keto Zucchini Roll-Ups................71
Cheesy Chicken Dish With Spinach And Tomatoes....72
Delicious Parmesan Chicken 72
Almond Chicken Cordon Bleu.....................72
Grilled Chicken Breast 73
Garlic Chicken Low-Carb 73
Chicken Nuggets With Fried Green Bean And Bbq-Mayo...............73
Chicken Fajitas Bake 74
Pie Keto Chicken Curry 74
Rotisserie-Style Roast Chicken 74
Lemon Herb Chicken Breasts 75
Coleslaw With Crunchy Chicken Thighs 75
Bacon-Wrapped Chicken Breasts Stuffed With Spinach...............75
Michigander-Style Turkey.......................76
Savoury And Sticky Baked Chicken Wings.........76
Low-Carb Chicken With Tricolore Roasted Veggies.76
Buffalo Drumsticks With Chili Aioli 77
Chubby And Juicy Roasted Chicken 77
Oven-Baked Chicken In Garlic 77
Keto Chicken With Herb Butter 78
Chicken With Mushrooms And Parmesan 78
Keto Fried Chicken With Broccoli...............78
Chicken With Coconut Curry 79
Simple Chicken Tonnato 79
Chicken With Tomato Cream 79
Lemon-Rosemary Roasted Cornish Hens............80
Roast Chicken With Broccoli And Garlic 80
Grilled Tandori Chicken Thighs 81
Delicious Fried Chicken With Broccoli 81
Rotisserie Chicken And Keto Chili-Flavored Béarnaise Sauce............82
Chicken Wings And Blue Cheese Dip..............82
Lime Chicken Ginger............................83
Caesar Salad 83
Chicken Provençale 84
Gravy Bacon And Turkey 84
Roasted Chicken Thighs And Cauliflower.........85
Chicken Breast Wrapped With Bacon And Cauliflower Purée............85

Chapter 7 Beef, Lamb and Pork.................. 86

Roasted Lamb Rack 87
Kalamata Parsley Tapenade And Salted Lamp Chops...............87
Braised Beef Brisket...........................87
Beef Chuck Roast 88
Saucy Pernil Pork..............................88
Creamy Pork Tenderloin 88

Simple Spicy Beef Brisket 88
Italian Sausage Satay 89
Seasoned Beef Roast 89
Seasoned Pork Chops 89
Garlicky Pork Roast...................................89
Cheese Stuffed Pork Chops 90
Spiced Pork Tenderloin.................................90
Marinated Steak Sirloin Kabobs 90
Basil-Rubbed Pork Chops 91
Creamy Pork Loin And Mushrooms.....................91
Cheesy Pork Chops And Bacon 91
Lemony Pork Bake 91
Beef Tenderloin Steaks Wrapped 92
Sloppy Joes 92
Sausage, Beef And Chili Recipe 92
Beef Mini Meatloaves 93
Keto Burgers..93
Pork Chops With Dijon Mustard 93
Beef And Buttered Brussels Sprouts 94
Garlicky Beef Steak 94
Spicy Lamb Meat 94
Baked Pork Gyros 94
Coconut Pork Chops 95
Spanish Beef Empanadas 95
Hearty Calf's Liver Platter 95
Bbq Party Pork Kabobs.................................96
Italian Metballs Parmigiana 96
Cheesy Lamb Sliders 96
Wine Braised Lamb Shanks 97
Keto Beef Burger 97
One-Pan Sausage & Broccoli 97
Lemony Pork Loin Roast 98
Pork Chops With Caramelized Onion 98
Pork Chops Stuffed With Cheese-Bacon Mix 98
Mint Oil Braised Lamb Chops 99
Thai Pork Meal.......................................99
Classic Sausage & Beef Meatloaf......................99
Roasted Vietnamese Lamb Chops 99
Herbed Lamb Leg.....................................100
Tangy Lamb Patties...................................100
Oven-Baked Lamb Leg.................................100
Zesty Lamb Leg 101
Sweet And Spicy Pork 101
Colorful Sausage & Bell Peppers Combo.................102
Baked Brussels Sprouts And Pine Nut With Bacon 102

Deviled Egg With Shrimp 105
Salmon Pie 105
Pan Seared Tilapia With Almond Crust....................105
Tasty Mahi Mahi Cakes 106
Keto Taco Fishbowl.....................................106
Grilled White Fish With Zucchini 106
Salmon With Tomato And Basil 107
Grilled Spicy Shrimp....................................107
Salmon Fillets With Dill And Lemon 107
Easy Salmon Steaks With Dill 107
Salmon Blackened Fillets 108
Crispy Keto Creamy Fish Casserole 108
Coconut Keto Salmon And Napa Cabbage 108
Parchment Baked Salmon 109
Classic Shrimp Scampi 109
Stuffed Mediterranean Swordfish 109
Low Carb Poached Eggs With Tuna Salad.............109
Cabbage Plate With Keto Salmon 110
Keto Maui Wowie Shrimp 110
Smoked Salmon And Lettuce Bites 110
Ahi Tuna Steaks.......................................111
Salmon With Garlic Dijon Mustard 111
Grilled Tuna Salad With Garlic Sauce 111
Asparagus Seared Salmon 111
Grilled Red Lobster Tails 112
Low Carb Seafood Chowder 112
Cheesy Broccoli With Keto Fried Salmon 112
Keto Chili-Covered Salmon With Spinach 113
Keto Egg Butter And Smoked Salmon 113
Keto Baked Salmon With Butter........................113
Cheesy Verde Shrimp 113
Best Marinated Grilled Shrimp 114
Cheesy Keto Tuna Casserole...........................114
Creamy Salmon Sauce Zoodles 114
Salmon Fillets Baked With Dijon........................115
Blackened Trout 115
Trout Fillets With Lemony Yogurt Sauce.................115
Delicious Keto Ceviche 115

Chapter 9 Soup and Stew.................................116

Cheesy Cauliflower Soup 117
Cauliflower Cream Soup................................117
Shrimp Mushroom Chowder 117
Egg Broth 118
Pork Tarragon Soup 118
Creamy Broccoli And Cauliflower Soup 118
Chicken Turnip Soup...................................119
Spinach Mushroom Soup 119
Garlicky Chicken Soup 119
Stewed Mahi Mahi 119
Cauliflower Curry Soup 120
Red Gazpacho Cream Soup 120

Chapter 8 Seafood and Fish 103

Lemony Grilled Calamari................................104
Browned Salmon Cakes.................................104
Snow Crab Clusters With Garlic Butter 104
Spiced Fish Curry 104

Sour And Spicy Shrimp Soup With Mushrooms.....120
Rich Beef Stew With Dumpling 121
Zucchini Cream Soup 121
Swiss Chard Egg Soup......................................121
Asparagus Cream Soup 122
Keto Beef Soup 122
Beef Taco Soup 122
Cheesy Zucchini Soup......................................122
Creamy Tomato Soup 123
Creamy Bacon And Tilapia Chowder 123
Zesty Double Beef Stew 123
Creamy Minty Spinach Soup...............................123
Lettuce Soup With Poached Egg 124
Sweet And Sour Chicken Soup With Celery 124
Zucchini Soup 124
Buttery Salmon And Leek Soup............................124
Broccoli Cheddar Soup 125
New England Clam Chowder 125
Spicy Shrimp And Chorizo Soup With Tomatoes And Avocado 125
Green Garlic And Cauliflower Soup.......................126
Bay Scallop And Bacon Chowder 126
Keto Beef Stew 126
Lamb Soup...126
Spicy Halibut In Tomato Soup 127
Sour Garlic Zucchini Soup 127
Creamy Beef And Broccoli Soup............................128
Cauliflower Leek Soup 128
Chicken And Mushroom Soup 128
Stewed Meat And Pumpkin 129
Creamy Crockpot Chicken Stew 129
Easy Green Soup 129
Creamy Veggie Soup...130
Sour Chicken And Kale Soup 130
Spicy Pork And Spinach Stew..............................131
Creamy Spinach Soup..131
Creamy Garlic Pork With Cauliflower Soup 131
Cheesy Sausage Soup With Tomatoes And Spinach .....
....132
Garlicky Pork Soup With Cauliflower And Tomatoes
....132
Creamy And Cheesy Spicy Avocado Soup 132
Cheesy Turkey And Bacon Soup With Celery And Parsley 133
Curried Shrimp And Green Beans Soup 133

Chapter 10 Appetizers and Snacks 134

Easy Enchilada Chicken Dip................................135
Keto Baked Eggs 135
Buttered Lobster And Cream Cheese Dip................135
Deviled Mayonnaise Eggs 135
Tasty Artichoke Dip 136
Grilled Portobello Mushrooms 136
Bacon-Wrapped Jalapeno Poppers 136
Tomatoes And Jalapeño Salsa 136
Keto Bacon-Wrapped Barbecue Shrimp 137
Balsamic Mushrooms 137
Keto Cheddar And Bacon Mushrooms 137
Red Pepper Roasted Dip 137
Easily Baked Buffalo Chicken Dip.........................138
Keto Smoked Salmon Fat Bombs 138
Baba Ghanoush...138
Mexican-Style Scrambled Eggs 138
Cheesy Cauliflower Crackers 139
Crab–Stuffed Avocado......................................139
Prosciutto And Asparagus Wraps 139
Hearty Bacon And Mushroom Platter 139
Low-Carb Cheesy Almond Biscuits 140
Cheesy Cauliflower Bake 140
Buttered Coconut Puffs....................................140
Deviled Eggs With Bacon And Cheese....................140
Baked Beef, Pork And Veal Meatballs.....................141
Almond Sausage Balls 141
Mediterranean Baked Spinach 141
Easy Parmesan Roasted Bamboo Sprouts 141
Stuffed Cheesy Mushrooms 142
Grilled Spicy Shrimp.......................................142
Spinach And Cheese Stuffed Mushrooms 142
Simple Broccoli Casserole..................................143
Low Carb Keto Sausage Balls..............................143
Buffalo Chicken And Cheese Dip 143
Almond Fritters With Mayo Sauce 143
Keto Broiled Bell Pepper 144
Cheddar Cheese Jalapeño Poppers 144
Fluffy Western Omelet......................................144
Cheesy Baked Jalapeño Peppers 145
Crispy Chicken 145
Easy Parmesan Chive And Garlic Crackers 145
Cheesy Crab Stuffed Mushrooms 146
Sweet And Zesty Chicken Wings 146
Homemade Cheddar Crackers 146
Cauliflower Bread Sticks With Cheese 147
Cheesy Keto Cupcakes......................................147
Chive Deviled Eggs And Savory Chorizo 147

Chapter 11 Desserts 148

Almond Meal Cupcakes 149
Keto Vanilla Ice Cream.....................................149
Almond Cinnamon Cookies 149
Egg Avocado Cups 149
Cream Cheese Chocolate Mousse 150
Vanilla Mug Cake...150
Cheesecake Strawberries...................................150
Keto Pumpkin Spice Fat Bombs...........................150

Chocolate Vanilla Cake 151
Chocolate Peanut Fudge 151
Mini Cheesecakes 151
Spicy Almond Fat Bombs............................ 152
Strawberries In Chocolate 152
Chocolate Granola Bars............................... 152
Raspberry And Chocolate Fat Bombs 152
Keto Lava Cake 153
Double Chocolate Brownies........................ 153
Frosted Snickerdoodle Cupcakes............... 153
Keto Mocha Ice Cream 154
Keto Chocolate-Coconut Bites.................... 154
Coco Avocado Truffles 154
Healthy Vanilla-Almond Ice Pops 154
Almond Flour Shortbread Cookies 155
Keto Almond Butter Fudge Slices 155
Low-Carb Raspberry Cheesecake 155
Cardamom Orange Bark............................... 155
Healthy Blueberry Fat Bombs 156
Low-Carb Chocolate Chip Cookies 156
Cream Cheese Brownies 156
Chia Pudding With Blueberries 156
Macadamia Nut And Chocolate Fat Bombs........... 157
Strawberry Popsicles 157
Easy Coconut Mounds 157
Easy Peanut Butter Cookies......................... 157
Almond And Cinnamon Truffles................. 158
Hemp Seeds And Chocolate Cookies.......... 158
Gooey Creamy Cake 158
Almond Snickerdoodle Cookies 158
Chocolate-Crusted Coffee Bites.................. 159
Keto Matcha Brownies With Pistachios................. 159
Gingersnap Nutmeg Cookies 159
Microwaved Rhubarb Cakes 160
Berry Tart... 160
Chocolate Tart 160
Almond Pumpkin Pie 161
Chilled Vanilla Ice Cream........................... 161
Keto Chocolate Cute Mug Cake................... 161
Smooth And Puffed Coconut Mousse....................... 162
Caramel And Cream With Coconut Panna Cotta ... 162
Chocolate And Blueberry Truffles 162
Chocolate-Strawberry Mousse.................... 163
Chocolate Marshmallows 163

Chapter 12 Salad....................................164

Watercress And Arugula Turkey Salad 165
Spinach Salad With Mustard Vinaigrette And Bacon
....165
Seared Rump Steak Salad 165
Sun-Dried Tomato And Feta Cheese Salad 166
Avocado, Cucumber And Bacon Salad................... 166

Chicken Salad With Parmesan Cheese.................... 166
Beef, Pork, And Vegetable Salad With Yoghurt
Dressing..166
Iceberg Lettuce Salad With Bacon And Gorgonzola
Cheese 167
Brussels Sprouts Citrus Bacon Dressing................ 167
Egg Salad With Mustard Dressing 167
Lettuce Wraps With Mackerel...................... 168
Green Chicken Salad 168
Bacon, Smoked Salmon And Poached Egg Salad...168
Brussel Sprouts And Spinach Salad 169
Easy Lunch Salad 169
Crabmeat And Celery Salad 169
Sumptuous Egg Salad................................... 169
Chicken, Cranberry, And Pecan Salad................... 170
Creamed Omega-3 Salad 170
Ranch Chicken And Bacon Salad 170
Simple Cauliflower Salad 170
Colorful Crab Ceviche Appetizer 171
Veggies And Calamari Salad 171
Easy Mediterranean Salad 171
Tasty Avocado Shrimp Salad 171
Green Salad With Baked Halibut 172
Shrimp Salad With Egg And Mayonnaise................ 172
Salmon And Almond Salad 172
Caprese Salad.. 172
Breaded Chicken Strips And Spinach Salad 173
Keto Lemon Dressing, Walnuts And Zucchini Salad
....173
Crispy Almonds With Brussels Sprout Salad 173
Feta Cheese And Cucumber Salad........................... 174
Delicious Steak Salad 174
Salmon Asparagus Pecan Salad........................... 174
Crab Salad.. 174
Kale And Avocado Salad With Lemon Dijon
Vinaigrette Dressing 175
Tasty Shrimp Salad 175
Mint And Tuna Salad................................... 175
Baked Salsa Chicken 175
Shrimp Salad With Avocado And Tomatoes........... 176
Green Anchovy Dressing 176
Lobster Salad 176
Keto Quick Caesar Dressing 176
Tuna Stuffed Avocados 177
Low-Carb Dressing.......................................177
Chicken Salad With Ranch Dressing.......................177
Grilled Salmon And Greek Salad 178
Cheesy Keto Chicken Broccoli Casserole 178
Appendix 1: Measurement Conversion Chart......... 179
Appendix 2:Index...180

INTRODUCTION

Ketogenic diet literally has dominated the dieting realm in recent decades, it may have been treated as a fad diet in the beginning, but with the passing of time, with thousands of Keto dieters experimenting, testing on this concept and this new way of life, and with plenty of scientific research endorsing, the Keto diet has undoubtedly been put to the dieting throne and accepted by thousands of people all over the world.

Yes, the Keto diet is highly beneficial and crazily popular, but one should not neglect the fact that it has also been dubbed as one of if not the most restrictive diets. Its core emphasis on cutting carbohydrates and adding fats into your diet may seem easy at first. But when I tell you, you should cut almost all sugar you put into your mouth; you may think, well, that's easy, I'll just toss out or give away all my honey and syrup in my pantry, and I am definitely on the fast lane towards Keto success. Well, not this easy, tiger! The food industry has developed to the extent where added sugar is almost ubiquitous in the foods you find in the grocery store, and foods you firmly believe are safe may present severe problems to your Keto success. So, if you are serious about Keto diet, take the food under your hands and start cooking by yourself.

You may ask:
I am super busy with my daily routines and my responsibilities, and cooking is so tedious, messy, and takes so much time. What do I do?

After a tour of my local whole foods, I find the Keto foods are expensive, and I don't trust my cooking skills with my 15 dollars per pound grass-fed sirloin. And I am not a kitchen savvy person, all the clumsiness and blundering in the kitchen will kill me if you have these doubts and insecurities.

Well, meal prepping is the answer.

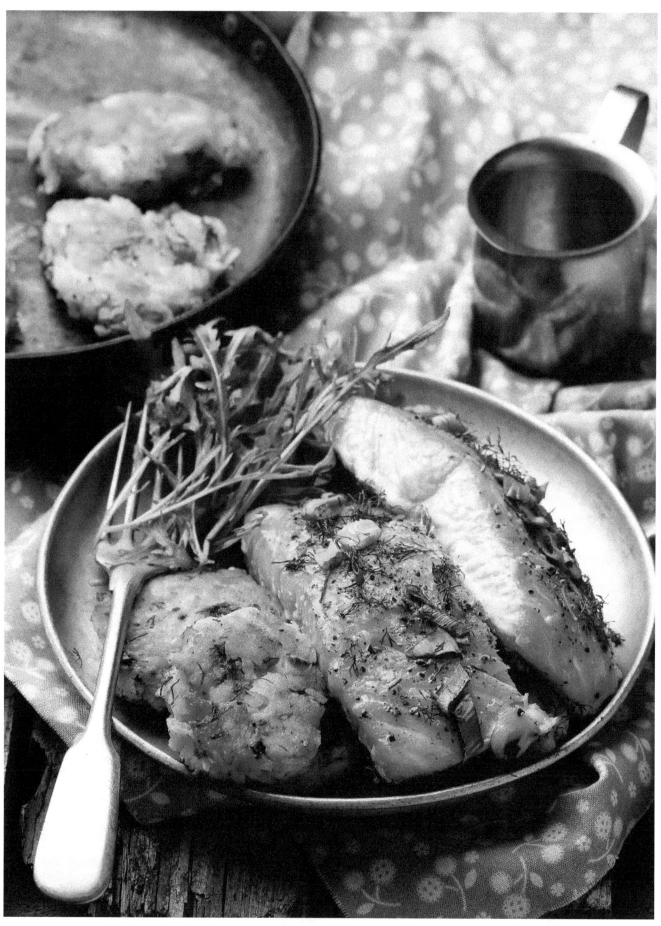

Chapter 1 Meal Prep for Keto Diet 101

Why Choose Keto Meal Prep

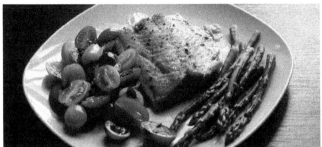

Meal prepping could bring us enormous benefits in our everyday Keto life.

① Reduce food cost: meal prepping undoubtedly can help save money. Except for avoiding food waste, smart shopping can significantly enhance your efficiency and decrease daily expenditure.
Tips for saving money:
- Purchasing items in bulk
- Shopping sales and using coupons
- Shopping seasonal produce (abundant, tasty and least expensive)

② Cut down cooking time and allow more time to enjoy life: this may be the most desirable benefit of meal prep. No one will stay in the kitchen for hours to cook every day, on top of that, you still need time to clean up the mess afterward.
Tips for solving this problem:
- Batching cooking is the top advice.
- Use simple staples and easy-to-find ingredients
- Precook the ingredients for recipes later in the week
- Purchase already cut and washed produce or use frozen foods
- Repeat meals during the week
- Use the same ingredients in multiple recipes

③ Keep the consistency of your Keto plan: You need to put in attention and energy into the keto diet to persist. Otherwise, giving up halfway through is almost a sure thing. When conducting meal prep for your Keto diet plan, you will make Keto meals for the following whole week, which means there is no need to concern about what to eat for each meal in the following week and just grab the containers in your refrigerator and go to work or study. Just imagine the freedom meal prepping gives you!

④ Control what you eat and the portion: as we all know, in the early stage of Keto diet, one would often encounter problems like craving for sweets, snacks or non-Keto foods, or eating the right food but the portion is probably out of control. Mealing planning can go a long way in resolving these problems, because you already know what to eat and how much to eat for each day and each meal of the week.

⑤ Break free of the kitchen: Without a meal plan, just imagine how you will spend 4 hours each day to prepare a Keto meal. What if there are missing ingredients for the recipe you are going to make? In busy days, spare time is limited. We can make our Keto-style life more comfortable by creating meal plans in advance and cook in batches. After all, Keto diet is not just about eating and cooking. Work, entertainment, exercise... there is definitely more to the keto life than obsessing over every calorie you eat.

The Keto Diet Principles

Understanding the principles guiding the Keto diet is crucial in your Keto journey. An easy and straightforward way to put it is to reduce your daily carb intake to 50 grams or even fewer. And significantly increase your fat intake.

Here to give you a picture of the card content in our everyday foods: a large potato 50 grams; a slice of pizza; 40 grams; a bagel; 30 grams; a medium apple; 21 grams. So you need to be careful and conscious about the food you put into your mouth, especially the carb-concentrated foods.

When talking about fat, the first thing that might pop into your head may be lard and oils. However, there are far more food choices that are fat-condensed, to name a few: an avocado has roughly 29 grams , an ounce of macadamia nuts contain 21 grams and an ounce of pecans contains, 20 grams. All in all, fat can be found everywhere, and your high-fat pursuit can be a breeze if you choose the right food.

Keto Diet Food Pyramid

So, when you apply Keto diet principles into your food selection, you will find there is a hierarchy among different foods.

There are foods that are the epitome of Keto diet, which contain high and healthy fat, and/or low carbs. And there are foods that should be consumed with careful calculation, and you may also need to put some foods into the no-fly zone.

KETO DIET FOOD PYRAMID

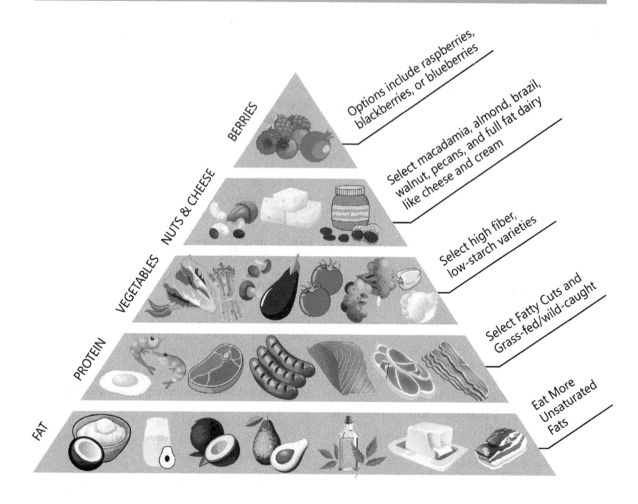

BERRIES — Options include raspberries, blackberries, or blueberries

NUTS & CHEESE — Select macadamia, almond, brazil, walnut, pecans, and full fat dairy like cheese and cream

VEGETABLES — Select high fiber, low-starch varieties

PROTEIN — Select Fatty Cuts and Grass-fed/wild-caught

FAT — Eat More Unsaturated Fats

BEVERAGES

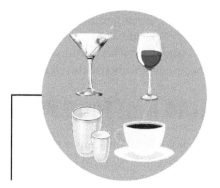

Dry wine, Spirits, coffee, tea and water are generally low-carb, always read nutrition labels

FOODS TO AVOID

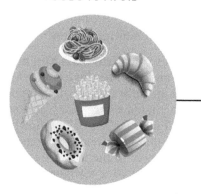

Avoid desserts, candy, pastas, cereals, breads and starches like corn and potatoes

THE MACROS RATIO OF KETO DIET

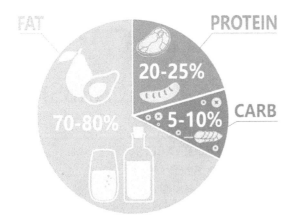

FAT   PROTEIN

20-25%

70-80%   5-10%   CARB

HIGH FAT   MODERATE PROTEIN   LOW CARB

Keto Diet Macros Ratio

The three categories of macros are fats, carbohydrates, and protein. The standard Keto diet features a macro ratio of about 70-80% fat, 20-25% protein, and 5-10% of carbohydrate.

Based on a standard 2000-calorie daily caloric intake, it requires daily fat consumption of around 150 grams to shift your metabolism so it burns fat as fuel, so you need to plan your meals around fat-condensed foods like avocados, butter, ghee, fatty fish, meats, olives and olive oil.

You also need to slash your carbs from about 300 grams per day to less than 50 grams per day, which means abandon breads and sugar and shift towards leafy greens, non-starchy veggies, and low-carb fruits like berries.

Finally, eat a moderate amount of protein, around 90 grams per day or 30 grams per meal (about 4 ounces of meat, fish or poultry).

How to Calculate Your Calories

Understanding the number of nutrients that sits in every ingredient per meal consumed is a daunting task. Thankfully, many nutrient calculators aid in determining these figures. Consider these tips:
❖ Find a highly rated nutrient calculator online or app and follow the guidelines for calculating nutrient counts per meal.
❖ Also, visit the USDA National Nutrient Database at http://ndb.nal.usda.gov/ndb/search/list and follow the guidelines provided for calculating nutrient counts.

Determining your basal metabolic value
The basal metabolic value (BMR) is the number of calories that your body requires to sustain its basic functions. Calculating BMR varies for men and women, and uses the weight, height, and age in years to determine.

The formula:
Women:
$BMR = 655 + (9.6 \times \text{weight in kg}) + (1.8 \times \text{height in cm}) - (4.7 \times \text{age in years})$
Men:
$BMR = 66 + (13.7 \times \text{weight in kg}) + (5 \times \text{height in cm}) - (6.8 \times \text{age in years})$

How to Set Calorie Goals

Knowing your BMR helps you gain, lose, or maintain weight. By establishing how many calories your body burns, it helps you know how many of them to consume.
- To maintain weight, eat the same calories as you burn.
- To lose weight, eat fewer calories than you burn.
- To gain weight, eat more calories than you burn.
Using this formula can help you determine the amount of calories found per meal.

Note that:
- 1 gram of carbs = 4 calories
- 1 gram of protein = 4 calories
- 1 gram of fat = 9 calories

Calculate your macro percentage per meal
- Total fat % = [Total fat (g) × 9 ÷ total calories] × 100%
- Total protein % = [Total protein (g) × 4 ÷ total calories] × 100%
- Total carbs % = [Net carbs (g) × 4 ÷ total calories] × 100%

Also, note:
- The total figures per macros without the percentile gauge gives you the amount of representing macro against total calories.
- Net carbs (per meal) = Total carbs − fiber

The Keto Food List

This cookbook aims to help you cultivate a friendly and healthy habit of meal prepping for your Keto diet plan. The core of meal prep is meal management. To achieve this target, keep your prep simple, which means you should use simple staples and easy-to-find ingredients without lowering your life quality. This is the basis of meal prep. However, it's not enough. How to mobilize the resource is the key. Later on in this chapter, the four progressive meal preps will empower you to have the ability of meal management. And here lists of Keto food to enjoy and food to avoid will bring some clarity to your keto food choices:

KETO FOODS TO ENJOY
HIGH FAT / LOW CARB (BASED ON NET CARBS)

MEATS & SEAFOOD
- Beef (ground beef, steak, etc.)
- Chicken
- Crab
- Crawfish
- Duck
- Fish
- Goose
- Lamb
- Lobster
- Mussels
- Octopus
- Pork (pork chops, bacon, etc.)
- Quail
- Sausage (without fillers)
- Scallops
- Shrimp
- Veal
- Venison

DAIRY
- Blue cheese dressing
- Burrata cheese
- Cottage cheese
- Cream cheese
- Eggs
- Greek yogurt (full-fat)
- Grilling cheese
- Halloumi cheese
- Heavy (whipping) cream
- Homemade whipped cream
- Kefalotyri cheese
- Mozzarella cheese
- Provolone cheese
- Queso blanco
- Ranch dressing
- Ricotta cheese
- Unsweetened almond milk
- Unsweetened coconut milk

VEGETABLES
- Alfalfa sprouts
- Asparagus
- Avocados
- Bell peppers
- Broccoli
- Cabbage
- Carrots (in moderation)
- Cauliflower
- Celery
- Chicory
- Coconut
- Cucumbers
- Garlic (in moderation)
- Green beans
- Herbs
- Jicama
- Lemons
- Limes
- Mushrooms
- Okra
- Olives
- Onions (in moderation)
- Pickles
- Pumpkin
- Radishes
- Salad greens
- Scallions
- Spaghetti squash (in moderation)
- Tomatoes (in moderation)
- Zucchini

NUTS & SEEDS
- Almonds
- Brazil nuts
- Chia seeds
- Flaxseeds
- Hazelnuts
- Macadamia nuts
- Peanuts (in moderation)
- Pecans
- Pine nuts
- Pumpkin seeds
- Sacha inchi seeds
- Sesame seeds
- Walnuts

FRUITS
- Blackberries
- Blueberries
- Cranberries
- Raspberries
- Strawberries

KETO FOODS TO AVOID
LOW FAT / HIGH CARB (BASED ON NET CARBS)

MEATS & MEAT ALTERNATIVES
- Deli meat (some, not all)
- Hot dogs (with fillers)
- Sausage (with fillers)
- Seitan
- Tofu

DAIRY
- Almond milk (sweetened)
- Coconut milk (sweetened)
- Milk
- Soy milk (regular)
- Yogurt (regular)

NUTS & SEEDS
- Cashews
- Chestnuts
- Pistachios

VEGETABLES
- Artichokes
- Beans (all varieties)
- Burdock root
- Butternut squash
- Chickpeas
- Corn
- Edamame
- Eggplant
- Leeks
- Parsnips
- Plantains
- Potatoes
- Sweet potatoes
- Taro root
- Turnips
- Winter squash
- Yams

FRUITS &
- Apples
- Apricots
- Bananas
- Boysenberries
- Cantaloupe
- Cherries
- Currants
- Dates
- Elderberries
- Gooseberries
- Grapes
- Honeydew melon
- Huckleberries
- Kiwifruits
- Mangos
- Oranges
- Peaches
- Peas
- Pineapples
- Plums
- Prunes
- Raisins
- Water chestnuts

KETO COOKING STAPLES
1. Pink Himalayan salt
2. Freshly ground black pepper
3. Ghee (clarified butter, without dairy; buy grass-fed if you can)
4. Olive oil
5. Grass-fed butter

KETO PERISHABLES
1. Eggs (pasture-raised, if you can)
2. Avocados
3. Bacon (uncured)
4. Cream cheese (full-fat; or use a dairy-free alternative)
5. Sour cream (full-fat; or use a dairy-free alternative)
6. Heavy whipping cream or coconut milk (full-fat; I buy the coconut milk in a can)
7. Garlic (fresh or pre-minced in a jar)
8. Cauliflower
9. Meat (grass-fed, if you can)
10. Greens (spinach, kale, or arugula)

Intermittent Fasting on Keto Diet

Some people may find it difficult to enter ketosis even though you are doing everything right, if you are one of them, then you should definitely consider trying intermittent fasting. Intermittent fasting (IF) is the practice of going 16-24 hours without food. It can help you ease into ketosis or help produce ketone if you are in ketosis, intermittent fasting is effortless if you are doing the right way.

Benefits of intermittent fasting include:
- Boost energy
- Improve mental clarity
- Increase blood ketones
- Intermittent fasting benefits include:
- weight loss without slowed metabolism
- Enhance insulin sensitivity and lowered insulin levels
- lower blood pressure, cholesterol levels and triglycerides

There are various ways of Intermittent fasting. The two most common ways are:

16-hour fast: you will eat all your meals within an 8-hour time period and fast the remaining 16 hours. This can be done 3-5 days a week. This method is easy to implement with little effort. It may not limit calories significantly; however, it leaves the body time to increase ketone and allow the digestive system a good break. Research has found that restricting eating to within 8 or 9 hours does not negatively impact your ability to maintain or build muscle.

20-hour fast: you will eat all your meals within a 4-hour eating window and fast the remaining 20 hours. This protocol will probably prevent muscle gain while increasing fat loss.

While fasting, staying fully hydrated is key. Approved liquids to drink while fasting include black coffee, tea and bone broth.

Nevertheless, some occasions are not suitable for fasting. For example, please don't fast when you are restricting calories, Combining fasting with calorie restriction may lead to health imbalance, which may slow down your progress to fat-adaption and make you feel miserable. Also, please don't fast when you have crappy sleep, endless hunger, high stress levels, reduced ketones (because of the stress we 're putting on our bodies), less energy, and imbalanced hormones.. A misconception many have is that the more and longer you fast, the better off you'll be. Well, that is not true, Fasting should be part of a balanced fat-fueled lifestyle. Don't force yourself to fast if you don't feel right. We should always slow down and listen to our bodies. They tell us everything when you need the information.

Chapter 2 Meal Prep Basics

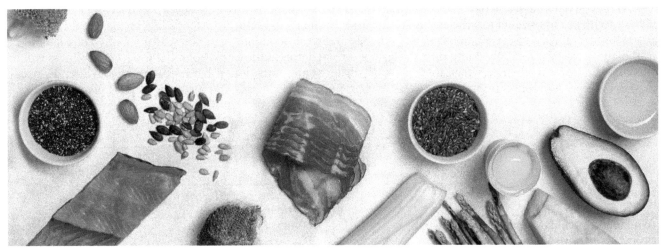

Grab-and-go Containers

Speak of meal prep, you need containers definitely, especially those that you can store in the fridge, put in your bags, and reheat in the microwaves. Below is a list of what to look for when purchasing your storage containers:

Leakproof: You definitely don't want to spill your sauce to stain your tote bag, especially when you are traveling or commuting. Choose a container that is durable and shatter-resistant with strong latches, so that even if it falls, it is still safe to use.

BPA-free: BPA (bisphenol A). BPA is an industrial chemical that has been used to make certain plastics and resins, and the plastics has long been used to produce food containers. Scientific research has shown that BPA can seep into the food or beverages. And exposure to BPA can lead to possible health damage to the brain, prostate gland of fetuses, infants and children. When storing your food, steer clear from the BPA and look for products labeled as BPA-free.

Stackable or nestable: In meal prepping, you will cook several servings all at once, and then you are going to store them in the fridge and then pack them in your bag. Stackable or nestable containers can save space both in your fridge and in your bag.

Microwave-, dishwasher- and freezer-safe: this one seem intuitive, since you need to store the containers in the fridge/ freezer, reheating them in the microwave before eating, and since you are cooking in batches, using the dishwasher will definitely cut out the annoying clean work.

When it comes to different materials of the containers, each has its advantages and disadvantages.

Plastic containers are durable and relatively cheaper, and they are also lightweight; however, the downside of plastics is that they absorb flavors and they exert adverse environmental impact.

Glass containers do not affect the taste, and they keep the food fresh and keep its flavours; however, glass containers are fragile, and this may bring safety issues, especially that the broken glass can get into your food.

Stainless steel can be resistant to fire and heat, and it retains strength at high temperatures. The main disadvantage is stainless steel containers are more expensive and they can't be reheated in the microwave.

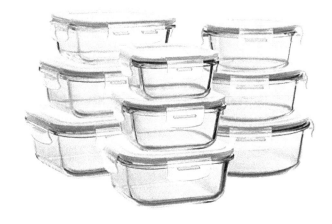

The Basic Storage Guideline

It's vital to always label and date the containers when you store food in the refrigerator and freezer. To minimize food spoilage, you should use the earliest dates first. In the refrigerator, raw foods like meats should be placed at the bottom. Ready-to-eat foods like cooked dishes and fresh food like vegetables, fruits and yogurt should be stored above the raw food. By doing this, the risk of cross-contamination and potential food-borne illness will be minimized. Use food when they're at their peak of freshness and nutrition or before the "best by " date. Here is a chart for freezer and refrigerator storage times of Keto popular foods (fats and meats in the first place):

FOOD STORAGE CHART

	FRIDGE	FREEZER
Salads: Egg Salad, Tuna Salad Chicken	3 TO 5 DAYS	DOES NOT FREEZE WELL
Hamburger, Meatloaf, And Other Dishes Made With Ground Meat(Raw)	1 TO 2 DAYS	3 TO 4 MONTHS
Steaks: Beef, Lamb Pork, (Raw)	3 TO 5 DAYS	3 TO 4 MONTHS
Chops: Beef, Lamb Pork, (Raw)	3 TO 5 DAYS	4 TO 6 MONTHS
Roasts: Beef, Lamb Pork, (Raw)	3 TO 5 DAYS	4 TO 12 MONTHS
Whole Chicken Turkey Or, (Raw)	1 TO 2 DAYS	1 YEAR
Pieces: Chicken Turkey Or, (Raw)	1 TO 2 DAYS	9 MONTHS
Soups And Stews With Vegetables And Meat	3 TO 4 DAYS	2 TO 3 MONTHS
Pizza	3 TO 5 DAYS	1 TO 2 MONTHS
Beef, Lamb Pork, Or Chicken(Cooked)	3 TO 5 DAYS	2 TO 6 MONTHS

FRESH MEATS	FRIDGE	FREEZER
Salads, Eggs, Fish	1 TO 2 DAYS	DOES NOT FREEZE WELL
Beef, Pork, Lamb	1 TO 2 DAYS	3 TO 4 MONTHS
Beacon	7 DAYS	1 MONTH
Poultry	1 TO 2 DAYS	9 TO 12 MONTHS

COOKED MEATS	FRIDGE	FREEZER
Salads, Eggs, Fish	3 TO 5 DAYS	DOES NOT FREEZE WELL
Beef, Pork, Lamb	3 TO 5 DAYS	3 TO 6 MONTHS(UP TO 12 MONTHS FOR ROASTS)
Beacon	7 DAYS	1 MONTH
Poultry	3 TO 5 DAYS	2 TO 4 MONTHS

Foods That Do Not Freeze Well

Most foods are suited to store in the refrigerator, but foods that can be stored in the freezer are not as many as that in the refrigerator. Foods that do not freeze well will lose flavor and original texture if stored in the freezer. Here I make a list of foods that do not freeze well:

Certain raw vegetables (such as cabbage, celery, watercress, cucumber, lettuce, and radishes)
- Cooked egg white
- Hard-boiled eggs
- Meringues
- Milk-based sauces (like for gravies and casseroles)
- Cheese or crumb toppings in casseroles
- Sour cream
- Mayonnaise and mayo-based salads (tuna salad, egg salad)
- Vinaigrette and guacamole
- Cream-based soups and sauces
- Fried foods (become soggy)
- Fully cooked rice
- Plain cooked pasta (can be frozen in dishes if undercooked)

TOP 4 Practical Storage Tips

Place perishable foods in the refrigerator and freezer once you get home: perishable foods should not be left outside the refrigerator or freezer for over 2 hours. If the temperature in your kitchen is above 90°F (32°C), food should not be left out at room temperature for over 1 hour. So once you get home, place them in the refrigerator and freezer as soon as possible.

Maintain proper temperatures: the refrigerator should be set at a maximum of 41°F (5°C) and the freezer should keep things frozen and be set around 32°F (0°C). Thermometers can double check whether your refrigerator and freezer are set at the correct temperatures.

Don't overcrowd the refrigerator and freezer: if the refrigerator and freezer are full of foods and items, air can't circulate and proper temperature can't be maintained. Keeping proper air circulation is as important as setting the proper temperature for the refrigerator and freezer.

Be watchful of food spoilage: when food starts to spoil, it has a bad odor and feels slimy. Mold will grow and threaten your health. When this happens, just toss it out unhesitatingly.

Smart labeling: labeling is the most useful method in any meal prep to manage food. It can take out the guesswork and help to save time. Label each container with the food item and the date you should eat it by. The chart on page 17 can help you label your foods with the correct use-by dates.

Thawing Method

The best method to thaw proteins like meat, poultry, and fish is to place it in the refrigerator from the freezer overnight. Some large-size proteins may need several days. For instance, for a whole chicken, it will need 1-2 days for complete thawing in the refrigerator. For small-size proteins, such as shrimp, you can put it into cool water for about 1.5 hours for proper thawing. However, never thaw cooked food in this way because it will give bacteria a perfect environment to grow. The correct way to handle cooked food is to use either the defrost setting or half power in the microwave. The drawback to this method, though, is that if some meats or seafood don't get even heating when thawing, it will begin to cook in the microwave. Under such circumstances, cook it right away after thawing. Don't thaw meats at room temperature, since this will allow bacteria to thrive and generate lots of unnecessary clean-up work.

The best way to thaw cooked dishes is to place them in the refrigerator in advance, thus the entire thawing is under a safe temperature. After that, thawed dished can be stored in the refrigerator for 3 to 4 days. Generally, the inner temperature of reheated dishes should reach 165°F (74°C), which could be measured in the thickest part with a thermometer.

Reheating Tips

Speaking of reheating foods, the golden rule is to "reheat the food in how it was cooked". However, it may be impossible for one who is busy at work or study during the daytime to have cookware at hand when you are going to eat your meals. Most of us use microwaves to reheat meals. The following tips may help improve the quality of your reheated meals in the microwave:

1) When reheating red meat and chicken in the microwave, add a little water (no more than 1 tablespoon) to help keep moisture.

2) For fish, in case that it pops and explodes all over the microwave, be sure to cover the container when reheating and use increasing heat levels, that is, start with low power for 10 seconds, then medium power for 10 seconds, then medium-high power for 30 seconds.

3) The best way to reheat baked, fried and roasted food is using an oven with aluminum foil covering the tray. If you use the microwave to reheat, put a cup of water in it besides the food to reduce the "sogginess" factor.

4) Sautéed, stir-fried, and steamed food usually is appropriate to be reheated in the microwave, but remember to stir it halfway to make sure even heating. Sprinkling the food with a bit of water can keep it from drying out.stir it halfway to make sure even heating. Sprinkling the food with a bit of water can keep it from drying out.

Leftovers Repurposing

No matter in daily cooking or in meal prepping, leftovers are inevitable. Leftovers don't have to be considered as kitchen waste with a destiny of being thrown away. This part will change your opinion on how to deal with leftovers and help you save energy, money and time by repurposing them. When it comes to repurposing leftovers, start thinking of them as ingredients, not leftovers. You might make an entirely new meal from the leftovers of a different meal. In fact, there are two types of leftovers: entire recipes and individual ingredients.

If you have an entire main dish or side dish 'leftover' you can:

1) Freeze unused portions of food for a future recipe.

2) If there isn't enough leftover to call it a full meal, use what you have as a side dish to your next meal.

3) Use side dishes as ingredients in a meal.

4) Eat dinner for breakfast or breakfast for dinner. Don't be get tied up to conventional norms of when certain foods should be eaten.

5) Have a leftover night where you eat the last little bits of whatever is left, clearing out the fridge.

And the second type of leftover is leftover ingredients:

1) Use the freezer when possible. Transfer them to a freezer-safe container, mark the item, amount left, and the date.

2) Fruit can be frozen for smoothies.

3) Wilting salad greens can be sautéed and added to eggs, ground meat, or even "hidden" in smoothies.

4) Leftover coconut milk or other milk can be frozen in ice cubes for smoothies.

5) we can throw Leftover veggies into an "everything but the kitchen sink" salad or soup.

Must-have Kitchen Equipment

1. Food Scale

Keto diet is a restrictive diet, so you should be conscious of the amount of food you put into your mouth. A food scale is your best pal to assist your carb planning and moderate your fat intake until you can estimate the macros by eyeballing portions.

2. Cast Iron Pan

There are plenty of benefits of a cast iron pan, not only are they nonstick, chemical-free, easy to clean, and with a long life span, they can also add iron to your food and can be used in the stove and oven.

3. Spiral Slicer

Jealous of the zucchini spaghetti you see on a magazine? Actually, with a spiral slicer, you can easily make those noodle shapes without a sweat. Pour on your favorite Keto-friendly sauce. This would make a fantastic low-carb meal.

4. Food Processor

This can make the smoothest nut butter, grate cauliflower, and pulse soaked/ roasted nuts and seeds into flour.

5. Electric Hand Mixer

You must have beaten an egg until your hands are stiff, then you must know how difficult it is, an electric hand mixer would save you a ton of effort and time, especially when you are mixing heavy ingredients.

6. Knife Sharpening Stone

Most of the prep work is cutting, and when you are dealing with a blunt knife, just imagine how frustrating it would be.

7. Silicone Molds and Sce Cube Trays

Use them to mold your excess bone broth for later use, or you could make a ton of fat bombs in different shapes.

8. A Good Set of Knives

When meal prepping, you are going to need to cut, slice and chop a lot of vegetables and meat, so a good set of knives would definitely be a good assist in your meal prepping journey.

9. Multi-cooker

It plays multiple roles in your meal prepping. you can use them to sauté, to pressure cook and to slow cook.

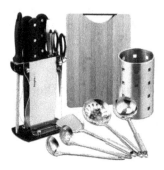

Chapter 3 Cook Once, Keto All Week

Keto Meal Prep Guideline

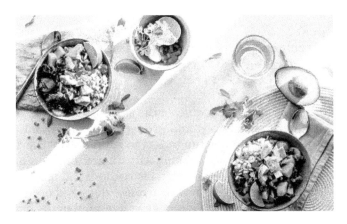

The goal of meal prepping is to get more done with less effort in limited time. You will naturally get faster at meal prepping the more you practice. Meal prep starts with planning. It's essential to make a plan and get everything ready for the meal prepping day. For most people, Sunday is the most appropriate day to prep meals. If Sundays are not your ideal prep day, then figure out which day works best for you. Here are general principles for a whole process of meal prep, but what you do depends on the dishes being made, so please adjust the following to make it your own:

Meal planning: Before the meal prep day, select recipes you will prep. Write down them and make a meal plan chart. Read through the recipes, write down a list of ingredients and pantry, and other things you need to make these recipes into tasty and ready meals.

Go shopping: Review the ingredients listed and make comparisons with what you already have in your pantry or refrigerator. Before going shopping, remember to eat something, because there is no greater enemy of a successful shopping trip than going while you are hungry.

Store ingredients: If you're shopping the day when you're prepping food, place cold items in the refrigerator to maintain their temperature until you start your meal prep. If you go shopping on a day or two before your meal prep day, make sure to store your food in the refrigerator or freezer immediately. Meats, fish, or chicken to be used within the next 48 hours should be portioned and stored in the refrigerator. The remaining raw proteins should be properly labeled and stored in the freezer.

Prep ingredients: the first step of meal prep should be prep ingredients. Read all recipes thoroughly to understand how to process corresponding ingredients. Then have all the ingredients prepped and measured to make cooking go as smoothly as possible. When the recipes call for them, there isn't much to do except add them in.

Slow cooker first: when making meal prep, work from the most time-consuming item to the least. In Keto diet the slow cooker is a great tool to make bone broth. It usually takes 4-6 hours to make a dish. What you need to do is just tossing the ingredients inside and press the "cook " bottom. When it works, you can move onto another recipe.

Recipes with long cooking times in the oven next: meat is the staple food of Keto diet. Roasting meat in bulk for the next week means it may cost a long time (depend on recipes). Put the marinated meat into the oven and in the meantime, you can take on other cooking tasks.

Hands-on stovetop recipes follow: in this step, separate ingredients for each recipe to be cooked on the stovetop, such as used Chicken and Mushrooms, Seared salmon with asparagus and hollandaise, and so on. Usually you can take the shortcut by stovetop—make one-pan meals. One-pan meals could enhance cooking efficiency and at the same time reduce cleanup work.

No-bake recipes are completed last: these are easy-to-make recipes, including sauces, dips, and dressings and require no or minimal cooking. Mayo, vinaigrette and guacamole are commonly used in Keto meals. They are quick and easy to make, and can last 2 weeks if you store them properly. You can make them as 1-cup portions, so they last a while. Remember to label each portion with "best by" date.

Put it together and box it up: once you have all the dishes prepped and cooked, it's time to put it all together. Toss them together to make the dish, or put the meal together by cooking the components together to make it, like a stir-fry. Then divide them into portions, make labels, and so you can grab and go. For a dish like meatballs, you may decide to divide it into two large containers, one for the refrigerator and one for the freezer.

4 Progressive Keto Meal Prep

In this cookbook, we created a 4-week meal prepping plan. The meals are for one person. The first week starts with only 1 breakfast and 2 lunch using 5 recipes, progressing to 2 breakfasts, 3 lunches/dinners and 1 snack using 9 recipes in the second week. One recipe for each breakfast or snack. Each lunch or dinner is made up of a main dish recipe and a side recipe. Recipes for lunches and dinners are pretty much interchangeable.

- ◆ **Meal prep 1: 1 breakfast and 2 lunches (1+2*2recipes)**
- ◆ **Meal prep 2: 1 breakfast, 3 lunches/dinners (1 +3*2recipes)**
- ◆ **Meal prep 3: 1 breakfast, 3 lunches/dinners, and 1 snack (1+3*2+1 recipes)**
- ◆ **Meal prep 4: 2 breakfast, 3 lunches/dinners, and 1 snack (2+3*2+1 recipe)**

People usually dine out for their breakfast and lunch during the workweek, which costs at least 15-20 dollars for each meal if you live in the major big cities in the US. A brief calculation would give you a picture of how much you can save if you are prepping meals at home. Saving $15 - $20 a day (up to $75 to $100 dollars every workweek) is a safe bet. To achieve that, you need time to become adept at multitasking with different recipes in the kitchen and finally master the art of meal-prepping. The meal plans and step-by-step instructions will provide you with examples and methods to learn about what is involved in the kitchen, how to arrange steps and orders and how long you need in prepping. Being successful early on can empower and motivate you to prep more and to prep a wider variety of dishes. After exploring progress, you will be able to create your own meal prep by using plentiful recipes of the cookbook and do what works best with your schedule and available meal prep time.

Inevitably, most Keto dieters will conduct fasting to help achieve their health goals. You can plan how often you will fast each week. But, generally, fasting or no fasting will be totally up to you. For instance, originally you may not have plans to fast on Monday, however, when you get up that morning, you feel good, get a good vibe for fasting and decide to skip the meals during fasting time frame. So what to do with these meals? Taking this into consideration, I design 5-day meal prep for each week and leave 2 days for fasting allowing for meal adjustment. Having ready meals on the table on work-off days, you can be free from cooking meals and get full rest. Or they can also be frozen or served to family members or guests.

Every meal prep includes a recipe plan, a shopping list, a meal plan chart and a step-by-step cooking instruction. Each recipe contains macros information, the number of servings, serving size, and nutrition breakdowns. You'll also find practical culinary tips or food-management tips that will help you enhance your cooking skills and secure the nutrition, taste and safety of your meals.

Meal plan 1

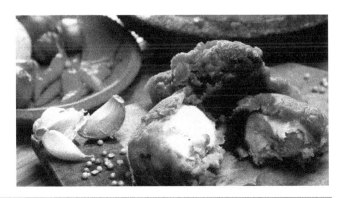

Recipe 1: Spiced Eggs And Bacon Breakfast
Recipe 2: Cheesy Garlic Chicken
Recipe 3: Garlicky Cauliflower Bake
Recipe 4: Beef Roast
Recipe 5: Coconut Cream Spinach

	BREAKFAST	LUNCH
DAY 1	Spiced Eggs And Bacon Breakfast	Cheesy Garlic Chicken; Garlicky Cauliflower Bake
DAY 2	Spiced Eggs And Bacon Breakfast	Beef Roast; Coconut Cream Spinach
DAY 3	Spiced Eggs And Bacon Breakfast	Cheesy Garlic Chicken; Garlicky Cauliflower Bake
DAY 4	Spiced Eggs And Bacon Breakfast	Beef Roast; Coconut Cream Spinach
DAY 5	Spiced Eggs And Bacon Breakfast	Beef Roast; Coconut Cream Spinach

SHOPPING LIST 1

PANTRY LIST:
- Olive oil (68 fl. oz. / 1.9 kg)
- Coconut oil (1 pack of 16 oz. / 454 g)
- Sea salt (1 pack of 10 oz. / 284 g)
- Black Pepper (1 pack of 6 oz. / 170 g)
- Garlic Powder (1 pack of 2.6 oz. / 74 g)
- Psyllium husk powder (1 pack of 10 oz. / 284 g)
- Italian herb seasoning (1 pack of 5 oz. / 142 g)
- Red pepper flake (1 pack of 8 oz. / 227 g)
- Paprika (1 pack of 8½ oz. / 241 g)
- Lemon juice (1 pack of 12½ fl. oz. / 354 g)
- Dijon mustard (1 pack of 8 oz. / 227 g)
- Dried Onion (1 pack of 2½ oz. / 71 g)
- Dried oregano (1 pack of 4 oz. / 113 g)
- Baking powder (1 pack of 4 oz. / 113 g)
- Coconut flour (1 pack of 1 lb. / 454 g)
- Almond flour (1 pack of 1 lb. / 454 g)
- Blanched slivered almonds (1 pack of 8 oz. / 227 g)
- Parmesan cheese (1 pack of 8 oz. / 227 g)
- Cream cheese (1 pack of 8 oz. / 227 g)
- Cheddar cheese (1 pack of 8 oz. / 227 g)
- Coconut aminos (1 bottle: 8fl. oz. / 227 g)
- Melted butter (1 bottle of 16 oz. / 454 g)
- Unsweetened butter (10 oz. / 284 g)

VEGETABLE:
- Arugula lettuce (1 oz. / 28 g)
- Green bell pepper (2), chive (1), garlic (6 cloves)
- Cauliflower (1 head), fresh parsley (1), spinach (1 package)
- Onion (1)

MEAT/POULTRY/FISH & SEAFOOD:
- Bacon (5 oz. / 142 g), Chicken Breast (4) (8 oz. / 227 g each)
- Beef tenderloin roast (3 lb. / 1.4 kg)

EGG /MILK:
- Egg (4)
- Coconut milk (1 bottle of 32 fl. oz. / 907 g)

Meal Prep Day Instruction 1

1. Preheat the oven to 425°F (220°C).
2. Begin by preparing ingredients of CHEESY GARLIC CHICKEN through step 2, step 3 and step 4. When the reheating temperature reached, place the chicken into the oven through step 5.
3. While CHEESY GARLIC CHICKEN is cooking, prepare the cauliflower through step 1 and 2 of GARLICKY CAULIFLOWER BAKE.
4. And prepare the ingredients of BEEF ROAST through step 2.
5. When CHEESY GARLIC CHICKEN is done, increase the oven temperature to 450°F (235°C). Once the oven is preheated, put the CAULIFLOWER in it and bake for about 25 minutes.
6. When GARLICKY CAULIFLOWER is baking, prepare COCONUT CREAM SPINACH through step 1 and 2, and finish preparing the dish through step 3.
7. After 25 minutes, scatter the parsley and Parmesan cheese on the CAULIFLOWER and bake for another 5 minutes, or until the cheese melts.
8. When GARLICKY CAULIFLOWER is completed, decrease the oven temperature to 350°F (180°C). Once the temperature is reached, place the BEEF into the oven and cook for 10 minutes. Finish preparing BEEF ROAST through step 3.
9. While the BEEF is roasting, prepare SPICED EGGS AND BACON BREAKFAST.

SPICED EGGS AND BACON BREAKFAST

Macros: Fat 84% | Protein 13% | Carbs 3%
Prep time: 5 minutes | Cook time: 10 minutes | Serves 2

It is a keto breakfast meal which is also perfect for lunch or dinner. The addition of the bell paper and walnuts brings crunchiness. The ingredients are not complicated and it only takes 15 minutes to prepare and cook.

5 ounces (142 g) bacon
4 eggs
1 ounce (28 g) walnuts
2 avocados, cubed

1 ounce (28 g) arugula lettuce, chopped
1 green bell pepper, chopped
Salt and freshly ground black pepper, to taste
1 tablespoon finely chopped fresh chives

1. Add the bacon to a frying pan over medium heat and fry for 2 minutes on each side until it buckles and curls. Set the cooked bacon aside. Leave the fat from the bacon in the pan.
2. Reduce the heat to medium-low, break the eggs into the frying pan and fry for 2 minutes or until the eggs reach your desired doneness.
3. Transfer the eggs to two serving plates. Top with bacon, nuts, avocado, arugula, and bell pepper. Sprinkle with the salt, pepper, and chives before serving.

STORAGE: Store in an airtight container in the fridge for up to 4 days or in the freezer for up to 1 month.
REHEAT: Microwave, covered, until the desired temperature is reached or reheat in a frying pan or air fryer / instant pot, covered, on medium.
SERVE IT WITH: To make this a complete meal, serve with kale and coconut shake.

PER SERVING
calories: 973 | fat: 88.0g | fiber: 15.0g | net carbs: 8.0g | protein: 26.0g

CHEESY GARLIC CHICKEN

Macros: Fat: 44% | Protein: 54% | Carbs: 1%
Prep time: 20 minutes | Cook time: 35 minutes | Serves 4

This cheesy garlic chicken is quick and easy to make. It is perfect for gatherings and dinners. Its crunchy bark and soft meat tell a story every taste bud should know.

¼ cup olive oil
2 cloves garlic, crushed
⅛ cup coconut flour
¼ cup Parmesan cheese, grated
4 skinless, boneless chicken breast halves

1. Start by heating the oven to 425°F (220°C).
2. Pour the olive oil and garlic into a pan over low heat to cook for 1 to 2 minutes until aromatic, then pour them into a small bowl.
3. Mix the flour and the cheese in another bowl and set aside.
4. Put the chicken into the garlic mixture with tongs, then coat it with the cheese mixture. Put the chicken on a baking dish and put it in the preheated oven.
5. Let it bake for 30 to35 minutes or until the juices are clear and the chicken has no pink.
6. Remove the chicken from the oven and serve warm.

STORAGE: Store in an airtight container in the fridge for up to 4 days or in the freezer for up to 1 month.
REHEAT: Microwave, covered, until the desired temperature is reached or reheat in air fryer / instant pot covered, on medium.
SERVE IT WITH: To make this a complete meal, serve it with some riced cauliflower.
PER SERVING
calories: 433 | fat: 21.4g | carbs: 1.7g | protein: 55.0g

GARLICKY CAULIFLOWER BAKE

Macros: Fat 79% | Protein 7% | Carbs 14%
Prep time: 15 minutes | Cook time: 25 minutes | Serves 6

This garlic cauliflower is oven roasted and is a great side dish. It's delicious and can also be used to top veggie bowls or salads.

4 tablespoons olive oil, divided
2 tablespoons garlic, minced
1 large head cauliflower, separated into florets
Salt and freshly ground black pepper, to taste
1 tablespoon fresh parsley, chopped
⅓ cup Parmesan cheese, grated

1. Start by preheating the oven to 450°F (235°C). Grease a casserole dish with 1 tablespoon olive oil.
2. In a large resealable bag, combine the remaining olive oil and garlic, then add the cauliflower. Toss to coat well. Pour them into the casserole dish, then sprinkle the pepper and salt to season.
3. Bake in the preheated oven for about 25 minutes, stirring once, until lightly browned.
4. Scatter the parsley and Parmesan cheese on top and bake for another 5 minutes, or until the cheese melts.
5. Remove the casserole dish from the oven. Allow to cool for 20 minutes before serving.

STORAGE: Store in an airtight container in the fridge for up to 3 days, or in a freezer for up to a month.
REHEAT: Microwave, covered, until the desired temperature is reached or reheat in a frying pan or air fryer / instant pot, covered, on medium.
SERVE IT WITH: To make this a complete meal, serve with crispy chicken thighs.
PER SERVING
calories: 119 | fat: 8.3g | carbs: 8.5g | protein: 4.8g

BEEF ROAST

Macros: Fat 67% | Protein 31% | Carbs 2%
Prep time: 5 minutes | Cook time: 45 minutes | Serves 6

One of the easiest and simplest beef roast recipes is here to add more flavors to your dinner table. The beef tenderloin roast is seasoned with coconut aminos to keep the meal low in sodium and carbs. When roasted with a butter glaze on top, the meat gets a soft and juicy taste every time.

1 (3 pounds / 1360 g) beef tenderloin roast
1/2 cup melted butter
3/4 cup coconut aminos

1. Preheat the oven to 350°F (180°C).
2. In a shallow baking dish, place the tenderloin and drizzle the melted butter and coconut aminos on top.
3. Place the baking dish in the oven and roast for 10 minutes. Flip the tenderloins then continue roasting for 40 minutes, or until the internal temperature reaches 145°F (63°C).
4. Allow to cool for 10 minutes before slicing.

STORAGE: Store in an airtight container in the fridge for up to 5 days or in the freezer for about 1 month.
REHEAT: Microwave, covered, until the desired temperature is reached or reheat in a frying pan or air fryer / instant pot, covered, on medium.
SERVE IT WITH: To add more flavors to this meal, serve the beef roast with a creamy spinach salad on the side.

PER SERVING
calories: 591 | fat: 33.1g | net carbs: 2.5g | protein: 66.8g

COCONUT CREAM SPINACH

Macros: Fat 37% | Protein 28% | Carbs 35%
Prep time: 10 minutes | Cook time: 15 minutes | Serves 4

Thinking of best recipe options for a holiday treat? Well creamed spinach is the best recipe choice to prepare for a family getting together for a party or celebration, accompanied by a nice roast.

½ cup unsweetened coconut milk
1 (10-ounce / 284-g) package frozen chopped spinach
¼ cup minced onion
½ teaspoon garlic powder
¼ teaspoon dried minced onion

1. Process the milk and spinach in a food processor until creamy and smooth.
2. Add the fresh onion, garlic powder, and dried onion, then mix well.
3. Transfer the mixture into a medium saucepan and cook over medium heat until it thickens, for 3 minutes. Allow to simmer over low heat for 10 minutes more.
4. Remove from the heat and serve warm.

STORAGE: Store in an airtight container in the fridge for up to 4 days.
REHEAT: Microwave, covered, until the desired temperature is reached or reheat in a frying pan or instant pot, covered, on medium.
PER SERVING
calories: 72 | fat: 3.0g | carbs: 7.8g | protein: 5.3g

Meal plan 2

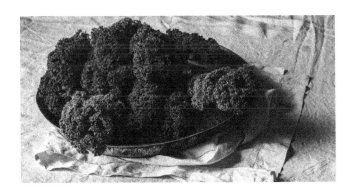

Recipe 1: Cheesy Keto Blueberry Pancake
Recipe 2: Pork Beef Italian Meatballs
Recipe 3: Simple Broccoli Raab
Recipe 4: Sauteed Sausage And Shrimp
Recipe 5: Simple Arugula Salad
Recipe 6: Spice-Roasted Chicken
Recipe 7: Lemon Broccoli With Almond Butter

	BREAKFAST	LUNCH	DINNER
DAY 1	Cheesy Keto Blueberry Pancake	Pork Beef Italian Meatballs; Simple Broccoli Rabe	Sauteed Sausage And Shrimp; Simple Arugula Salad
DAY 2	Cheesy Keto Blueberry Pancake	Spice-Roasted Chicken; Lemon Broccoli With Almond Butter	Pork Beef Italian Meatballs; Simple Broccoli Rabe
DAY 3	Cheesy Keto Blueberry Pancake	Sauteed Sausage And Shrimp; Simple Arugula Salad	Spice-Roasted Chicken; Lemon Broccoli With Almond Butter
DAY 4	Cheesy Keto Blueberry Pancake	Spice-Roasted Chicken; Lemon Broccoli With Almond Butter	Sauteed Sausage And Shrimp; Simple Arugula Salad
DAY 5	Cheesy Keto Blueberry Pancake	Pork Beef Italian Meatballs; Simple Broccoli Rabe	Spice-Roasted Chicken; Lemon Broccoli With Almond Butter

SHOPPING LIST 2

VEGETABLE:
- Lemon 2
- Onion 2
- Red bell pepper 1
- Asparagus (1 lb. / 454 g)
- Shallot (6 cloves)
- Micro greens (10 oz. / 284 g)
- Avocado (1)
- Broccoli (1 head)

MEAT/POULTRY/FISH, SEAFOOD/EGG:
- Chorizo sausage (6 oz. / 170 g)
- Shrimp (½ lb. / 227 g)
- Eggs (10)
- Whole chicken (1)

FRUIT:
- Fresh blueberries (10 oz. / 284 g)

NUT:
- Sunflower seeds (10 oz. / 284 g)

Meal Prep Day Instruction 2

1. Begin by preparing the coconut milk of PORK BEEF ITALIAN MEATBALLS through step 2. During soaking, prepare onions through step 3, prepare the meat mixture through step 4 and step 5. Then put the ingredient in the refrigerator for 1 hour.
2. Prepare CHEESY KETO BLUEBERRY PANCAKE. Make the egg mixture through step 1 and the flour mixture through step 2, combine with the two and let stand for 2 minutes. And then cook the pancake through step 3 and 4, until the batter has finished.
3. Prepare the shrimp and sausage of SAUTEED SAUSAGE AND SHRIMP through step 1 to 4, and sauté the ingredients through step 5 and 6.
4. prepare LEMON BROCCOLI WITH ALMOND BUTTER by starting firstly boiling a pot of water, and meanwhile prepare the ingredients, and then cook them through step 2, 3 and 4.
5. Prepare boiling water through step 1 of SIMPLE BROCCOLI RABE. At the same time, prepare the broccoli through step 2 and 3, and cook it through step 4 and 5. complex the dish through step 5.
6. The last dish is SIMPLE ARUGULA SALAD. Make seasoning mixture by step 1 and 2. then make a Dijon mustard dressing see step 3. Prepare arugula and micro greens through step 4 and at the last combine all these ingredients well by step 5 to complete the dish.
7. The meatball mixture of PORK BEEF ITALIAN MEATBALLS is done now. Preheat the oven to 425°F (220°C), meanwhile make the baking sheet ready. And move the mixture from the refrigerator and make the meatballs through step 7 and cook it through step 8.
8. While the meatballs are baking, prepare ingredients of SPICE-ROASTED CHICKEN by step 2.
9. When PORK BEEF ITALIAN MEATBALLS is done, place the seasoned chicken in the oven and roast for 1 hour though step 3 and roast for 1 hour.

CHEESY KETO BLUEBERRY PANCAKE

Macros: Fat: 82% | Protein: 12% | Carbs: 6%
Prep time: 5 minutes | Cook time: 10 minutes | Serves 4

Pancakes have always been a favorite of adults and kids through the ages. This is because it can be customized according to anyone's preferences. This pancake is the perfect low-carb breakfast dish for every occasion. Grab a fork and dive in!

6 eggs
3 ounces (85 g) melted butter
4 ounces (113 g) cream cheese
⅔ cup almond flour
2 teaspoons baking powder

⅔ cup oat fiber
½ lemon, the zest
1 pinch salt
3 ounces (85 g) fresh blueberries

1. Whisk the eggs, butter, and cream cheese in a bowl.
2. Mix the flour, baking powder, oat fiber, lemon zest, and salt in another bowl then pour them over the egg mixture. Mix until smooth, then let stand for 2 minutes.
3. Pour ⅓ cup of the batter into a small frying pan over medium heat to make a pancake.
4. Fry for 4 minutes or until lightly browned. Flip the pancake halfway through and top with ⅓ of the blueberries.
5. Repeat until the batter has finished, then serve it on a plate.

STORAGE: Store in an airtight container in the fridge for up to 4 days or in the freezer for up to 1 month.
REHEAT: Microwave, covered, until the desired temperature is reached or reheat in a frying pan or air fryer / instant pot, covered, on medium.
SERVE IT WITH: To make this a complete meal, serve it with whipped cream and a cup of black tea.
PER SERVING
calories: 476 | fat: 43.0g | net carbs: 6.0g | fiber: 13.0g | protein: 14.0g

PORK BEEF ITALIAN MEATBALLS

Macros: Fat 62% | Protein 34% | Carbs 3%
Prep time: 20 minutes | Cook time: 35 minutes | Serves 10

A mixture of pork and beef is just the perfect delight for all the meat lovers. This protein-rich meatball recipe makes the best use out of the basic kitchen ingredients and pork and beef mince. Seasoned with dried herb seasonings, spices the meatballs are also loaded Parmesan cheese.

1 teaspoon olive oil, for greasing
⅛ cup coconut flour
½ cup unsweetened coconut milk
2 tablespoons olive oil
1 onion, diced
1 pound (454 g) ground pork
1 pound (454 g) ground beef
2 eggs

¼ bunch fresh parsley, chopped
1 teaspoon ground black pepper
2 teaspoons salt
3 garlic cloves, crushed
2 tablespoons Parmesan cheese, grated
1 teaspoon dried Italian herb seasoning
½ teaspoon red pepper flakes

1. Line a baking sheet with foil and lightly grease it with a teaspoon of olive oil.
2. Add the coconut flour to a small bowl and pour in the milk. Set aside and leave this flour soaked for 20 minutes.
3. Take a suitable skillet and place it over medium heat. Add the oil to heat, then toss in the onions. Sauté for about 20 minutes until translucent.
4. Transfer the sautéed onion to a large bowl and add the pork, beef, eggs, parsley, black pepper, salt, garlic, Parmesan cheese, Italian herb seasoning, and red pepper flakes.
5. Use a rubber spatula to mix all these ingredients well and cover with plastic wrap to refrigerate for 1 hour.
6. Meanwhile, preheat the oven to 425°F (220°C).
7. Remove the mixture from the refrigerator. Using a small cookie scoop to scoop portions of the mixture and roll into 1 ½-inch meatballs.
8. Place these meatballs on the prepared baking sheet and bake for approximately 20 minutes until browned.
9. Remove from the oven and serve while still warm.

STORAGE: Store in an airtight container in the fridge for up to 2 days or in the freezer for about 1 month.
REHEAT: Microwave, covered, until the desired temperature is reached or reheat in a frying pan or air fryer / instant pot, covered, on medium.
SERVE IT WITH: To make this a complete meal, serve the meatballs with broccoli rabe as a side dish.
PER SERVING
calories: 82 | fat: 5.5g | net carbs: 1.7g | protein: 6.2g

SIMPLE BROCCOLI RABE

Macros: Fat 80% | Protein 9% | Carbs 11%
Prep time: 20 minutes | Cook time: 20 minutes | Serves 4

B roccoli rabe is an easy meal to prepare. In less than 20 minutes, you will have your broccoli full of flavors and nutritional value. A sprinkle of cheese makes the meal tasty and soft. You can add more minced garlic to improve the taste to your preference.

1 pound (454 g) trimmed broccoli rabe
5 tablespoons extra virgin olive oil
1 minced garlic clove

1 chopped onion
1 tablespoon grated Parmesan cheese

1. Put a large pot with lightly salted water on medium-high heat to boil.
2. Meanwhile, make an X in the bottom of the broccoli rabe stems on your cutting board, then put in the boiling water.
3. Cook for 5 minutes until tender. Remove from the heat and drain the water. Set aside.
4. Put a large heavy skillet over medium heat, and heat the oil to fry the garlic and onion for 2 minutes until tender.
5. Add the broccoli rabe and fry for 15 minutes until soft. Sprinkle with Parmesan cheese.
6. Remove from the heat and serve on a plate.

STORAGE: Store in an airtight container in the fridge for up to 5 days.
REHEAT: Microwave, covered, until the desired temperature is reached or reheat in a frying pan, covered, on medium.
SERVE IT WITH: To make this a complete meal, serve the broccoli rabe with your juicy meatballs.
PER SERVING
calories: 192 | fat: 17.3g | carbs: 5.7g | protein: 4.6g

SAUTEED SAUSAGE AND SHRIMP

Macros: Fat 70% | Protein 25% | Carbs 5%
Prep time: 15 minutes | Cook time: 20 minutes| Serves: 4

Ever thought of enjoying a perfect meal at your table? Think of baked shrimp and sausage. With a wide range of essential ingredients, you are assured of a better seafood packed with deliciousness at the comfort of your home.

2 tablespoons olive oil
6 ounces (170 g) diced chorizo sausage
½ pound (227 g) shrimp, peeled and deveined
1 chopped red bell pepper

½ small chopped sweet onion
2 teaspoons minced garlic
¼ cup chicken stock
1 pinch red pepper flakes

1. Melt 2 tablespoons of olive oil in a large skillet over medium-high heat.
2. Add the sausage and sauté for 6 minutes until warmed through.
3. Stir in the shrimp and cook until they turn opaque, about 4 minutes.
4. Put the cooked shrimp and sausage into a bowl and set aside
5. Put the red bell pepper, onion, and garlic to the skillet and sauté until tender.
6. Add the ¼ cup chicken stock, cooked shrimp and sausage. Cook over medium-low heat for about 3 minutes until the liquid is reduced.
7. Serve with red pepper flakes sprinkled on top.

STORAGE: Store in an airtight container in the fridge for up to 5 days or in the freezer for up to 1 month.
REHEAT: Microwave, covered, until the desired temperature is reached.
SERVE IT WITH: To make this a complete meal, serve the cooked sausage and shrimp with a bowl of green salad.
PER SERVING
calories: 323 | fat: 24.0g | total carbs: 8.0g | fiber: 2.0g | net carbs: 6.0g | protein: 20.0g

SIMPLE ARUGULA SALAD

Macros: Fat 80% | Protein 15% | Carbs 5%
Prep time: 5 minutes | Cook time: 20 minutes | Serves 2

The combination of Arugula, shallots, and asparagus makes a tasty salad. When added lemon flavors and Dijon mustard, you will enjoy the salad until you can't get enough of it.

1 tablespoon olive oil
20 stalks asparagus, rinsed, trimmed and sliced
Salt and freshly ground black pepper, to taste
¼ teaspoon Dijon mustard
½ teaspoon shallot, diced
2 tablespoons olive oil

1 tablespoon lemon juice
2 cups fresh arugula
1 cup micro greens
2 tablespoons toasted sunflower seeds
2 hard-boiled eggs, sliced
½ avocado

1. Pour the oil in a large skillet then heat over medium high heat.
2. Add the asparagus, pepper, and salt to cook for 4 minutes. Remove from heat and put aside.
3. In the meantime, make a dressing by whisking together the Dijon mustard, pepper, salt, shallot, olive oil, and lemon juice until well combined. Put aside.
4. Divide the arugula and micro greens equally between 2 serving bowls.
5. Add the cooked asparagus, sunflower seeds, sliced eggs, and avocado.
6. Pour the dressing over the greens and serve.

STORAGE: Store in separate airtight containers in the fridge for up to 3 days or in the freezer for up to 1 month.
SERVE IT WITH: Sautéed shrimp will accompany the green salad nicely.
PER SERVING
calories: 434 | fat: 39.0g | carbs: 12.8g | fiber: 8.2g | protein: 16.0g

SPICE-ROASTED CHICKEN

Macros: Fat: 54% | Protein: 43% | Carbs: 3%
Prep time: 15 minutes | Cook time: 1 hour 15 minutes | Serves 6

Spicy chicken dishes can never be underrated and the same can be said for this absolutely delicious spice roasted chicken dish. Coated with a blend of spices, your taste buds are taken on a wild ride with every bite.

1 tablespoon olive oil
1 whole chicken, cut into 8 pieces
1 teaspoon salt
1 teaspoon ground black pepper

1 teaspoon ground paprika
1 teaspoon garlic powder
1 teaspoon dried oregano

1. Start by preheating the oven to 425°F (220°C). Coat a baking pan with olive oil.
2. Lay the chicken in the baking pan, then sprinkle the salt, pepper, paprika, oregano, and garlic powder on both sides of the chicken.
3. Put the pan in the oven and roast for 1 hour until the juices are clear and a meat thermometer inserted in the center of the chicken reaches at least 165°F (74°C).
4. Remove the chicken from the oven and serve on plates.

STORAGE: Store in an airtight container in the fridge for up to 4 days or in the freezer for up to 1 month.
REHEAT: Microwave, covered, until the desired temperature is reached or reheat in a frying pan or air fryer/instant pot, covered, on medium.
SERVE IT WITH: To make this a complete meal, serve it with tender butter broccoli.

PER SERVING
calories: 430 | fat: 25.6g | carbs: 0.8g | protein: 45.9g

LEMON BROCCOLI WITH ALMOND BUTTER

Macros: Fat 80% | Protein 9% | Carbs 11%
Prep time: 5 minutes | Cook time: 10 minutes | Serves 4

The broccoli tastes better with a combination of lemons and almonds. Enjoy the tasty meal, but do not overcook the broccoli to retain the nutritional values. For best results, use melted butter.

1 head fresh broccoli, cut into florets
¼ cup butter, melted
¼ cup blanched slivered almonds

2 tablespoons lemon juice
1 teaspoon lemon zest

1. Bring a large pot of lightly salted water to a boil. Add the broccoli florets and cook for about 4 minutes until fork-tender.
2. Remove the broccoli florets from the pot. Drain the water and place on a platter.
3. Melt the butter in a small saucepan on medium-low heat. Add the almonds, lemon juice, and lemon zest. Stir to combine well.
4. Pour the mixture over the broccoli and serve immediately.

STORAGE: Store in an airtight container in the fridge for up to 4 days or in the freezer for up to 1 month.
REHEAT: Microwave, covered, until the desired temperature is reached or reheat in a frying pan or air fryer / instant pot, covered, on medium.
SERVE IT WITH: To make this a complete meal, serve the lemon broccoli and almonds with baked salmon.

PER SERVING
calories: 170 | fat: 15.3g | carbs: 7.0g | protein: 3.8g

Meal plan 3

Recipe 1: Low-Carb Kale With Pork And Eggs
Recipe 2: Coconut Baked Lobster
Recipe 3: Massaged Collard And Avocado Salad
Recipe 4: Easy Stewed Salmon
Recipe 5: Easy Grilled Asparagus
Recipe 6: Pecan Crusted Pork Chops
Recipe 7: Easy Broccoli And Cheese
Recipe 8: Amazing Brussel Sprouts Salad

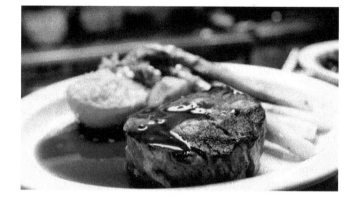

	BREAKFAST	LUNCH	DINNER	SNACK
DAY 1	Low-Carb Kale With Pork And Eggs	Coconut Baked Lobster; Massaged Collard And Avocado Salad	Easy Stewed Salmon;Easy Grilled Asparagus	Amazing Brussel Sprouts Salad
DAY 2	Low-Carb Kale With Pork And Eggs	Easy Stewed Salmon;Easy Grilled Asparagus	Pecan Crusted Pork Chops;Easy Broccoli And Cheese	Amazing Brussel Sprouts Salad
DAY 3	Low-Carb Kale With Pork And Eggs	Pecan Crusted Pork Chops;Easy Broccoli And Cheese	coconut Baked Lobster; Massaged Collard And Avocado Salad	Amazing Brussel Sprouts Salad
DAY 4	Low-Carb Kale With Pork And Eggs	Easy Stewed Salmon;Easy Grilled Asparagus	Pecan Crusted Pork Chops;Easy Broccoli And Cheese	Amazing Brussel Sprouts Salad
DAY 5	Low-Carb Kale With Pork And Eggs	coconut Baked Lobster; Massaged Collard And Avocado Salad	Pecan Crusted Pork Chops;Easy Broccoli And Cheese	Amazing Brussel Sprouts Salad

Shopping List 3

VEGETABLE

- Kale (½ lb. / 227 g)
- Green onion (5 oz. / 142 g)
- Fresh dill (3 oz. / 85 g)
- Collard greens (8 oz. / 227 g)
- Onion (1)
- Asparagus (1 lb. / 454 g)
- Broccoli (1 head) (10½ oz. / 298 g)
- Brussels sprout (6)
- Avocado (1)

MEAT/POULTRY/FISH, SEAFOOD/ EGG

- Smoke pork belly (6 oz. / 170g)
- Egg (10)
- Lobster meat (0.8 lb. / 363 g)
- Salmon fillet (1 lb. / 454 g)
- Pork loin (4)
- Fish broth (1 pack of 8 oz. / 227 g)

FRUIT:

- Cranberry (3 oz. / 85 g)

Nut:

- Pecan (10 oz. / 284 g)
- Pumpkins seeds (10 oz. / 284 g)

Meal Prep Day Instruction 3

1. Preheat the oven to 400°F (205°C).
2. Start by making the filling and the toppings of COCONUT BAKED LOBSTER through step 2, 3, 4 and 5. and then spread ingredients over the lobster, see step 6 and bake for 25 minutes.
3. Prepare the coconut milk and egg mixture and the pecan and cheese mixture through step 1 and step2 of PECAN CRUSTED PORK CHOPS. Combine the seasoned pork chops with the two mixtures through step 2. finish cooking through step 3.
4. Prepare LOW-CARB KALE WITH PORK AND EGGS.
5. Prepare EASY STEWED SALMON.
6. Start preparing EASY GRILLED ASPARAGUS by preheating the grill to high heat, and cook the ingredients through step 2 and 3.
7. When preparing EASY BROCCOLI AND CHEESE, firstly boil the water, at the same time prepare the ingredients see step 2 and 3. finally put into Microwave see step 4 and finish cooking.
8. Prepare MASSAGED COLLARD AND AVOCADO SALAD. Firstly, the massaged greens through step 1 and 2 and make the avocado mixture through step 3, finally combine them together see step 4.
9. Prepare AMAZING BRUSSEL SPROUTS SALAD.

LOW-CARB KALE WITH PORK AND EGGS

Macros: Fat 87% | Protein 11% | Carbs 2%
Prep time: 5 minutes | Cook time: 15 minutes | Serves 2

It is a delicious meal. The nuts bring about the crunchiness and together with the crisp pork flavor and texture is added into the meal.

3 ounces (85 g) butter
½ pound (227 g) kale, rinsed, trimmed, and chopped into square
6 ounces (170 g) smoked pork belly

1 ounce (28 g) pecans or walnuts
1 ounce (28 g) frozen cranberries
4 eggs, whisked
Salt and freshly ground black pepper, to taste

1. In a nonstick skillet, add ⅔ of the butter and melt over high heat. Add the kale and fry for 2 minutes or until they slightly turn to brown at the edges. Remove from the skillet and set aside.
2. Put the pork belly in the skillet and sear for 60 seconds or until lightly browned.
3. Reduce the heat then place the kale back to the skillet. Add the walnuts and cranberries. Stir for another 2 minutes until cooked through, then transfer them into a bowl.
4. Melt the remaining butter in the skillet and fry the whisked eggs over medium heat for 3 minutes, then sprinkle with salt and pepper.
5. Transfer the eggs to two serving plates and top with divided pork belly and kale mixture before serving.

STORAGE: Store in an airtight container in the fridge for up to 4 days or in the freezer for up to 1 month.
REHEAT: Microwave, covered, until the desired temperature is reached or reheat in a frying pan or air fryer / instant pot, covered, on medium.
SERVE IT WITH: To make this a complete meal, serve with sugar-free chocolate coconut keto smoothie.
PER SERVING
calories: 1032 | fat: 98.0g | net carbs: 7.0g | fiber: 5.0g | protein: 25.0g

COCONUT BAKED LOBSTER

Macros: Fat: 62% | Protein: 24% | Carbs: 14%
Prep time: 15 minutes | Cook time: 35 minutes | Serves: 6

Prepare the filling from measured amounts of basic ingredients first. You are in need of your friends enjoying the whole deliciousness from a lobster, get straight to kitchen, and try each step. Enjoy!

FILLING:

¼ cup coconut oil
2 cups chopped green onion, green parts only,
¼ cup unsweetened coconut milk

⅛ cup chopped fresh dill
½ teaspoon ground gray sea salt
2½ cups chopped cooked lobster meat

TOPPING:

4 tablespoons unsweetened coconut milk
2 tablespoons coconut oil
½ teaspoon ground gray sea salt

½ teaspoon ground black pepper
3 large egg yolks

1. Start by preheating the oven to 400°F (205°C).
2. To make the filling: Put ¼ cup coconut oil and green onions in a large frying pan. Fry the onions for 5 minutes until translucent.
3. Add the cooked lobster meat, dill, ¼ cup coconut milk, and ½ teaspoon salt, then cook for 2 minutes more.
4. Pour the mixture to a shallow casserole dish. Set aside.
5. To make the toppings: Put 4 tablespoons coconut milk, salt, 2 tablespoons coconut oil, and pepper in a food processor. Blend until almost mashed, then add the egg yolk to mix.
6. Spread the mashed mixture over the lobster in the casserole dish.
7. Bake in the preheated oven until the top turns golden brown, for about 25 minutes.
8. Remove from the oven and serve warm.

STORAGE: Store in an airtight container in the fridge for up to 3 days.
REHEAT: Microwave, covered, until the desired temperature is reached or place in a covered casserole dish and reheat in a preheated 300°F (150°C) oven for 15 minutes, until warmed through. Or reheat in a frying pan, on medium
SERVE IT WITH: To make this a complete meal, serve the coconut baked lobster on a bed of greens.
PER SERVING
calories: 301 | fat: 20.6g | carbs: 10.4g | fiber: 2.5g | protein: 18.4g

MASSAGED COLLARD AND AVOCADO SALAD

Macros: Fat 83% | Protein 10% | Carbs 7%
Prep time: 5 minutes | Cook time: 20 minutes | Serves 4

Nothing beats the combination of collard greens and avocado. It is a salad match that everyone should try out. Make this quick salad for lunch or dinner then serve with your favorite keto-friendly dressing.

SALAD:

4 cups collard greens, stem removes and roughly sliced
1 tablespoon avocado oil

1 tablespoon fresh lemon juice
¼ teaspoon sea salt

DRESSING:

1 mashed avocado
1 tablespoon avocado oil
1 tablespoon fresh lemon juice
1 teaspoon nutritional yeast

¼ teaspoon sea salt
¼ teaspoon pepper
3 tablespoons pumpkin seeds

1. Put the collard greens into a large bowl, then add avocado oil, lemon juice, and salt.
2. Massage the greens until they are coated well, for about 2 minutes. Set aside.
3. In a small bowl, whisk together the avocado oil, lemon juice, pepper, avocado, salt, and nutritional yeast until creamy and smooth.
4. Pour the avocado mixture over the massaged greens, then garnish with pumpkin seeds to serve.

STORAGE: Store in an airtight container in the fridge for up to 4 days or in the freezer for up to 1 month.
PER SERVING
calories: 188 | fat: 17.4g | carbs: 7.7g | fiber: 4.6g | protein: 4.8g

EASY STEWED SALMON

Macros: Fat: 47% | Proteins: 47% | Carbs: 6%
Prep time: 20 minutes | Cook time: 15 minutes | Serves 3

Follow the given steps to get a mouth-watering stew from salmon that will leave friends yearning for more. Personally, I love having it while steaming hot. Perhaps, you love that too. Get it while hot, sit right back at the comfort of your table and enjoy a meal enriched with essential nutrients.

1 pound (454 g) cubed salmon fillet
1 tablespoon butter
1 medium chopped onion
1 cup homemade fish broth
Salt and freshly ground black pepper, to taste

1. On a plate, rub the salmon with black pepper and salt on both sides. Set aside.
2. Melt the butter in a skillet over medium-high heat, then sauté the onions until soft, about 3 minutes.
3. Add the salmon and cook for 2 minutes each side until opaque.
4. Pour in the fish broth and stir well.
5. Cook covered for about 7 minutes, or until the fish is cooked through.
6. Serve while still hot.

STORAGE: Store in an airtight container in the fridge for up to 3 days.
REHEAT: Microwave the salmon, covered, until the desired temperature is reached or reheat in a frying pan or instant pot, covered, on medium.
SERVE IT WITH: To make this a complete meal, serve the stewed salmon with grilled keto-friendly vegetables

PER SERVING
calories: 272 | fat: 14.2g | carbs: 4.4g | protein: 32.1g

EASY GRILLED ASPARAGUS

Macros: Fat 72% | Protein 24% | Carbs 4%
Prep time: 15 minutes | Cook time: 3 minutes | Serves 4

If you need a quick fix meal, then roasted asparagus is the right one. It is crunchy and full of delicious flavors. This quick and easy recipe for oven grilled asparagus is the perfect spring side dish.

1 pound (454 g) asparagus spears, trimmed and fresh
1 tablespoon olive oil
Salt and ground black pepper, to taste

1. Start by preheating the grill to high heat.
2. Brush the asparagus with olive oil. Sprinkle the salt and ground black pepper to season.
3. Arrange the asparagus on the grill grate and grill for about 3 minutes, or until lightly charred.
4. Let them cool for about 2 minutes and serve.

STORAGE: Store in an airtight container in the fridge for up to 3 days, or in a freeze for up to 3 months.
REHEAT: Microwave, covered, until the desired temperature is reached or reheat in a frying pan or air fryer / instant pot, covered, on medium.
SERVE IT WITH: This meal is eaten as a side or dessert. It can be served alongside salmon.

PER SERVING
calories: 44 | fat: 3.5g | net carbs: 0.4g | fiber: 2.6g | protein: 2.7g

PECAN CRUSTED PORK CHOPS

Prep time: 15 minutes | Cook time: 24 minutes | Serves 4
Macros: Fat: 76% | Protein: 22% | Carbs: 2%

An easy and delicious recipe of pork chops that will be a wonderful addition in your dinner menu list... The richness of the pecans teams up greatly with the pork chops.

2 tablespoons unsweetened coconut milk
2 eggs
1½ cups pecans, chopped finely
¼ cup Parmesan cheese, grated
4 (4-ounce / 113-g) ½-inch thick pork loin chops
Sea salt and ground black pepper, to taste
2 tablespoons olive oil

1. In a shallow bowl, place the coconut milk and eggs, then beat until just combined. In a separate bowl, mix together the pecans and Parmesan cheese.
2. Season the pork chops with salt and black pepper evenly. Now, dip each pork chop into the egg mixture and then coat with pecan mixture fully.
3. In a large nonstick skillet, heat the oil over medium heat. Add the pork chops and cook for about 10 to 12 minutes per side until cooked through.
4. Remove from the heat and serve on plates.

STORAGE: Store in an airtight container in the fridge for up to 3 days.
REHEAT: Microwave, covered, until the desired temperature is reached or reheat in a frying pan or air fryer / instant pot, covered, on medium.
SERVE IT WITH: Roasted broccoli will accompany these chops nicely.
TIP: Pecans can be replaced with walnuts too.
PER SERVING
calories: 577 | fat: 49.0g | net carbs: 2.1g | fiber: 5.0g | protein: 32.0g

EASY BROCCOLI AND CHEESE

Macros: Fat 80% | Protein 14% | Carbs 6%
Prep time: 5 minutes | Cook time: 15 minutes | Serves 4

Even if you are a beginner, you will find this recipe quite easy to prepare. With readily available ingredients, you can be sure to prepare the recipe within a few minutes. Use melted butter for best results.

1 (10-ounce / 284-g) package frozen broccoli, cut into florests
3 tablespoons melted butter
Salt and freshly ground pepper, to taste
½ cup shredded Cheddar cheese

1. Bring a large pot of lightly salted water to a rapid boil. Add the broccoli florets and cook for 1 to 2 minutes until fork-tender but firm.
2. Remove from the pot and drain the water. Put the broccoli florets on a microwave-safe dish.
3. Add the melted butter and toss well. Season as desired with salt and pepper, then sprinkle the cheese on top.
4. Microwave on high until the cheese is melted, about 1 minute.
5. Let cool for about 5 minutes before serving.

STORAGE: Store in an airtight container in the fridge for up to one week.
REHEAT: Microwave, covered, until the desired temperature is reached or reheat in a frying pan or instant pot, covered, on medium.
SERVE IT WITH: To make this a complete meal, serve the broccoli and cheese with sauce made from cheese.
PER SERVING
calories: 152 | fat: 13.6g | carbs: 3.7g | protein: 5.7g

AMAZING BRUSSEL SPROUTS SALAD

Macros: Fat 80% | Protein 13% | Carbs 7%
Prep Time: 10 minutes | Cook Time: 0 minute | Serves 2

It's no secret that Brussels sprouts are extremely good for your body. But if you're struggling with this super food taste, look no further. This amazing Brussels sprout salad is nutritious, delicious, and easy to make.

6 Brussels sprouts
½ teaspoon apple cider vinegar
1 teaspoon olive oil

Salt, to taste
1 tablespoon Parmesan cheese, freshly grated

1. Clean and rinse the Brussels sprouts under running cold water.
2. Cut off the Brussels sprouts roots and discard.
3. Half the Brussels sprouts lengthwise then slice the halves in the opposite direction.
4. Add the Brussels sprouts in a medium mixing bowl then add the apple cider vinegar, olive oil, and salt to taste. Toss until well mixed.
5. Sprinkle with the grated cheese. Stir until well mixed.
6. Let it chill in the fridge for 5 minutes, then serve.

STORAGE: Store in an airtight container in the fridge for about 4.
SERVE IT WITH: To make this a delicious complete meal, serve it with sirloin steak or chicken veggie skewers.
PER SERVING
calories: 112 | fat: 9.9g | carbs: 1.9g | protein: 3.9g

Meal plan 4

Recipe 1: Cheesy Bacon Pancake With Parsley
Recipe 2: Buttered Eggs With Avocado And Salmon
Recipe 3: Low-Carb Buttered Sirloin Steak
Recipe 4: Keto Green Beans
Recipe 5: Divine Stuffed Pork Chops
Recipe 6: Easy Asparagus With Parmesan
Recipe 7: Exotic Flounder With Lemon Sauce
Recipe 8: Simple Baked Salmon Salad

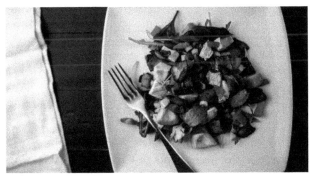

	BREAKFAST	LUNCH	DINNER	SNACK
DAY 1	Cheesy Bacon Pancake With Parsley	Low-Carb Buttered Sirloin Steak; Keto Green Beans	Exotic Flounder With Lemon Sauce	Simple Baked Salmon Salad
DAY 2	Buttered Eggs With Avocado And Salmon	Exotic Flounder With Lemon Sauce	Divine Stuffed Pork Chops; Easy Asparagus With Parmesan	Simple Baked Salmon Salad
DAY 3	Cheesy Bacon Pancake With Parsley	Divine Stuffed Pork Chops; Easy Asparagus With Parmesan	Low-Carb Buttered Sirloin Steak; Keto Green Beans	Simple Baked Salmon Salad
DAY 4	Buttered Eggs With Avocado And Salmon	Exotic Flounder With Lemon Sauce	Divine Stuffed Pork Chops; Easy Asparagus With Parmesan	Simple Baked Salmon Salad
DAY 5	Cheesy Bacon Pancake With Parsley	Low-Carb Buttered Sirloin Steak; Keto Green Beans	Divine Stuffed Pork Chops; Easy Asparagus With Parmesan	Simple Baked Salmon Salad

Shopping List 4

VEGETABLE
- **Yellow onion (1)**
- **Fresh parsley (5 oz. / 142 g)**
- **Avocado (2)**
- **Green beans (1 lb. / 454 g)**
- **Frozen spinach (1 pack of 10 oz. / 284 g)**
- **Mint leaves (3 oz. / 85 g)**
- **Salad leave (3 oz. / 85 g)**
- **Cucumber (1)**

MEAT/POULTRY/FISH, SEAFOOD/EGG
- **Bacon (3½ oz. / 99 g)**
- **Egg (4)**
- **Smoker salmon (4 oz. / 113 g)**
- **Beef steaks (1 lb. / 454 g)**
- **Chicken broth (1 pack of 5 oz. / 142 g)**
- **Pork chop (4) (4 oz. / 113 g each)**
- **Boneless flounder fillet 4 (4 oz. / 113 g)**
- **Salmon fillet (10 oz. / 284 g)**

CHEESE:
- **Heavy whipping cream (1 pack of 8 oz. / 227 g)**
- **Feta cheese (1 pack of 8 oz. / 227 g)**
- **Greek yogurt (1 pack of 8 oz. / 227 g)**

SAUCE:
- **Rice vinegar**
- **Mayonnaise**

Meal Prep Day Instruction 4

1. Preheat the oven to 350°F (180°C).
2. Prepare the ingredients of CHEESY BACON PANCAKE WITH PARSLEY through step 2, 3, and 4, and then bake for 20 to 25 minutes.
3. While the BACON is baking, prepare the pork chops through step 2, and make the filling through step 3. Sear the chops in a saucepan see step 4 and set aside, ready for baking.
4. Then prepare the salmon fillet of the recipe SIMPLE BAKED SALMON SALAD through step 2, ready for baking.
5. Prepare LOW-CARB BUTTERED SIRLOIN STEAK.
6. When the CHEESY BACON PANCAKE is completed, increase the oven temperature to 400°F (205°C). Once the temperature is reached, place the pork chops in the oven and bake for about 20 minutes.
7. While the pork chops are baking, prepare EXOTIC FLOUNDER WITH LEMON SAUCE. Make the sauce through step 1. Prepare the flounder fillet through step 2. And complete the dish through step 3.
8. Once the PORK CHOPS are cooked, put the salmon fillet in the oven because the two dishes share the same temperature. And bake for 15 minutes.
9. While the salmon fillet is cooking, prepare BUTTERED EGGS WITH AVOCADO AND SALMON. Begin by boiling eggs, during this period of time, get parsley, salmon and avocados ready. And then chop the eggs and combine with sessions and these ingredients.
10. Then prepare KETO GREEN BEAN.
11. The last dish is EASY ASPARAGUS WITH PARMESAN.

CHEESY BACON PANCAKE WITH PARSLEY

Macros: Fat: 84% | Protein: 12% | Carbs: 4%
Prep time: 10 minutes | Cook time: 30 minutes | Serves 4

Looking for the perfect low-carb pancakes? This "Cheesy bacon pancake" dish is a healthy low-carb pancake recipe of your dreams. Made deliciously with the keto-friendly psyllium husk powder, it is a buttery melt-in-your tongue option that will make your taste buds come alive.

2 tablespoons butter
3½ ounces (99 g) bacon, sliced
½ yellow onion, sliced
½ cup cottage cheese
4 eggs
1 cup heavy whipping cream

½ cup almond flour
1 tablespoon ground psyllium husk powder
1 teaspoon salt
1 teaspoon baking powder
1 tablespoon chopped fresh parsley, for garnish

1. Start by preheating the oven to 350°F (180°C).
2. Put the butter in a frying pan over medium heat to melt. Add the sliced bacon and onions in the frying pan and fry until the onion is translucent and the bacon curls.
3. Whisk the cheese, eggs, and cream in a small bowl, then add the almond flour, psyllium husk, salt, and baking powder. Mix thoroughly to form a smooth batter.
4. Pour the batter into a greased baking pan and smooth the top with a spatula. Evenly spread the fried bacon and onions over it.
5. Place the pan in the oven and bake for 20 to 25 minutes until the pancake is completely set.
6. Serve warm garnished with parsley.

STORAGE: Store in an airtight container in the fridge for up to 4 days or in the freezer for up to 1 month.
REHEAT: Microwave, covered, until the desired temperature is reached or reheat in a frying pan or air fryer / instant pot, covered, on medium.
SERVE IT WITH: To make this a complete meal, serve it with a cup of black tea.
PER SERVING
calories: 545 | fat: 49.0g | net carbs: 4.0g | fiber: 1.0g | protein: 15.0g

BUTTERED EGGS WITH AVOCADO AND SALMON

Macros: Fat 88% | Protein 10% | Carbs 2%
Prep time: 5 minutes | Cook time: 15 minutes | Serves 2

It is a breakfast specially made for champions. Are you a champion? The meal keeps you in game for several hours. What makes it even better is that it is keto-friendly. What are you waiting for? Grab your ingredients and get going.

4 eggs
5 ounces (142 g) butter, at room temperature
¼ teaspoon ground black pepper
½ teaspoon sea salt

1 tablespoon chopped fresh parsley
4 ounces (113 g) smoked salmon
2 diced avocados

1. Put the eggs in a pot of water, then bring to a boil.
2. Reduce the heat and allow to simmer for about 7 minutes. Remove the eggs from the pot, then place the eggs in a bowl of cold water to cool.
3. Peel the egg shells then chop the eggs finely. In a separate bowl, mix the eggs together with butter using a fork. Sprinkle the pepper and salt to season.
4. Transfer to two serving plates and top with finely chopped parsley, slices of the salmon and avocados.

STORAGE: Store in an airtight container in the fridge for up to 4 days or in the freezer for up to 1 month.
REHEAT: Microwave the salmon, covered, until the desired temperature is reached or reheat in a frying pan or air fryer / instant pot, covered, on medium.
SERVE IT WITH: To make this a complete meal, serve it with mocha keto coffee shake.
PER SERVING
calories: 1147 | fat: 113.0g | net carbs: 4.0g | fiber: 13.0g | protein: 27.0g

LOW-CARB BUTTERED SIRLOIN STEAK

Macros: Fat 48% | Protein 51% | Carbs 1%
Prep time: 10 minutes | Cook time: 10 minutes | Serves 3

It is a keto-friendly delicacy with low-gluten content that will satisfy your beef craving. It is very easy to cook and has an amazing taste and flavor.

3 tablespoons butter
1 pound (454 g) sirloin beef top steaks
½ teaspoon garlic powder
1 minced garlic clove
Salt and freshly ground black pepper, to taste

1. In a frying pan over medium heat, add the butter and beef steaks. Sear the steaks for 2 minutes on each side until lightly browned.
2. Add the garlic powder, minced garlic clove, black pepper and salt to the steaks. Cook for about 3 minutes more until desired doneness.
3. Transfer to serving plates and serve while hot.

STORAGE: Store in an airtight container in the refrigerator for up to 4 days.
REHEAT: Microwave, covered, until the desired temperature is reached or reheat in a frying pan or air fryer / instant pot, covered, on medium.
SERVE IT WITH: To make this a complete meal, serve with keto green beans on the side.
PER SERVING
calories: 245 | fat: 13.0g | total carbs: 1.9g | protein: 31.4g

KETO GREEN BEANS

Macros: Fat 60% | Protein 20% | Carbs 20%
Prep time: 5 minutes | Cook time: 15 minutes | Serves 3

This is one of the easiest recipes you can prepare and it takes less than half an hour to be ready. You will love every bit of it!

1 tablespoon olive oil
1 tablespoon sesame seeds
1 pound (454 g) green beans, fresh, cut into 2-inch pieces
Freshly ground black pepper, to taste
¼ teaspoon salt
¼ cup chicken broth

1. In a nonstick skillet over medium heat, heat the olive oil. Add the sesame seeds and cook until it starts to darken.
2. Add the green beans and cook for 5 minutes. Keep stirring during the cooking.
3. Add the pepper, salt and chicken broth. Cover the lid and cook for about 6 minutes or until the green beans are tender.
4. Remove the lid and continue cooking for about 2 minutes to evaporate the liquid. Transfer to a platter and serve warm.

STORAGE: Store in an airtight container in the fridge for up to 3 days. It is not recommended to freeze.
REHEAT: Microwave, covered, until the desired temperature is reached or reheat in a frying pan or instant pot, covered, on medium.
SERVE IT WITH: To make this a complete meal, serve this dish with fried beef steak.
PER SERVING
calories: 92 | fat: 6.2g | carbs: 5.0g | protein: 5.0g

DIVINE STUFFED PORK CHOPS

Macros: Fat: 66% | Protein: 32% | Carbs: 2%
Prep time: 20 minutes | Cook time: 30 minutes | Serves 4

A delicious way to enjoy pork chops with a fabulous stuffing... This fabulous stuffing of spinach, olives and feta cheese brightens the taste of pork chops.

4 (4-ounce / 113-g) 2-inch thick center pork chops
¾ cup chopped frozen spinach, thawed and squeezed
3 tablespoons Kalamata olives, pitted and chopped

4 ounces (113 g) feta cheese, crumbled
Sea salt and ground black pepper, to taste
3 tablespoons olive oil

SPECIAL EQUIPMENT:
Toothpicks, soaked for at least 30 minutes

1. Preheat the oven to 400°F (205°C).
2. Arrange 1 pork chop onto a cutting board. Hold a sharp knife parallel to work surface, slice the pork chop horizontally to create a pocket, without cutting all the way through. Repeat with the remaining pork chops.
3. Make the filling: In a small bowl, place the spinach, olives and feta cheese and mix until well combined. Stuff each pork chop with the filling evenly. Then, secure the slit of each chop with toothpicks. Season the stuffed chops with salt and black pepper lightly.
4. In a large saucepan, heat the oil over medium-high heat and sear the chops for about 10 minutes or until golden brown on both sides. Transfer the saucepan to the oven and bake for about 20 minutes or until done completely.
5. Remove from the oven to serving plates. Let the chops rest for about 10 minutes before serving.

STORAGE: Store in an airtight container in the fridge for up to 4 days or in the freezer for up to 1 month.
REHEAT: Microwave, covered, until the desired temperature is reached or reheat in a frying pan or air fryer / instant pot, covered, on medium.
SERVE IT WITH: These stuffed chops are great with Parmesan asparagus.
PER SERVING
calories: 342 | fat: 25.0g | net carbs: 2.1g | fiber: 1.0g | protein: 27.0g

EASY ASPARAGUS WITH PARMESAN

Macros: Fat 77% | Protein 15% | Carbs 8%
Prep time: 5 minutes | Cook time: 10 minutes | Serves 4

This recipe is so crispy and filled with flavor. It is one of the easiest recipes to make as it takes only 10 minutes. The combination of asparagus and cheese is popular and will definitely make you love this recipe!

1 tablespoon butter
¼ cup olive oil
1 pound (454 g) fresh asparagus spears, trimmed

Kosher salt and freshly ground black pepper, to taste
¾ cup Parmesan cheese, grated

1. In a large nonstick skillet, heat the butter with olive oil over medium heat until the butter melts.
2. Add the asparagus spears and sauté for 10 minutes or until the asparagus is soft.
3. Drain the extra oil and then sprinkle with pepper, salt and cheese. Cook for 2 minutes more or until the cheese melts.
4. Transfer to a serving plate. Allow to cool before serving.

STORAGE: Store in an airtight container in the fridge for up to 3 days. It is not recommended to freeze.
REHEAT: Microwave, covered, until the desired temperature is reached or reheat in a frying pan or air fryer / instant pot, covered, on medium.
SERVE IT WITH: To make this a complete meal, serve it with pork, beef, and fish fillets.
PER SERVING
calories: 201 | fat: 17.8g | carbs: 3.8g | protein: 7.6g

EXOTIC FLOUNDER WITH LEMON SAUCE

Macros: Fat 53% | Protein 46% | Carbs 1%
Prep time: 10 minutes | Cook time: 10 minutes | Serves 4

A healthy and elegant recipe of flounder fish for dinner. Lemony buttered sauce gives flounder fillets a richly delicious taste.

SAUCE:
½ cup unsalted butter, cut into pieces
2 tablespoons fresh lemon juice

Sea salt and ground black pepper, to taste

FLOUNDER:
¼ cup almond flour
4 (4-ounce / 113-g) boneless flounder fillets
Sea salt and ground black pepper, to taste

2 tablespoons olive oil
1 tablespoon fresh parsley, chopped

1. To make the sauce: In a medium saucepan, place the butter over medium heat and cook for about 4 minutes or until golden brown, stirring frequently. Remove the saucepan from heat and stir in the lemon juice, salt and black pepper. Set aside.
2. In a shallow bowl, place the almond flour. With paper towels, pat dry the flounder fillets and then, season with salt and black pepper lightly. Now, coat each flounder fillet with almond flour evenly. In a large skillet, heat the oil over medium-high heat, and cook the flounder fillets for about 2 to 3 minutes per side or until golden brown.
3. Remove from the heat to serving plates. Drizzle each fillet with sauce and serve immediately with the garnishing of parsley.

STORAGE: Store in an airtight container in the fridge for up to 4 days or in the freezer for up to 1 month.
REHEAT: Microwave, covered, until the desired temperature is reached or reheat in a frying pan or air fryer / instant pot, covered, on medium.
TIP: Garnishing of lemon zest will add a refreshingly tasty touch in flounder fillets.
PER SERVING
calories: 240| fat: 14.1g | net carbs: 0.7g | fiber: 0.8g | protein: 27.5g

SIMPLE BAKED SALMON SALAD

Prep time: 10 minutes | Cook time: 15 minutes | Serves 2
Macros: Fat 70% | Protein 12% | Carbs 18%

B akes salmon and a salad made up of a variety of vegetables if a perfect choice for dinner. Add the plain Greek yogurt to the salad to improve the taste and flavors.

10 ounces (284 g) salmon fillet
2 tablespoons olive oil
1 tablespoon plain Greek yogurt
Black pepper, to taste
1 tablespoon rice vinegar
Salt, to taste
1 tablespoon finely chopped mint leaves

1 teaspoon mayonnaise, keto-friendly
1 tablespoon olive oil
½ cup baby spinach
1 cup mixed salad leaves
1 sliced cucumber
½ cup chopped parsley

1. Start by preheating the oven to 400°F (205°C).
2. Put the fillet on a baking sheet, then rub with olive oil on both sides.
3. Place in the oven and bake until cooked through, about 15 minutes.
4. Remove from the oven to a plate and keep warm.
5. Meanwhile, combine the yogurt, pepper, rice wine vinegar, salt, mint, mayonnaise, and oil in a mixing bowl. Set aside for 5 minutes to blend the flavors.
6. Place the spinach and the salad leaves on a serving plate, then add the cucumber, and parsley on top. Add the cooked fillet and pour over the yogurt mixture. Serve immediately.

STORAGE: Store in separate airtight containers in the fridge for up to 3 days.
REHEAT: Microwave the fish, covered, until the desired temperature is reached.
PER SERVING
calories: 270 | fat: 20.0g | total carbs: 11.8g | fiber: 8.5g | protein: 32.0g

Chapter 4
Breakfast

PUMPKIN BREAD AND SALMON SANDWICH

Macros: Fat 80% | Protein 17% | Carbs 3%
Prep time: 5 minutes | Cook time: 1 hour 10 minutes | Serves 2

It is a keto sandwich that is perfect for brunch with fellow friends. It can be a holiday breakfast, too. It is simple to prepare the meal. The salmon sandwich never fails to impress.

SPICY PUMPKIN BREAD:

1 tablespoon melted coconut oil, for greasing the pan	husk powder
2 tablespoons pumpkin pie spice	1¼ cups almond flour
1 teaspoon salt	1 tablespoon baking powder
⅓ cup chopped walnuts	½ cup flaxseed
⅓ cup pumpkin seeds, plus more for topping	3 eggs
	14 ounces (397 g) pumpkin purée
1¼ cups coconut flour	¼ cup melted coconut oil
2 tablespoons ground psyllium	½ cup unsweetened apple sauce

TOPPINGS:

2 tablespoons heavy whipping cream	2 tablespoons melted butter
4 eggs	1 ounce (28 g) leafy lettuce greens
Salt and freshly ground black pepper, to taste	3 ounces (85 g) smoked salmon
2 ounces (57 g) butter, for frying	1 tablespoon chopped fresh chives
1 pinch chili flakes	

MAKE THE SPICY PUMPKIN BREAD:

1. Preheat the oven to 400°F (205°C). Grease a bread pan with melted coconut oil and set aside.
2. In a bowl, add pumpkin pie spice, salt, walnuts, pumpkin seeds, coconut flour, husk powder, almond flour, baking powder, and flaxseed and mix.
3. In a separate bowl, whisk together eggs, pumpkin purée, oil and apple sauce until smooth. Add the dry ingredients to the bowl of wet ingredients. Stir well with a fork until it forms a smooth batter.
4. Pour the batter into the greased baking dish and smooth the top with a spatula. Scatter the top with a tablespoon of pumpkin seeds.
5. Bake in the preheated oven for 1 hour or until a toothpick inserted in the center comes out clean.
6. Allow to cool for 8 minutes before slicing and set aside.

MAKE THE SANDWICH:

1. In a bowl, add the cream and eggs and whisk to combine. Sprinkle pepper and salt to season.
2. In a frying pan, add the butter and melt over medium high heat. Add the egg mixture and cook for about 4 minutes until scrambled, stirring occasionally. Remove from the heat to a plate, then sprinkle with chili flakes. Set aside.
3. Lay the pumpkin bread slices on a clean work surface and brush with melted butter.
4. Top with scrambled eggs, lettuce leaves, salmon and chopped chives, then serve.

STORAGE: Store in an airtight container in the fridge for up to 4 days. It is not recommended to freeze.
REHEAT: Microwave, covered, until the desired temperature is reached or reheat in a frying pan or air fryer / instant pot, covered, on medium.
SERVE IT WITH: To make this a complete meal, serve the dish with a cup of strawberry avocado smoothie.
PER SERVING
calories: 571 | fat: 51.0g | total carbs: 10.0g | fiber: 6.0g | protein: 24.0g

PANCAKES WITH CREAM AND RASPBERRIES

Macros: Fat 84% | Protein 13% | Carbs 3%
Prep time: 5 minutes | Cook time: 5 minutes | Serves 4

These are delicious keto pancakes. When you try this pancake, you will never look back to the ordinary pancakes. The berry topping gives it the sweetness and flavor. You should definitely try out this recipe.

PANCAKES:

4 eggs	7 ounces (198 g) cottage cheese
1 tablespoon ground psyllium husk powder	2 ounces (57 g) coconut oil

TOPPINGS:

1 cup heavy whipping cream	2 ounces (57 g) fresh raspberries

1. Whisk the eggs in a bowl and add psyllium husk and cottage cheese. Stir to combine until you get a smooth batter.
2. In a large skillet, melt the coconut oil over medium heat.
3. Pour the batter into the skillet and tilt the pan so it spreads all over. Cook for about 2 to 3 minutes until golden brown. Carefully flip it over and cook for 1 minute more.
4. Transfer the pancake to a plate. Serve topped with heavy cream and raspberries.

STORAGE: Store in an airtight container in the fridge for up to 4 days. It is not recommended to freeze.
REHEAT: Microwave the pancakes, covered, until the desired temperature is reached or reheat in a frying pan or air fryer / instant pot, covered, on medium.
SERVE IT WITH: To make this a complete meal, serve the dish with a cup of green keto smoothie.
PER SERVING
calories: 428 | fat: 40.0g | total carbs: 7.0g | fiber: 4.0g | protein: 14.0g

SPICY EGGS WITH CHEESE

Macros: Fat 73% | Protein 24% | Carbs 3%
Prep time: 5 minutes | Cook time: 10 minutes | Serves 1

It is an easy to prepare low-carb and keto-friendly breakfast. One can take it as lunch or dinner. The oregano spicing up the color and flavor sums up the deliciousness of the meal.

½ tomato	2 eggs
Salt and freshly ground black pepper, to taste	2 ounces (57 g) cubed Cheddar cheese
½ tablespoon butter	½ teaspoon dried oregano

1. In a bowl, season the tomato with salt and pepper.
2. Melt the butter in a frying pan over medium heat. Add the tomato, cut side down, and break the eggs into the pan.
3. Fry them for about 4 minutes, flipping the eggs and tomato halfway through the cooking time, or until cooked to your desired doneness. Season with salt and pepper.
4. Transfer the eggs to a serving plate. Top with fried tomato, cheese and oregano before serving.

STORAGE: Store in an airtight container in the fridge for up to 4 days. It is not recommended to freeze.
REHEAT: Microwave the eggs and tomato, covered, until the desired temperature is reached or reheat in a frying pan or air fryer / instant pot, covered, on medium.
SERVE IT WITH: To make this a complete meal, serve with sugar-free chocolate butter smoothie.
PER SERVING
calories: 396 | fat: 32.0g | total carbs: 5.0g | fiber: 2.0g | protein: 24.0g

SCRAMBLED EGGS WITH SALMON

Macros: Fat 73% | Protein 25% | Carbs 2%
Prep time: 2 minutes | Cook time: 10 minutes | Serves 1

The meal takes less time as it is simple to prepare and cook. The meal is rich in nutrients and flavors. Addition of the chives and pepper adds flavor and taste to the food.

2 eggs, whisked	chives
2 tablespoons butter	Salt and freshly ground black
¼ cup heavy whipping cream	pepper, to taste
1 tablespoon chopped fresh	2 ounces (57 g) cured salmon

1. In a frying pan, add butter and heat until it melts. Pour the eggs and cream into the pan and stir until scrambled.
2. Lower the heat and allow the mixture to simmer for a few minutes. Continue stirring the mixture until creamy. Sprinkle with the chives, pepper, and salt.
3. Transfer the egg mixture to a platter and serve with cured salmon on the side.

STORAGE: Store in an airtight container in the fridge for up to 4 days. It is not recommended to freeze.
REHEAT: Microwave, covered, until the desired temperature is reached or reheat in a frying pan or air fryer / instant pot, covered, on medium.
SERVE IT WITH: To make this a complete meal, serve with lemon cucumber smoothie.
PER SERVING
calories: 749 | fat: 61.0g | total carbs: 3.0g | fiber: 0g | protein: 47.0g

CREAMY BAGEL OMELET

Macros: Fat: 71% | Protein: 28% | Carbs: 1%
Prep time: 5 minutes | Cook time: 10 minutes | Serves 1

Do you want to make a quick and easy breakfast? Look no further than this bagel omelet dish. Guaranteed to taste delicious, it is perfect for kids and adults alike. It is the perfect recipe for all your busy weekdays.

3 large eggs	2 ounces (57 g) smoked salmon
1 tablespoon heavy whipping	1 tablespoon fresh dill, minced
cream or coconut cream	1 shaved scallion, divided
1 tablespoon butter	1 teaspoon bagel seasoning

1. Heat a medium frying pan over medium heat until it warms.
2. Whisk the eggs and whipping cream in a small bowl.
3. Put the butter in the pan, when the butter melts, tilt the pan so it covers the bottom evenly. Pour in the egg mixture and spread it all over the pan.
4. Use a spatula to mix the eggs, making sure not to scramble them.
5. Turn off the heat, then put the smoked salmon, dill, and ¾ of the scallions in the middle of the egg, then use the spatula to lift one edge of the egg to cover the filling. Roll it over until it is shaped like a tube.
6. Serve the omelet on a plate garnished with the bagel seasoning and the remaining scallions.

STORAGE: Store in an airtight container in the fridge for up to 4 days. It is not recommended to freeze.
REHEAT: Microwave, covered, until the desired temperature is reached or reheat in a frying pan or air fryer / instant pot, covered, on medium.
SERVE IT WITH: To make this a complete meal, serve it with some berries and a cup of coffee.
PER SERVING
calories: 391 | fat: 31.0g | total carbs: 1.0g | fiber: 0g | protein: 27.0g

CHEESY BACON EGG CUPS

Macros: Fat: 58% | Protein: 39% | Carbs: 3%
Prep time: 5 minutes | Cook time: 15 minutes | Serves 3

This cheesy bacon egg cup dish is perfect for any busy weekday. Loved by kids and adults, kick things up a notch with this delicious variation of the standard breakfast recipe and you won't regret it.

3 ounces (85 g) bacon, in slices	Salt and freshly ground black
3 ounces (85 g) Cheddar cheese,	pepper, to taste
shredded	Thinly sliced fresh basil, for
6 large eggs	garnish

SPECIAL EQUIPMENT:
A 6-cup muffin tin, lightly greased with coconut oil

1. Start by preheating the oven to 400°F (205°C).
2. Put a bacon slice in each muffin cup, making sure it curves around the well to form a bowl. Add 2 tablespoons of cheese into every bacon cup.
3. Break an egg into each cup and sprinkle with salt and pepper.
4. Put the muffin cups in the oven and bake for 12 to 14 minutes until the egg whites are set.
5. Serve hot garnished with basil.

STORAGE: Store in an airtight container in the fridge for up to 4 days or in the freezer for up to 1 month.
REHEAT: Microwave, covered, until the desired temperature is reached or reheat in an air fryer or instant pot, covered, on medium.
SERVE IT WITH: To make this a complete meal, serve it with a cup of black tea.
PER SERVING
calories: 154 | fat: 10.0g | total carbs: 1.0g | fiber: 0g | protein: 15.0g

BUTTERY EGGS WITH AVOCADO ANG SPINACH

Macros: Fat: 84% | Protein: 12% | Carbs: 4%
Prep time: 5 minutes | Cook time: 7 minutes | Serves 1

Looking for a light egg breakfast? Look no further than this buttery egg with avocado and spinach dish. Get those important greens in every bite with this egg recipe. It is perfect for adults with busy weekdays and for kids.

½ ounce (14 g) butter	½ avocado, scooped out and cut
2 eggs	into wedges
Salt and freshly ground black	1 (3-ounce / 85-g) tomato, sliced
pepper, to taste	½ cup baby spinach

1. Melt the butter in a frying pan over medium heat.
2. Break the eggs into the pan and let it fry on one side for 2 minutes for sunny-side-up eggs. For well-cooked eggs, fry for 1 minute on each side. Season with salt and pepper.
3. Transfer the fried eggs to a plate. Serve topped with avocado wedges, sliced tomatoes, and baby spinach.

STORAGE: Store in an airtight container in the fridge for up to 4 days. It is not recommended to freeze.
REHEAT: Microwave the eggs, covered, until the desired temperature is reached or reheat in a frying pan or air fryer / instant pot, covered, on medium.
SERVE IT WITH: To make this a complete meal, serve it with a cup of coffee with some cream.
PER SERVING
calories: 481 | fat: 45.0g | total carbs: 12.0g | fiber: 7.0g | protein: 14.0g

VINAIGRETTE AND MUSHROOM FRITTATA

Macros: Fat 86% | Protein 12% | Carbs 2%
Prep time: 15 minutes | Cook time: 40 minutes | Serves 4

This recipe is versatile as you can take during any meal session. And it is also easy to prepare. Famously referred to as the Italy's open-faced omelet. It is a keto classic meal with the excellent complement to the eggs.

VINAIGRETTE:

4 tablespoons olive oil

1 tablespoon white wine vinegar

FRITTATA:

1 pound (454 g) sliced mushrooms

4 ounces (113 g) butter

6 chopped scallions

1 teaspoon salt

½ teaspoon ground black pepper

1 tablespoon fresh parsley

10 eggs

8 ounces (227 g) shredded cheese

1 cup keto-friendly mayonnaise

½ teaspoon salt

¼ teaspoon ground black pepper

4 ounces (113 g) leafy greens

1. Preheat the oven to 350°F (180°C).
2. Make the vinaigrette: In a bowl, combine the olive oil and vinegar. Stir well to combine. Set aside.
3. Make the frittata: Melt the butter in a nonstick skillet over medium-high heat, then add and sauté the mushrooms until lightly browned. Remove from the heat and reserve the melted butter to grease a baking dish.
4. On a plate, combine the scallions with fried mushrooms, then sprinkle with salt and pepper. Fold in the parsley.
5. In another bowl, whisk together the eggs, cheese, mayonnaise, salt and pepper.
6. Add the mushroom mixture to the egg mixture. Stir to combine well.
7. Pour the mixture into the greased baking dish. Arrange the dish in the preheated oven and bake for about 40 minutes until lightly browned and puffed.
8. Transfer to four serving plates. Allow to cool for 5 minutes, then serve with the vinaigrette and leafy greens.

STORAGE: Store in an airtight container in the fridge for up to 4 days or in the freezer for up to 1 month.
REHEAT: Microwave, covered, until the desired temperature is reached or reheat in a frying pan or air fryer / instant pot, covered, on medium.
SERVE IT WITH: To make this a complete meal, serve with keto vanilla milkshake.
PER SERVING
calories: 1084 | fat: 104.0g | total carbs: 8.0g | fiber: 3.0g | protein: 32.0g

GOAT CHEESE AND ASPARAGUS OMELET

Macros: Fat 74% | Protein 22% | Carbs 4%
Prep time: 10 minutes | Cook time: 15 minutes | Serves 2

With fresh spring vegetables, the omelet is a pleasant choice in every energetic breakfast. The meal is full of flavor and the simplicity in making it tops it all. The meal is versatile as you can take it with almost every other meal.

4 large eggs

2 tablespoons heavy whipping cream

1 tablespoon butter

4 chopped green asparagus, cut into 1-inch pieces

Salt and freshly ground black pepper, to taste

2 ounces (57 g) goat cheese, shredded

1 ounce (28 g) baby spinach

½ chopped scallion

1. Whisk all the eggs in a bowl, then add the cream. Mix well until foamy, then set the mixture aside.
2. Melt the butter in a skillet over medium heat. Add the asparagus and sauté for approximately 4 minutes until fork-tender.
3. Transfer the asparagus to a plate and leave the melted butter in the skillet.
4. Make the omelet: Lower the heat, then pour the egg mixture into the skillet. Tilt the pan so the mixture covers the bottom of the skillet evenly. Cook for 1 minute and sprinkle with salt and pepper in the last 30 seconds. Top the omelet with cheese, asparagus and spinach on the omelet. Flip the omelet, then let it cook for 2 minutes more.
5. Divide and transfer to two serving plates. Top with the scallion and allow to cool for 5 minutes before serving.

STORAGE: Store in an airtight container in the fridge for up to 4 days. It is not recommended to freeze.
REHEAT: Microwave, covered, until the desired temperature is reached or reheat in a frying pan or air fryer / instant pot, covered, on medium.
SERVE IT WITH: To make this a complete meal, serve with turmeric keto smoothie.
PER SERVING
calories: 327 | fat: 27.0g | total carbs: 5.0g | fiber: 2.0g | protein: 18.0g

EASY SAUSAGE, EGG, AND CHEESE CASSEROLE

Macros: Fat 81% | Protein 17% | Carbs 2%
Prep time: 15 minutes | Cook time: 35 minutes | Serves 4

Here's a scrumptious breakfast casserole that the entire family will love. The meal is quick and easy to prepare for a crowd. Bacon can also be used in place of sausage according to your preference.

2 tablespoons coconut oil

1 tablespoon butter, unsalted

⅓ cup yellow onions, chopped

1 pound (454 g) bulk breakfast sausage

6 whisked eggs

1 pressed clove garlic

⅓ cup heavy whipping cream

½ teaspoon ground black pepper

1 teaspoon salt

1 cup Cheddar cheese, shredded

1. Preheat the oven to 350°F (180°C) and coat a baking dish lightly with coconut oil.
2. In a skillet, add the butter and heat to melt. Add the onions then sauté for about 4 minutes until soft.
3. Add the sausage, then cook for about 5 minutes until browned evenly. Drain excess butter and set aside until ready to use.
4. In a bowl, add the whisked eggs, garlic, cream, pepper, and salt, then whisk together thoroughly.
5. Evenly spread the sausage on the baking dish, then top with cheese. Add the egg mixture.
6. Bake for about 35 minutes until the edges begin to brown.
7. Transfer to serving plates to cool for about 5 minutes before serving.

STORAGE: Store in an airtight container in the fridge for up to 4 days or in the freezer for up to 1 month.
REHEAT: Microwave, covered, until it reaches the desired temperature.
SERVE IT WITH: To make this a complete meal, serve it with a cup of unsweetened coconut milk.
PER SERVING
calories: 977 | fat: 88.2g | total carbs: 5.0g | fiber: 0.2g | protein: 41.1g

CRUNCHY CINNAMON FRENCH TOAST

Macros: Fat: 83% | Protein: 14% | Carbs: 3%
Prep time: 5 minutes | Cook time: 15 minutes | Serves 2

French toast has never tasted better. This low-carb alternative is perfect for busy weekdays. It is very delicious and is perfect for breakfast or brunch.

MUG BREAD:

1 teaspoon melted butter
1½ teaspoons baking powder
1 pinch salt
2 tablespoons almond flour

2 tablespoons coconut flour
2 eggs, beaten
2 tablespoons heavy whipping cream

BATTER:

2 eggs
2 tablespoons heavy whipping cream

½ teaspoon ground cinnamon
1 pinch salt
2 tablespoons butter

1. Preheat the oven to 350°F (180°C). Grease a glass dish with melted butter and set aside.
2. In a bowl, mix the baking powder, salt, almond flour, and coconut flour with a spoon, then add the eggs and the whipping cream. Stir well until it is smooth.
3. Pour the mixture into the greased dish then put it in the microwave to cook on high pressure for 2 minutes or until a knife inserted in the middle comes out clean.
4. Remove the bread from the microwave and let cool. Slice the bread in half and set aside.
5. Mix the batter ingredients together in a bowl. Soak the bread in the bowl to coat well.
6. Arrange the bread in a baking dish and put in the oven to toast for 5 minutes on each side until golden brown.
7. Remove the bread from the oven. Let rest for 5 minutes before serving.

STORAGE: Store in an airtight container in the fridge for up to 4 days. It is not recommended to freeze.
REHEAT: Microwave, covered, until it reaches the desired temperature.
SERVE IT WITH: To make this a complete meal, serve it with a cup of green tea.

PER SERVING
calories: 392 | fat: 36.0g | total carbs: 6.0g | fiber: 3.0g | protein: 14.0g

SPICY CHEESY EGGS WITH AVOCADO AND CILANTRO

Macros: Fat: 79% | Protein: 12% | Carbs: 9%
Prep time: 15 minutes | Cook time: 20 minutes | Serves 4

Only for the spiciest of them all, this dish is the perfect blend of cheesy deliciousness and healthy low-carb ingredients. Perfect for adults and kids who love taking bites on the wild side. The cheesy eggs dish will be your favorite.

½ cup olive oil, divided
2 fresh jalapeños, minced
1 white onion, minced
2 garlic cloves, minced

2 cups crushed tomatoes
Salt and freshly ground black pepper, to taste
8 eggs

TOPPINGS:

1 avocado, sliced
2 ounces (57 g) shredded queso fresco

4 tablespoons fresh cilantro, chopped

1. Pour ⅓ of the olive oil into a large skillet over medium heat, then add the jalapeños to cook until slightly tender. Mix in the onions and garlic and keep stirring until the onions become translucent.
2. Pour the crushed tomatoes into the pan and reduce the heat. Let it cook until the sauce has thickened, then season with salt and pepper. Remove the tomato mixture from the heat to a plate. Set aside.
3. Pour the remaining oil into the skillet over medium heat.
4. One at a time, crack the eggs into the skillet. Fry for 2 minutes or until the egg white has set but the yolk is still runny. Sprinkle with salt and pepper. Stir in the tomato mixture and cook for 1 minute more.
5. Divide the egg mixture among four plates. Top each plate evenly with sliced avocado, queso fresco, and cilantro. Serve warm.

STORAGE: Store in an airtight container in the fridge for up to 4 days. It is not recommended to freeze.
REHEAT: Microwave the egg mixture, covered, until the desired temperature is reached or reheat in a frying pan or air fryer / instant pot, covered, on medium.
SERVE IT WITH: To make this a complete meal, serve it with a glass of sparkling water.

PER SERVING
calories: 513 | fat: 45.0g | total carbs: 17.0g | fiber: 6.0g | protein: 16.0g

HEALTHY HEMP SEED PORRIDGE

Macros: Fat 82% | Protein 16% | Carbs 2%
Prep time: 2 minutes | Cook time: 5 minutes | Serves 2

Made with seeds, nuts, vanilla extract and cinnamon, hemp seed porridge is keto-friendly. Taste very similar to oatmeal but is low in carbs and high in protein and fat. Takes a very short time to prepare.

PORRIDGE:

1 cup unsweetened almond milk
½ cup hemp seeds, hulled
1 tablespoon chia seeds
2 tablespoons flaxseeds, roughly ground

2 tablespoons coconut oil
1 tablespoon erythritol
¾ teaspoon vanilla extract
¾ teaspoon ground cinnamon
¼ cup almond meal

TOPPINGS:

4 raw Brazil nuts, roughly chopped
2 tablespoons hemp seeds,

hulled
Fresh berries, optional

1. In a saucepan, add the milk, hemp seeds, chia seeds, flaxseeds, coconut oil, erythritol, vanilla, and cinnamon. Stir well to combine. Heat over medium-high heat and bring to a boil.
2. As it bubbles, stir well and cover. Cook for about 2 minutes.
3. Remove the mixture from the heat, then add almond meal and stir. Divide equally between 2 bowls. Top each of bowls equally with the Brazil nuts, hemp seeds, and berries before serving.

STORAGE: Store in an airtight container in the fridge for up to 4 days or in the freezer for up to 1 month.
REHEAT: Microwave, covered, until it reaches the desired temperature.
SERVE IT WITH: To make this a complete meal, serve with low-carb strawberry smoothie.
PER SERVING
calories: 610 | fat: 55.6g | total carbs: 15.2g | fiber: 12.4g | protein: 24.6g

COFFEE CHIA SMOOTHIE

Macros: Fat: 92% | Protein: 6% | Carbs: 2%
Prep time: 5 minutes | Cook time: 0 minutes | Serves 2

A smoothie with health benefits of coffee, chia seeds, flaxseed meal, coconut oil, almond, coconut milk compliments coffee and seeds will bring you a pleasant morning or add a soft flavor for your dinner.

2 cups unsweetened strong-brewed coffee, frozen in cubes
1 cup unsweetened almond milk
1 cup unsweetened coconut milk
2 tablespoons coconut oil

2 tablespoons chia seeds
2 tablespoons flaxseed meal
1 to 2 tablespoons granulated monk fruit sweetener
⅛ teaspoon ground cinnamon

1. Add all ingredients in a high-power blender and pulse until creamy and smooth.
2. Pour the smoothie into two glasses and serve immediately.

STORAGE: Store brewed coffee in ice cube trays and freeze for 1 to 2 weeks.
SERVE IT WITH: Serve this smoothie with the topping of heavy cream.
PER SERVING
calories: 430 | fat: 44.2g | total carbs: 6.6g | fiber: 4.5g | protein: 6.0g

SAUSAGE BREAKFAST

Macros: Fat 76% | Protein 22% | Carbs 2%
Prep time: 10 minutes | Cook time: 50 minutes | Serves 8

The sausage breakfast is filled with a delicious egg mixture over a crescent crust. The meal is easy to prepare and takes a short time to cook.

2 tablespoons olive oil, divided
1 pound (454 g) homemade sausage
8 large eggs
1 tablespoon fresh oregano, chopped

2 cups cooked spaghetti squash
Sea salt and ground black pepper to taste
½ cup Cheddar cheese, shredded

1. Preheat the oven to 375°F (190°C) and grease a casserole dish with 1 tablespoon of olive oil.
2. Heat the remaining olive oil in a skillet. Add the sausages and cook for 5 minutes or until they are browned.
3. In a bowl, break the eggs and whisk well. Add oregano and squash, then mix well. Add salt and pepper to season. Add the sausage, then stir to mix.
4. Pour the sausage mixture in the casserole dish.
5. Scatter the cheese over the mixture and cover loosely with an aluminum foil.
6. Bake in the preheated oven for about 30 minutes. Remove the aluminum foil, then bake for 15 minutes more.
7. Allow the casserole to cool for about 8 minutes before serving.

STORAGE: Store in an airtight container in the fridge for up to 4 days or in the freezer for up to 1 month.
REHEAT: Microwave, covered, until it reaches the desired temperature.
SERVE IT WITH: To make this a complete meal, serve with chocolate peanut butter smoothie.
PER SERVING
calories: 297 | fat: 25.0g | total carbs: 4.0g | fiber: 2.0g | protein: 18.0g

KETO KALE AND BACON WITH EGGS

Macros: Fat: 68% | Protein: 22% | Carbs: 10%
Prep time: 5 minutes | Cook time: 20 minutes | Serves 2

Need to stock up on healthy and nutritious veggies? Or you just don't want to eat your veggies without some meat. This is the best combination of vegetables and other healthy food sources. This delicious dish is perfect for adults and kids.

4 ounces (113 g) bacon, chopped into bite-sized pieces
¾ pound (340 g) kale, chopped

2 eggs
Salt and freshly ground black pepper, to taste

1. Put the bacon in a large frying pan over medium heat. Cook for 4 minutes on each side or until it is crispy. Remove from the pan to a bowl and set aside.
2. Put the kale in the pan and sprinkle salt and pepper, and then cook for 2 minutes. Remove from the pan to two plates and set aside.
3. Break the eggs straight into the pan and cook for 2 minutes or until the egg white has set but the yolk is still runny. Season with salt and pepper.
4. Top each plate of kale with bacon and fried egg, then serve.

STORAGE: Store in an airtight container in the fridge for up to 4 days. It is not recommended to freeze.
REHEAT: Microwave, covered, until the desired temperature is reached or reheat in a frying pan or air fryer / instant pot, covered, on medium.
SERVE IT WITH: To make this a complete meal, serve it with a glass of sparkling water.
PER SERVING
calories: 355 | fat: 27.0g | total carbs: 14.0g | fiber: 5.0g | protein: 19.0g

EVERYTHING BAGEL SEASONED EGGS

Macros: Fat: 67% | Protein: 26% | Carbs: 7%
Prep time: 10 minutes | Cook time: 5 minutes | Serves 2

One of the simplest and easiest breakfast of boiled eggs! Spice mixture gives a deliciously spicy kick to boiled eggs.

4 eggs
3 tablespoons white sesame seeds
1 tablespoon black sesame seeds

2 teaspoons poppy seeds
1 tablespoon onion flakes
1 teaspoon garlic flakes
1 teaspoon coarse sea salt

1. In a medium saucepan of water, place the eggs over medium-high heat and bring to a boil. Boil for about 1 minute. Cover the saucepan and immediately remove from the heat. Set the pan aside, covered for about 10 minutes. Drain the eggs and transfer the eggs into a bowl of cold water to cool completely.
2. Meanwhile, in a bowl, mix the remaining ingredients for seasoning.
3. When cooled, peel the eggs and transfer to serving plates. Sprinkle the eggs with some seasoning mixture and serve immediately.

STORAGE: Store this seasoning in the sealed jar in the fridge for up to six months.
SERVE IT WITH: Serve these eggs with avocado slices on the side.
PER SERVING
calories: 230 | fat: 17.2g | total carbs: 6.0g | fiber: 2.0g | protein: 14.9g

WALNUT GRANOLA

Macros: Fat 84% | Protein 11% | Carbs 5%
Prep time: 10 minutes | Cook time: 1 hour | Serves 8

The nut granola is a versatile meal. The addition of nuts makes it a nutritious keto diet. You can omit or add other ingredients to suit your preference.

1 cup raw sunflower seeds	½ cup raw pumpkin seeds
2 cups shredded coconut, unsweetened	½ teaspoon nutmeg, ground
	10 drops liquid stevia
½ cup walnuts	½ cup coconut oil, melted
1 cup almonds, sliced	1 teaspoon cinnamon, ground

1. Preheat the oven to 250°F (120°C) and line two baking sheets with parchment paper.
2. In a bowl, add the sunflower seeds, shredded coconut, walnuts, almonds, and pumpkin seeds. Toss well to mix.
3. Add the nutmeg, stevia, coconut oil, and cinnamon in a small bowl, and stir thoroughly to blend.
4. Make the granola mixture: Pour the nutmeg mixture into the sunflower seed mixture and blend well to coat the nuts.
5. Spread the granola mixture on the baking sheets. Arrange the sheets in the preheated oven.
6. Bake for 1 hour or until the granola is crispy and lightly browned. Stir the granola every 15 minutes to break the large pieces.
7. Transfer to serving bowls to cool for 8 minutes before serving.

STORAGE: Store in an airtight container in the fridge for up to 4 days or in the freezer for up to 1 month.
REHEAT: Microwave, covered, until it reaches the desired temperature.
SERVE IT WITH: To make this a complete meal, serve with a cup of unsweetened coffee.
PER SERVING
calories: 397 | fat: 37.0g | total carbs: 10.0g | fiber: 5.0g | protein: 11.0g

CHICKEN AND EGG STUFFED AVOCADO

Macros: Fat 71% | Protein 24% | Carbs 5%
Prep time: 10 minutes | Cook time: 20 minutes | Serves 4

Avocado and chicken blend in well in eggs. Salt and pepper add spice to the dish. The meal is perfect for breakfast.

2 peeled and pitted avocados, halved lengthwise	¼ cup Cheddar cheese, shredded
4 eggs	Sea salt and freshly ground black pepper, to taste
1 (4-ounce / 113-g) cooked chicken breast, shredded	

1. Preheat the oven to 425°F (220°C).
2. Double the size of the hole in each avocado half with a spoon and arrange on a baking dish, hollow parts facing up.
3. In every hole, crack an egg and divide the chicken breast between every half of the avocado. Sprinkle with the Cheddar cheese and add salt and pepper to season.
4. Bake for about 20 minutes or until the eggs are cooked through.
5. Transfer to four serving plates and serve while warm.

STORAGE: Store in an airtight container in the fridge for up to 4 days or in the freezer for up to 1 month.
REHEAT: Microwave, covered, until it reaches the desired temperature.
SERVE IT WITH: To make this a complete meal, serve with strawberry zucchini chia smoothie.
PER SERVING
calories: 330 | fat: 26.0g | total carbs: 8.0g | fiber: 4.0g | protein: 20.0g

EGGS & SPINACH FLORENTINE

Macros: Fat: 60% | Protein: 36% | Carbs: 4%
Prep time: 10 minutes | Cook time: 5 minutes | Serves 2

A classic egg Florentine that is perfect for an indulgent breakfast! This classic Eggs Florentine recipe is made with Parmesan spinach with poached eggs.

1 cup fresh spinach leaves, washed completely	Sea salt and ground black pepper, to taste
2 tablespoons Parmesan cheese, grated freshly	1 tablespoon white vinegar
	2 eggs

1. In a microwave-safe dish, place the spinach and microwave on High for about 1 to 2 minutes. Remove the bowl from microwave and cut the spinach into bite-sized pieces. Transfer the spinach onto 2 serving plates and sprinkle with Parmesan cheese, salt and black pepper.
2. In a pan of simmering water, add the vinegar and with a spoon, stir quickly. Carefully, break an egg into the center of simmering water. Turn off the heat and cover the pan until the egg is set. Repeat with the remaining egg.
3. Top each plate of spinach with 1 egg and serve.

STORAGE: Transfer the steamed spinach in a container and store in the refrigerator for 1 to 2 days.
REHEAT: Reheat the spinach in microwave and top with poached eggs before serving.
SERVE IT WITH: Serve it with bacon slices.
PER SERVING
calories: 87 | fat: 5.8g | total carbs: 1.1g | fiber: 0.3g | protein: 7.9g

SCRAMBLED EGGS WITH CHEESE AND CHILI

Macros: Fat 68% | Protein 29% | Carbs 3%
Prep time: 5 minutes | Cook time: 5 minutes | Serves 2

The scrambled eggs with chili is a magnificent way to start the day, they're packed with flavor and contain nutrients that offer a hearty southern breakfast. The best part is they take a short time to prepare.

4 large eggs	½ sliced avocado
1½ teaspoons butter, unsalted	¼ cup sour cream
½ cup warm homemade chili	¼ cup Cheddar cheese, shredded
Salt and ground black pepper, to taste	

1. Whisk the eggs in a bowl.
2. In a skillet, add the butter and heat to melt. Add the eggs then sauté until scrambled. Add the chili, then stir to mix.
3. Add salt and pepper to season.
4. Transfer to serving plates and serve with avocado, sour cream, and cheese.

STORAGE: Store in an airtight container in the fridge for up to 4 days or in the freezer for up to 1 month.
REHEAT: Microwave, covered, until it reaches the desired temperature.
SERVE IT WITH: To make this a complete meal, serve with cinnamon raspberry breakfast smoothie.
PER SERVING
calories: 496| fat: 37.6g | total carbs: 8.2g | fiber: 4.0g | protein: 35.3g

KETO CEREAL

Macros: Fat: 85% | Protein: 11% | Carbs: 4%
Prep time: 15 minutes | Cook time: 15 minutes | Serves 6

Have you finally gotten tired of walking around your supermarket or grocery store and seeing only sugar-filled cereal? Look no further than this low-carb alternative that is suitable for adults and kids. Say hello to this delicious cereal that is packed with only nutritious goodness for you and your family.

1 tablespoon golden flaxmeal
1 teaspoon ground cinnamon
1 cup almond flour
2 tablespoons sunflower seeds

1 teaspoon vanilla extract
¼ teaspoon salt
2 tablespoons water
1 tablespoon coconut oil

TO SERVE:
6 cups unsweetened almond milk

1. Start by preheating the oven to 350°F (180°C).
2. Pour the golden flaxmeal, cinnamon, flour, sunflower seeds, vanilla extract, and salt into a food processor and process until the mixture is smooth.
3. Add the water and the coconut oil to the food processor and pulse until a dough is formed.
4. Transfer the dough to a parchment paper on a flat work surface, then press until it is flat. Cover the dough with another parchment paper and roll the dough until it is 1.5 to 3 mm thick.
5. Remove the top parchment paper and cut the dough into 1-inch squares with a pizza cutter or knife.
6. Arrange the squares with the bottom layer of parchment paper on a baking sheet. Bake for 10 to 15 minutes until the edges are golden brown and crispy.
7. Let cool for 5 minutes, then serve it with unsweetened almond milk.

STORAGE: Store in an airtight container in the fridge for up to 4 days or in the freezer for up to 1 month.
REHEAT: Microwave, covered, until the desired temperature is reached or reheat in an air fryer or instant pot, covered, on medium.
SERVE IT WITH: To make this a complete meal, serve it with a glass of sparkling water.
PER SERVING
calories: 181 | fat: 17.0g | total carbs: 2.0g | fiber: 0g | protein: 5.0g

KETO CINNAMON FLAXSEED BUN MUFFINS

Macros: Fat 86% | Protein 11% | Carbs 3%
Prep time: 10 minutes | Cook time: 15 minutes | Serves 12

The keto cinnamon buns are a marvellous way to start your day. Naturally high in fiber, low in carbohydrates, sugar-free and paleo-friendly. They are gluten-free, dairy-free and sugar-free, hence provide a healthier option.

2 cups flaxseeds, roughly ground
2 tablespoons ground cinnamon
⅓ cup erythritol
½ teaspoon gray sea salt, finely ground
1 tablespoon baking powder

5 large whisked eggs
⅓ cup melted coconut oil
½ cup water
¼ teaspoon liquid stevia
2 teaspoons vanilla extract

SPECIAL EQUIPMENT:
A 12-cup muffin pan

1. Preheat the oven to 350°F (180°C) and line a muffin pan with 12 paper liners. Set aside.
2. In a bowl, add the flaxseeds, cinnamon, erythritol, salt, and baking powder, then stir to combine.
3. Add the eggs, oil, water, stevia, and vanilla in a blender, then pulse until bubbly.
4. Pour the egg mixture into the flaxseed mixture and stir with a spatula until the batter becomes very fluffy. Allow the batter to sit for about 3 minutes.
5. Divide the batter into the muffin cups. Bake in the preheated oven for about 15 minutes.
6. Remove the pan from the oven to a wire rack to cool for about 20 minutes before serving.

STORAGE: Store in an airtight container in the fridge for up to 4 days or in the freezer for up to 1 month.
REHEAT: Microwave, covered, until it reaches the desired temperature.
SERVE IT WITH: To make this a complete meal, serve with sugar-free chocolate sea salt smoothies.
PER SERVING
calories: 254 | fat: 24.2g | total carbs: 8.8g | fiber: 6.4g | protein: 6.7g

SHRIMP AND CHIVES OMELET

Macros: Fat 86% | Protein 13% | Carbs 1%
Prep time: 5 minutes | Cook time: 15 minutes | Serves 2

It is a keto meal that is delicious and only takes 15 minutes to cook. The folds of the omelet bring together the flavors in the recipe. The dressings are simple to prepare. Why not try it today?

FILLING:
4 tablespoons olive oil, divided
5 ounces (142 g) cooked shrimp, shelled and deveined
1 red chili pepper
2 garlic cloves, minced
½ teaspoon fennel seeds

Salt and freshly ground black pepper, to taste
½ teaspoon ground cumin
1 tablespoon fresh chives
½ cup keto-friendly mayonnaise

OMELET:
6 eggs
Salt and freshly ground black pepper, to taste

1. Heat 2 tablespoons olive oil in a skillet until it shimmers.
2. Add the shrimp, chili pepper, minced garlic, fennel seeds, pepper, salt, and cumin to the skillet, then cook for 3 to 4 minutes. Transfer the mixture to a bowl to cool.
3. Add the chives and mayonnaise to the mixture. Stir to combine well and set aside.
4. In a bowl, whisk all the eggs, then sprinkle salt and pepper to season.
5. Make the omelet: In a large skillet, heat the remaining olive oil. Pour the eggs to the skillet, tilting the pan to spread it evenly. Cook for 1 to 2 minutes or until the bottom is set.
6. Pour the shrimp mixture over the omelet. Using a spatula, gently fold the omelet in half to enclose the filling. Reduce the heat, then allow the omelet to set completely.
7. Divide the omelet between two plates and serve while warm.

STORAGE: Store in an airtight container in the fridge for up to 4 days. It is not recommended to freeze.
REHEAT: Microwave, covered, until the desired temperature is reached or reheat in a frying pan or air fryer / instant pot, covered, on medium.
SERVE IT WITH: To make this a complete meal, serve the omelet with veggie salad.
PER SERVING
calories: 880 | fat: 84.0g | total carbs: 5.0g | fiber: 2.0g | protein: 28.0g

WAFFLE SANDWICHES

Macros: Fat 78% | Protein 18% | Carbs 5%
Prep time: 10 minutes | Cook time: 20 minutes | Serves 2

This is a wonderful combination for a breakfast sandwich that is savory. You can play around by swapping the waffle sandwich ingredients, like going for ham instead of bacon!

WAFFLES:
2 large eggs, whisked
¼ teaspoon baking powder
½ tablespoon coconut flour
⅓ cup almond flour, blanched
Pinch of salt
4 drops liquid stevia
¼ teaspoon vanilla extract

SANDWICH FILLING:
4 slices bacon
2 eggs
2 slices Cheddar cheese, shredded
½ sliced avocado
Salt and ground black pepper, to taste

SPECIAL EQUIPMENT:
A waffle maker

1. Preheat a waffle maker to medium-high heat.
2. Make the waffles: In a mixing bowl, add the whisked eggs, baking powder, coconut flour, almond flour, salt, stevia, and vanilla and whisk well until smooth.
3. Transfer the batter into the waffle maker and cook for about 5 minutes until golden brown and a little crisp.
4. Meantime, make the sandwich filling: In a nonstick skillet, fry the bacon over medium-high heat for 8 minutes until crispy. Remove the bacon from the skillet and leave the bacon grease in the skillet.
5. Crack the eggs in the skillet, and cook to make the yolks runny.
6. Flip the eggs, then top each egg with a slice of the Cheddar cheese. Cover the skillet to allow the cheese to melt.
7. Make the sandwich: Quarter the waffle with a knife. Lay the quarters on two serving plates, then top each waffle with 2 bacon slices and the egg with cheese toppings, finished by avocado slices. Add salt and pepper to season.
8. Top each sandwich with the remaining quarters and serve.

STORAGE: Store in an airtight container in the fridge for up to 4 days or in the freezer for up to 1 month.
REHEAT: Microwave, covered, until it reaches the desired temperature.
SERVE IT WITH: To make this a complete meal, serve with keto coffee.
PER SERVING
calories: 666 | fat: 57.9g | total carbs: 10.7g | fiber: 3.4g | protein: 28.9g

BEEF & VEGGIE HASH

Macros: Fat: 64% | Protein: 27% | Carbs: 9%
Prep time: 15 minutes | Cook time: 35 minutes | Serves 4

One of the best ways to enjoy beef and veggies in your breakfast. This beef and veggie hash alongside eggs give you a healthy choice to start your day.

2 tablespoons olive oil
½ pound (227 g) ground beef
½ of zucchini, chopped
½ of red bell pepper, seeded and chopped
¼ of onion, chopped
2 teaspoons garlic, minced
1½ cups sugar-free tomato sauce
1 tablespoon dried basil, crushed
1 teaspoon dried oregano, crushed
Sea salt and ground black pepper, to taste
4 eggs

1. In a large deep saucepan, heat the oil over medium-high heat and cook the beef for about 10 minutes or until browned, stirring occasionally.
2. Add the zucchini, bell pepper, onion and garlic to cook for about 3 minutes, stirring frequently.
3. Stir in the tomato sauce, dried herbs, salt and black pepper, then bring to a gentle boil. Cook for about 10 minutes, stirring occasionally.
4. With the back of a spoon, make 4 wells in the beef mixture. Carefully, crack 1 egg into each well. Reduce the heat to medium-low and cook covered for about 9 to 10 minutes or until desired doneness.
5. Remove from the heat and serve warm.

STORAGE: Transfer the cooked beef and veggie mixture into a large container and refrigerate for 1 to 2 days.
SERVE IT WITH: Fresh green salad goes great with this dish.
PER SERVING
calories: 268 | fat: 19.2g | total carbs: 8.0g | fiber: 2.0g | protein: 17.8g

BACON QUICHE

Macros: Fat 71% | Protein 24% | Carbs 5%
Prep time: 20 minutes | Cook time: 50 minutes | Serves 8

The bacon quiche can be prepared ahead of time. They are highly recommended for breakfast. The bacon quiche will definitely become a family favorite. Ingredients can be adjusted to your liking.

CRUST:
2 tablespoons melted lard, plus more for greasing the tart pans
2 cups almond flour, blanched
1 large egg
⅛ teaspoon gray sea salt, finely ground

FILLING:
6 strips (6-ounce / 170-g) bacon
1⅓ cups unsweetened coconut milk
¼ cup plus 2 tablespoons nutritional yeast
4 large beaten eggs
⅛ teaspoon ground nutmeg
¼ teaspoon ground black pepper
¼ teaspoon gray sea salt, finely ground

1. Preheat the oven to 350°F (180°C) and lightly grease the tart pans with melted lard. Set aside.
2. Make the crusts: In a bowl, add the almond flour, lard, egg, and salt and whisk well to form a dough.
3. Divide the dough into 4 pieces, then lay each piece in the tart pan. Use a rounded spatula to press the dough into ⅛ inch.
4. Lay the tart pans on the baking sheet and bake in the preheated oven until the crusts become lightly golden for about 15 minutes.
5. Make the filling: In a frying pan, add the bacon and cook over medium-high heat until crispy. Remove from the pan, then roughly chop the bacon.
6. In another bowl, add coconut milk, yeast, eggs, nutmeg, pepper, and salt. Add the bacon then whisk well to combine.
7. Remove the crusts from oven and adjust the temperature to 325°F (160°C). Fill the crusts evenly with the filling.
8. Return the crusts to the oven. Bake for about 30 minutes until the tops turn lightly golden.
9. Transfer to a wire rack to cool before serving.

STORAGE: Store in an airtight container in the fridge for up to 4 days or in the freezer for up to 1 month.
REHEAT: Microwave, covered, until it reaches the desired temperature.
SERVE IT WITH: To make this a complete meal, serve with keto collagen smoothie.
PER SERVING
calories: 387 | fat: 30.6g | total carbs: 11.0g | fiber: 6.0g | protein: 22.8g

CREAMY BACON OMELET

Macros: Fat 81% | Protein 15% | Carbs 4%
Prep time: 10 minutes | Cook time: 10 minutes | Serves 4

The meal is easy to prepare and takes a short time to cook. The bacon and pepper add taste and flavor to the meal. You should definitely try out this recipe.

6 eggs	¼ cup onion, chopped
8 cooked and chopped bacon slices	½ cup canned artichoke hearts, chopped
2 tablespoons heavy whipping cream	Sea salt and ground black pepper, to taste
1 tablespoon olive oil	

1. In a bowl, whisk the eggs. Add the bacon and cream, then mix well to blend.
2. Heat the olive oil in a skillet over medium-high heat.
3. Sauté the onion in the skillet for 3 minutes or until tender.
4. Make the omelet: Pour the egg mixture into the skillet and swirl the pan so the mixture covers the bottom evenly.
5. Cook the omelet for about 2 minutes. Lift the edges with a spatula to allow the uncooked egg below spread.
6. Sprinkle the artichoke on the omelet, then flip. Cook for an additional 4 minutes or until the omelet becomes firm. Flip again to keep the artichoke on top. Sprinkle salt and pepper to season.
7. Transfer to serving plates to cool before serving.

STORAGE: Store in an airtight container in the fridge for up to 4 days or in the freezer for up to 1 month.
REHEAT: Microwave, covered, until it reaches the desired temperature.
SERVE IT WITH: To make this a complete meal, serve with a light salad.
PER SERVING
calories: 422 | fat: 38.0g | total carbs: 6.0g | fiber: 2.0g | protein: 16.0g

SIMPLE SCRAMBLED EGGS

Macros: Fat 68% | Protein 31% | Carbs 1%
Prep time: 10 minutes | Cook time: 15 minutes | Serves 2

Scrambled eggs provide a scrumptious breakfast option. The scrambled eggs are easy to prepare and take a short time to cook.

1 tablespoon unsalted butter	2 fresh chopped basil leaves
1 cup white mushrooms, sliced	⅓ cup chopped bacon, cooked
4 large scrambled eggs	Salt and freshly ground black pepper, to taste
⅓ cup crumbled goat cheese	

1. In a skillet, add the butter and heat to melt. Add the mushrooms and sauté for about 5 minutes or until soft.
2. Break the eggs in the skillet and sauté for about 5 minutes or until scrambled.
3. Add the cheese, basil, and bacon over the mushroom mixture and sauté for 2 minutes or until the cheese melts. Add salt and pepper to season.
4. Transfer to serving plates and serve warm.

STORAGE: Store in an airtight container in the fridge for up to 4 days or in the freezer for up to 1 month.
REHEAT: Microwave, covered, until it reaches the desired temperature.
SERVE IT WITH: To make this a complete meal, serve with sautéed spinach on the side.
PER SERVING
calories: 384 | fat: 29.0g | total carbs: 3.0g | fiber: 1.6g | protein: 29.4g

BASIC CAPICOLA EGG CUPS

Macros: Fat 74% | Protein 23% | Carbs 3%
Prep time: 5 minutes | Cook time: 14 minutes | Serves 3

Capicola egg cups offer a variety as far as eggs go. They are super delicious and ensures an excellent breakfast to kick-start your day. Prepare the egg cups easily and in a brief period.

1 tablespoon olive oil	6 large eggs
6 slices capicola	Salt and freshly ground black pepper, to taste
¾ cup Cheddar cheese, shredded	Thinly sliced basil, for garnish

SPECIAL EQUIPMENT:
A 6-cup muffin pan

1. Preheat the oven to 400°F (205°C) and grease the muffin cups with olive oil.
2. Put each slice of the capicola into each cup to form a bowl shape.
3. Sprinkle 2 tablespoons of cheese into every cup.
4. In every cup, crack an egg, then add salt and pepper to season.
5. Bake for about 14 minutes, or until eggs are set.
6. Garnish with the basil, then serve warm.

STORAGE: Store in an airtight container in the fridge for up to 4 days or in the freezer for up to 1 month.
REHEAT: Microwave, covered, until it reaches the desired temperature.
SERVE IT WITH: To make this a complete meal, serve with keto green lemon smoothie.
PER SERVING
calories: 307 | fat: 25.3g | total carbs: 2.3g | fiber: 0g | protein: 17.4g

STEVIA CHOCOLATE WAFFLE

Macros: Fat 71% | Protein 23% | Carbs 6%
Prep time: 5 minutes | Cook time: 5 minutes | Serves 1

The stevia chocolate waffle provides the solution for morning carb cravings. The ingredients are easily found on hand and make a fantastic breakfast or brunch option.

1 tablespoon olive oil	2 large eggs, beaten
⅓ cup almond flour, blanched	¼ teaspoon baking powder
½ tablespoon coconut flour	¼ teaspoon vanilla extract
4 drops liquid stevia	1 tablespoon chocolate chips

SPECIAL EQUIPMENT:
A waffle maker

1. Preheat the waffle maker to medium-high heat and grease the waffle maker with olive oil.
2. In a bowl, add the almond flour, coconut flour, stevia, eggs, baking powder, and vanilla. Blend well until it achieves the desired smooth consistency. Fold in the chocolate chips.
3. Pour the mixture into the waffle maker. Cook for about 5 minutes or until lightly browned.
4. Transfer to serving plates to cool before serving.

STORAGE: Store in an airtight container in the fridge for up to 4 days or in the freezer for up to 1 month.
REHEAT: Microwave, covered, until it reaches the desired temperature.
SERVE IT WITH: To make this a complete meal, serve with plain Greek yogurt.
PER SERVING
calories: 409 | fat: 32.0g | total carbs: 14.0g | fiber: 7.8g | protein: 24.0g

BACON AND BROCCOLI EGG MUFFINS

Macros: Fat 66% | Protein 31% | Carbs 3%
Prep time: 20 minutes | Cook time: 15 minutes | Serves 3

The broccoli egg muffins are packed with protein and low net carb which provides a healthy diet. The meal is recommended for breakfast because it sustains your energy for the whole day.

1 cup broccoli, chopped
3 slices bacon
6 beaten eggs
½ teaspoon black pepper, ground

¼ teaspoon garlic powder
½ teaspoon salt
A few drops of Sriracha hot sauce
1 cup Cheddar cheese, shredded

SPECIAL EQUIPMENT:
A 6-cup muffin pan

1. Preheat the oven to 350°F (180°C) and line 6 cups of muffin pan with silicone liners. Set aside.
2. Boil the broccoli in a pot of water for 6 to 8 minutes or until tender, then chop into ¼-inch pieces. Set aside.
3. In a nonstick skillet, fry the slices of bacon for about 8 minutes until crispy, then lay on a paper towel to drain.
4. In a bowl, pour the beaten eggs. Add pepper, garlic, hot sauce, and salt. Whisk well to mix.
5. Put the broccoli into the muffin cups. Top with the bacon, Cheddar cheese, and the egg mixture.
6. Bake in the preheated oven for 25 minutes or until eggs are set.
7. Transfer to serving plates to cool before serving.

STORAGE: Store in an airtight container in the fridge for up to 4 days or in the freezer for up to 1 month.
REHEAT: Microwave, covered, until it reaches the desired temperature.
SERVE IT WITH: To make this a complete meal, serve with coconut blackberry mint smoothie.
PER SERVING
calories: 296 | fat: 21.6g | total carbs: 6.5g | fiber: 4.0g | protein: 23.0g

STRAWBERRY SMOOTHIE BOWL

Macros: Fat 58% | Protein 30% | Carbs 12%
Prep time: 15 minutes | Cook time: 0 minutes | Serves 2

The smoothie bowl is a simple and easy to treat. It requires few ingredients and can be prepared for breakfast or as a snack. Toppings of your choice can also be added.

1 cup frozen strawberries
½ cup plain Greek yogurt
¼ cup almond milk, unsweetened

½ tablespoon whey protein powder, unsweetened
1 tablespoon chopped walnuts

1. In a blender, add the strawberries. Process until it has a smooth consistency.
2. Add the yogurt, almond milk, and protein powder, then process for 2 minutes more to combine well.
3. Equally divide the mixture into 2 bowls, and top with the walnuts before serving.

STORAGE: Store in an airtight container in the fridge for up to 4 days or in the freezer for up to 1 month.
SERVE IT WITH: To make this a complete meal, serve with healthy keto green smoothie.
PER SERVING
calories: 140 | fat: 9.0g | total carbs: 6.0g | fiber: 1.8g | protein: 10.5g

ALMOND CREAM CHEESE PANCAKES

Macros: Fat 77% | Protein 18% | Carbs 5%
Prep time: 15 minutes | Cook time: 15 minutes | Serves 1

The cream cheese pancakes are tender and fluffy, offering a perfect low-carb diet. They are super delicious and extra fluffy.

2 medium eggs
2 ounces (57 g) cream cheese
¼ cup almond flour, blanched
½ teaspoon vanilla extract

¼ teaspoon baking powder
1 teaspoon Swerve
1 tablespoon coconut oil
Salted butter, optional

1. In a blender, break the eggs and add cheese, almond flour, vanilla, baking powder, and Swerve. Process until the mixture is smooth and foamy.
2. Make the pancakes: Grease a skillet with coconut oil and heat. Drop one-third of the batter into the skillet and cook for 6 minutes. Flip the pancake halfway through the cooking time. Repeat with the remaining batter.
3. Transfer to serving plates and top with the salted butter, if desired.

STORAGE: Store in an airtight container in the fridge for up to 4 days or in the freezer for up to 1 month.
REHEAT: Microwave, covered, until it reaches the desired temperature.
SERVE IT WITH: To make this a complete meal, serve with pumpkin spice smoothie.
PER SERVING
calories: 481 | fat: 41.0g | total carbs: 12.0g | fiber: 6.0g | protein: 22.0g

SPANISH EGG FRITTATA

Macros: Fat 86% | Protein 12% | Carbs 2%
Prep time: 6 minutes | Cook time: 40 minutes | Serves 2

The effort required in making frittata is similar to scrambled eggs. The dish provides an appropriate choice for brunch. Quantity of ingredients can be altered depending on the number of people you're serving.

1 tablespoon olive oil
½ tablespoon butter
1½ ounces (42 g) bacon
2 ounces (57 g) fresh spinach
2 whisked eggs

¼ cup heavy whipped cream
1½ ounces (42 g) shredded Cheddar cheese
Salt and freshly ground black pepper, to taste

1. Preheat the oven to 375°F (190°C) and grease a baking dish with olive oil. Set aside.
2. In a skillet, add the butter and heat to melt, then add the bacon. Cook the bacon until crispy, about 8 minutes. Add the spinach and cook until tender. Remove from the heat to a large bowl.
3. Add the eggs, cream, cheese, salt and pepper into the large bowl, then stir to combine. Transfer the mixture to the baking dish.
4. Bake in the preheated oven for 30 minutes. Cut a small slit in the center, if raw eggs run into the cut, baking for another few minutes.
5. Transfer to serving plates to cool before serving.

STORAGE: Store in an airtight container in the fridge for up to 4 days or in the freezer for up to 1 month.
REHEAT: Microwave, covered, until it reaches the desired temperature.
SERVE IT WITH: To make this a complete meal, serve with strawberry avocado keto smoothie.
PER SERVING
calories: 643 | fat: 61.7g | total carbs: 2.9g | sugars: 0.6g | protein: 19.7g

BASIC CREAM CREPES

Macros: Fat 82% | Protein 11% | Carbs 7%
Prep time: 5 minutes | Cook time: 20 minutes | Serves 2

This is an exquisite breakfast with a very rich nutrient content. The dish is simple and easy to prepare. Cream crepes is also appropriate for a low-carb diet.

2 tablespoons melted coconut oil, divided
2 whisked eggs
Sea salt, to taste

1 teaspoon Swerve
2 tablespoons coconut flour
½ cup heavy whipping cream

1. In a bowl, add 1 tablespoon coconut oil, eggs, salt, and Swerve, then whisk to mix.
2. Slowly mix in the coconut flour, then fold in the cream until the mixture is smooth.
3. Heat the remaining oil in a skillet over medium heat. Pout half of the mixture into the skillet. Cook for 2 minutes on each side and repeat the process with the remaining mixture.
4. Transfer to serving plates and serve while warm.

STORAGE: Store in an airtight container in the fridge for up to 4 days or in the freezer for up to 1 month.
REHEAT: Microwave, covered, until it reaches the desired temperature.
SERVE IT WITH: To make this a complete meal, serve with keto cinnamon smoothie.
PER SERVING
calories: 390 | fat: 35.3g | total carbs: 7.4g | fiber: 0g | protein: 10.6g

LOW CARB JAMBALAYA WITH CHICKEN

Macros: Fat 76% | Protein 20% | Carbs 4%
Prep time: 25 minutes | Cook time: 25 minutes | Serves 4

Jambalaya is easy to make and allows you to experiment with your favorite protein. The meal is full of tasty flavors that brings everyone together.

⅓ cup lard
4 (8-ounce / 227-g) cooked and chopped sausage
1 cup cubed skinless chicken thighs, cooked
½ cup green onions, chopped
1¼ cups diced celery

2 tablespoons Cajun seasoning
½ cup chicken broth
2½ cups riced cauliflower
¼ cup diced tomatoes
Handful of freshly chopped parsley

1. In a frying pan, add the lard and heat to melt. Add the sausage, chicken thighs, green onions, celery, and Cajun seasoning. Cook for about 10 minutes until the celery softens, stirring occasionally.
2. Add the chicken broth and riced cauliflower. Cover and cook for about 5 minutes until the cauliflower is tender.
3. Add the diced tomatoes and stir. Increase the heat and cook uncovered for about 7 minutes, or until the liquid has evaporated.
4. Remove from heat to four bowls, then top with the parsley. Allow to cool for 5 minutes before serving.

STORAGE: Store in an airtight container in the fridge for up to 4 days.
REHEAT: Microwave, covered, until it reaches the desired temperature.
SERVE IT WITH: To make this a complete meal, serve with slow-cooked mushroom and chicken soup.
PER SERVING
calories: 446 | fat: 37.7g | total carbs: 7.6g | fiber: 3.4g | protein: 22.5g

CREAMY SPANISH SCRAMBLED EGGS

Macros: Fat 85% | Protein 10% | Carbs 5%
Prep time: 10 minutes | Cook time: 10 minutes | Serves 2

Spanish scramble is the best scrambled eggs that can easily be prepared for breakfast. Pepper is added to spice it up.

¼ cup heavy whipping cream
2 tablespoons finely chopped cilantro
4 large whisked eggs
Salt and black pepper, to taste

3 tablespoons butter
1 Serrano chili pepper
1 small chopped tomato
2 tablespoons sliced scallions

1. In a bowl, add the cream, cilantro, eggs, pepper, and salt and mix well.
2. In a pan, add the butter and heat to melt. Mix in Serrano pepper and tomatoes then sauté for 2 minutes over medium heat. Add cream mixture to the pan and sauté for 4 minutes or until scrambled.
3. Top with the scallions for garnish before serving.

STORAGE: Store in an airtight container in the fridge for up to 4 days or in the freezer for up to 1 month.
REHEAT: Microwave, covered, until it reaches the desired temperature.
SERVE IT WITH: To make this a complete meal, serve with mocha keto coffee shake.
PER SERVING
calories: 278 | fat: 26.3g | total carbs: 4.1g | fiber: 0.8g | protein: 7.0g

CLASSIC OMELET

Macros: Fat 73% | Protein 22% | Carbs 5%
Prep time: 10 minutes | Cook time: 30 minutes | Serves 6

Classic is just an example. We can inject it with our own preference and make it become our own 'classic'. The soft and creamy texture will enlighten your appetite and give you an excellent mood for a delightful working day.

9 eggs
½ cup unsweetened coconut milk
½ cup sour cream
1 teaspoon salt

2 green onions, chopped
1 teaspoon butter, melted
¼ cup Cheddar cheese, shredded

1. Start by preheating the oven to 350°F (180°C).
2. Whisk together the eggs, coconut milk, sour cream, and salt in a bowl, then fold in the green onions.
3. Coat a baking pan with the melted butter and tilt the pan so the butter covers the bottom evenly. Pour the egg mixture in the pan.
4. Arrange the pan in the preheated oven and bake for 25 minutes. You can check the doneness by cutting a slit in the center of the frittata, if raw eggs run into the cut, then baking for another few minutes. Sprinkle with the cheese and continue baking for an additional 2 minutes until the cheese melts.
5. Remove the omelet from the oven and serve warm.

STORAGE: Keep in the fridge for up to 3 to 4 days, or wrap in plastic and keep in the fridge for up to 4 weeks.
REHEAT: Microwave, covered, until the desired temperature is reached or reheat in a frying pan or air fryer / instant pot, covered, on medium.
SERVE IT WITH: To make this a complete meal, serve it with something crispy such as avocado sticks.
PER SERVING
calories: 287 | fat: 23.1g | total carbs: 4.3g | fiber: 0.5g | protein: 15.9g

SAUSAGE AND SPINACH HASH BOWL

Macros: Fat 84% | Protein 12% | Carbs 4%
Prep time: 25 minutes | Cook time: 25 minutes | Serves 2

Sausage and spinach hash bowl offers a satisfying and scrumptious brunch that will keep you going throughout the day. It is fast to cook and good for your health because of all the vegetables ingredients.

HASH:
⅔ cup peeled radishes, cut into ½-inch cubes
2 tablespoons lard
¼ cup green onions, chopped
(green parts only)
2 (4-ounce / 113-g) precooked sausages, cut into ½-inch cubes

FOR THE BOWLS:
2 cups fresh spinach
½ large sliced Hass avocado
2 cooked bacon, chopped into
½-inch strips
1 teaspoon fresh parsley, chopped

1. Steam the radishes until tender for about 10 minutes.
2. Make the hash: In a frying pan over medium-high heat, add the lard and heat to melt. Add the radishes then cook until the radishes turn brown, about 10 minutes.
3. Add the green onions and sausages then cook until the sausages turn brown, about 5 minutes.
4. Assemble the bowls: Equally divide the spinach into 2 serving bowls. Once the hash cooked through, divide between the bowls equally, laying them on top of the spinach bed.
5. Top with equal amounts of the avocado, bacon, and parsley before serving.

STORAGE: Store in an airtight container in the fridge for up to 4 days.
REHEAT: Microwave, covered, until it reaches the desired temperature.
SERVE IT WITH: To make this a complete meal, serve with vanilla milkshake.

PER SERVING
calories: 536 | fat: 49.8g | total carbs: 10.4g | fiber: 5.0g | protein: 16.5g

LEMON ALLSPICE MUFFINS

Macros: Fat 84% | Protein 13% | Carbs 3%
Prep time: 15 minutes | Cook time: 25 minutes | Serves 12

Allspice muffins are a delicious buttery, crumbly and sweet treat. The muffins are light and tender and get a kick from the allspice batter. The simplicity of the recipe and process produces delicious results.

1½ cups almond flour, blanched
½ cup flaxseeds, roughly ground
½ cup erythritol
2 teaspoons baking powder
1 tablespoon plus 1 teaspoon ground allspice
½ teaspoon ground gray sea salt
6 large whisked eggs
½ cup unsweetened coconut milk
½ cup melted coconut oil
1 teaspoon vanilla extract
Grated zest 1 lemon

TOPPING:
¼ cup walnut pieces, raw

SPECIAL EQUIPMENT:
A 12-cup muffin pan

1. Preheat the oven to 350°F (180°C) and line a muffin pan with 12 paper liners. Set aside.

2. In a bowl, add the almond flour, flaxseeds, erythritol, baking powder, allspice, and salt, then mix to blend.
3. In another bowl, add the eggs, coconut milk, coconut oil, vanilla, and lemon zest, then mix well. Add the almond flour mixture, then stir well with a spatula.
4. Divide the batter into the muffin cups, then sprinkle the walnuts on top.
5. Bake in the preheated oven until the top becomes golden for about 25 minutes.
6. Transfer to a wire rack to cool for about 10 minutes before serving.

STORAGE: Store in an airtight container in the refrigerator for up to 4 days or in the freezer for up to 1 month.
REHEAT: Microwave, covered, until it reaches the desired temperature.
SERVE IT WITH: To make this a complete meal, serve with perfect keto Frappuccino.

PER SERVING
calories: 260 | fat: 24.2g | total carbs: 5.8g | fiber: 3.4g | protein: 8.2g

PALEO OMELET MUFFINS

Macros: Fat 61% | Protein 31% | Carbs 8%
Prep time: 15 minutes | Cook time: 20 minutes | Serves 4

Small, cute, and easy made muffins. Its golden color will bring you dynamic to the keto diet. It's just like a little egg flower which holds the bacon up and raises your value on judging a good recipe.

8 eggs
8 ounces (227 g) cooked ham, crumbled
1 cup red bell pepper, diced
1 cup onion, diced
¼ teaspoon salt
⅛ teaspoon ground black pepper
2 tablespoons water

SPECIAL EQUIPMENT:
An 8-cup muffin pan, greased with olive oil

1. Start by preheating the oven to 350°F (180°C).
2. Whisk together the eggs, ham, red bell pepper, onion, salt, ground black pepper, and water in a large bowl.
3. Gently pour the mixture into the muffin cups, then arrange the cups in the preheated oven.
4. Bake for 18 minutes or until the tops of muffins spring back when lightly touched with your finger.
5. Remove from the oven. Let stand for a few minutes before serving.

STORAGE: Store in an airtight container for 1 to 2 days or keep in the fridge for up to 1 week.
REHEAT: Microwave, covered, until the desired temperature is reached or reheat in a frying pan or air fryer / instant pot, covered, on medium.
SERVE IT WITH: To make this a complete meal, serve it with a dollop of plain Greek yogurt or other drinks you like.

PER SERVING
calories: 357 | fat: 24.3g | total carbs: 8.3g | fiber: 1.7g | protein: 27.9g

NUT-FREE GRANOLA WITH CLUSTERS

Macros: Fat 79% | Protein 17% | Carbs 4%
Prep time: 20 minutes | Cook time: 50 minutes | Serves 12

The granola recipe is nut-free but is rich with a burst of flavor. The crunchy granola is simple and easy to make and is ready for the oven in a short time. Nut-free granola provides an excellent alternative for people allergic to nuts.

GRANOLA:

½ cup melted coconut oil, plus more for greasing the pan
1 large whisked egg
½ cup collagen peptides
3 tablespoons ground cinnamon
¼ teaspoon liquid stevia
2 teaspoons vanilla extract

¼ teaspoon finely ground gray sea salt
2 cups shredded coconut, unsweetened
1 cup hemp seeds, hulled
¼ cup chia seeds
1 cup sesame seeds

TOPPING:

Unsweetened coconut milk, as needed

Fresh berries, as needed

1. Preheat the oven to 300°F (150°C) and grease a baking pan with coconut oil. Set aside.
2. Make the granola: In a bowl, pour the egg, coconut oil, collagen, cinnamon, stevia, vanilla, and salt and whisk to combine.
3. In another bowl, add the shredded coconut, hemp seeds, chia seeds, and sesame seeds and mix well. Pour in the egg mixture and stir using a spatula to coat all the seeds.
4. Transfer to the greased baking pan and firmly press the mixture down with a spatula.
5. Bake for about 30 minutes until the corners and top start to turn golden.
6. Using a spatula to split granola into pieces. Flip them over, then bake for 20 minutes more until they turn golden.
7. Let the clusters cool for about 30 minutes. Transfer to serving bowls and pour in the coconut milk. Top with the berries and serve.

STORAGE: Store in an airtight container in the fridge for up to 4 days or in the freezer for up to 1 month.
REHEAT: Microwave, covered, until it reaches the desired temperature.
SERVE IT WITH: To make this a complete meal, serve with minty green protein smoothie.

PER SERVING
calories: 351 | fat: 31.0g | total carbs: 9.9g | fiber: 6.4g | protein: 14.5g

HAM AND VEGGIE OMELET IN A BAG

Macros: Fat 67% | Protein 28% | Carbs 5%
Prep time: 15 minutes | Cook time:13 minutes | Serves 1

This recipe shows us a unique way to make an omelet. But I believe the significance of this recipe is far more than an omelet, because it shows us a creative way of making food.

2 eggs
2 slices ham, chopped
1 tablespoon green bell pepper, chopped
2 tablespoons fresh tomato, chopped

2 fresh mushrooms, sliced
1 tablespoon onion, chopped
½ cup Cheddar cheese, shredded
1 tablespoon salsa

1. Whisk the eggs in a bowl, then add the whisked eggs, ham, green bell pepper, tomato, mushroom, onion, cheese, and salsa into a Ziploc bag. Shake the bag to combine well. You can prepare 4 more omelet bags at a time.
2. Bring a pot of water to a boil. Squeeze the air out of the bag and seal. Place the bag into the boiling water and cook for 13 minutes.
3. Remove the bag from the water. Open the bag and serve the omelet on a platter.

STORAGE: Keep in the fridge for up to 3 to 4 days, or wrap in plastic and keep in the fridge for up to 4 weeks.
REHEAT: Microwave, covered, until the desired temperature is reached or reheat in a frying pan or air fryer / instant pot, covered, on medium.
SERVE IT WITH: To make this a complete meal, serve it with something crispy such as avocado sticks.
PER SERVING
calories: 625 | fat: 46.6g | total carbs: 9.3g | fiber: 2.2g | protein: 44.4g

BREADLESS EGG SANDWICH

Macros: Fat 79% | Protein 19% | Carbs 2%
Prep time: 5 minutes | Cook time:16 minutes | Serves 2

We can try to use our imagination to create more ways of making a gluten-free or 'bread-free' sandwich or other keto-friendly breakfast. Making something wrapped in something have many possibilities to find.

4 slices bacon
2 eggs
Salt and freshly ground black

pepper, to taste
⅓ cup Cheddar cheese, shredded

1. Cook the bacon in a nonstick skillet over medium-high heat for 3 to 4 minutes. When it buckles and curls, loosen and flip the bacon slices so they brown evenly and cook for 3 to 4 minutes more.
2. Turn off the heat and crumble the bacon into pieces with a spatula. Transfer to a plate lined with paper towels. Set aside. Leave the bacon grease in the skillet.
3. Gently crack the eggs into the skillet, and sprinkle with salt and pepper.
4. Cook the eggs for 3 minutes until the egg whites are firm. Flip and scatter the eggs with bacon pieces and shredded cheese, then cook for 3 minutes more until the cheese melts.
5. Remove the eggs from the skillet and serve warm.

STORAGE: Store in an airtight container in the fridge for up to 2 days or keep in the freezer for up to 1 month.
REHEAT: Microwave, covered, until the desired temperature is reached or reheat in a frying pan or air fryer / instant pot, covered, on medium.
SERVE IT WITH: To make this a complete meal, you can serve it with plain Greek yogurt for an enjoyable morning.

PER SERVING
calories: 426 | fat: 37.4g | total carbs: 1.7g | fiber: 0g | protein: 20.7g

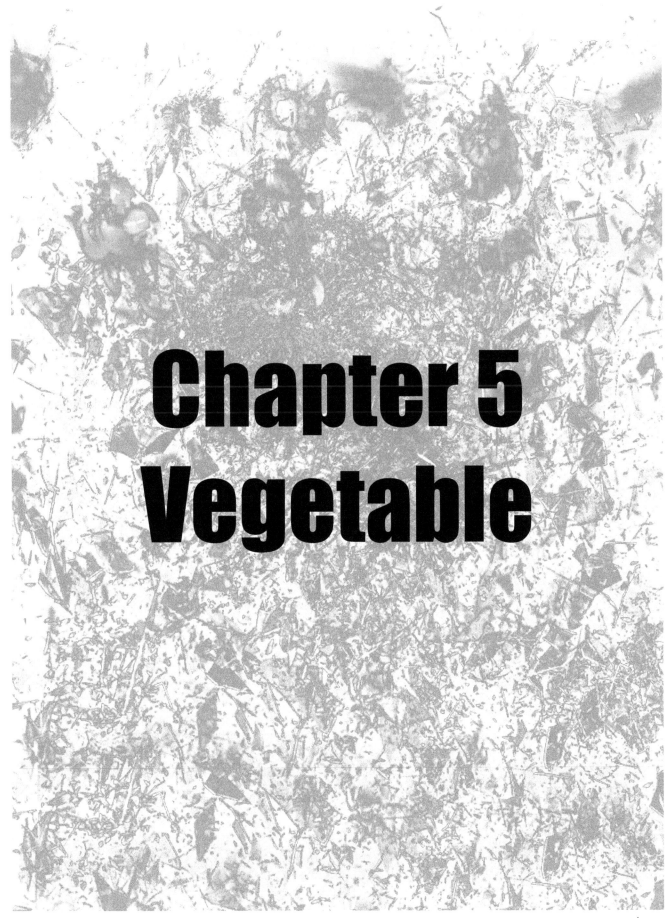

Chapter 5
Vegetable

SAUTEED MUSHROOM

Macros: Fat 66% | Protein 19% | Carbs 15%
Prep time: 5 minutes | Cook time: 10 minutes | Serves 2

Filled with different flavors, sautéed mushrooms are a perfect idea when you are stuck at what to prepare for dinner. You can enjoy the delicious meal full of flavors with juicy steak to fulfill your dinner.

½ tablespoon olive oil
2 tablespoons butter
1 pound (454 g) sliced button mushrooms
½ tablespoon balsamic vinegar

⅛ teaspoon dried oregano
1 minced garlic clove
Salt and freshly ground black pepper, to taste

1. Put a large skillet over medium heat, heat the oil and butter until melted.
2. Add the mushrooms, vinegar, balsamic vinegar, oregano, garlic, salt, and black pepper. Stir to combine well.
3. Fry for about 10 minutes, stirring occasionally, or until the mushrooms are tender and lightly browned.
4. Transfer to a plate and serve warm.

STORAGE: Store in an airtight container in the fridge for up to 4 days. It is not recommended to freeze.
REHEAT: Microwave, covered, until the desired temperature is reached or reheat in a frying pan or instant pot, covered, on medium.
SERVE IT WITH: To make this a complete meal, serve the mushrooms with a steak full of juices especially for dinner.
PER SERVING
calories: 163 | fat: 11.9g | total carbs: 8.6g | fiber: 2.3g | protein: 7.6g

SPINACH AND MUSHROOM ITALIAN-STYLE

Macros: Fat 74% | Protein 12% | Carbs 14%
Prep time: 20 minutes | Cook time: 10 minutes | Serves 4

Do not overcook the mushrooms and spinach. The white wine and balsamic vinegar give this dish a unique taste. You can enjoy with your friends and relatives for dinner, or use more onions as per your preference.

2 tablespoons olive oil
2 chopped garlic cloves
1 chopped scallion
14 ounces (397 g) sliced mushrooms
10 ounces (284 g) clean fresh spinach, roughly chopped

2 tablespoons balsamic vinegar
½ cup white wine
Salt and freshly ground black pepper, to taste
Chopped fresh parsley, for garnish

1. Put a large skillet over medium-high heat, then heat the oil.
2. When the oil is hot, fry the garlic and scallion to a tender texture, then add the mushrooms and cook for 4 minutes until they shrink.
3. Add the spinach and fry as you stir until it wilts, for a few minutes.
4. Add the vinegar as you stir until it is fully absorbed.
5. Pour in the white wine and cook on low until the wine has absorbed.
6. Season as desired with salt and pepper, then sir well.
7. Top with a sprinkle of fresh parsley and serve hot on a platter.

STORAGE: Store in an airtight container in the fridge for up to 4 days or in the freezer for up to 1 month.
REHEAT: Microwave, covered, until the desired temperature is reached or reheat in a frying pan or instant pot, covered, on medium.
SERVE IT WITH: To make this a complete meal, serve the mushroom and spinach with your favorite chicken.
PER SERVING
calories: 172 | fat: 14.1g | total carbs: 8.6g | fiber: 2.7g | protein: 5.3g

TASTY COLLARD GREENS

Macros: Fat 74% | Protein 20% | Carbs 6%
Prep time: 15 minutes | Cook time: 40 minutes | Serves 4

Enjoy this veggies for dinner. Cook the bacon and the greens until tender. When serving, you can add a sprinkle of chili flakes to improve the taste. It is a perfect recipe for the entire family.

6 slices bacon
Salt and freshly ground black black pepper, to taste
1 (1½- to 2-pound / 680- to

907-g) bunch collard greens, rinsed and trimmed
Cayenne pepper, to taste
⅓ cup vinegar

1. Put the bacon slices in a large skillet over medium-high heat. Cook for about 4 minutes on each side until browned evenly. Remove from the heat to a plate.
2. Bring a pot of water to a boil over low heat. Add the cooked bacon, black pepper, collard greens, cayenne pepper, salt, and vinegar. Stir well. Cook for 30 minutes until the greens become tender, stirring occasionally.
3. Transfer to a serving bowl and serve warm.

STORAGE: Store in an airtight container in the fridge for up to one week.
REHEAT: Microwave, covered, until the desired temperature is reached or reheat in a frying pan or instant pot, covered, on medium.
SERVE IT WITH: To make this a complete meal, serve the tasty collard greens with smoked turkey especially for dinner.
PER SERVING
calories: 199 | fat: 16.4g | total carbs: 9.7g | fiber: 6.9g | protein: 10.1g

SIMPLE PARMESAN ZUCCHINI FRIES

Macros: Fat 62% | Protein 25% | Carbs 13%
Prep time: 15 minutes | Cook time: 30 minutes | Serves 4

Zucchini are soft veggies. When added different flavors, they become delicious and tasty. Use the favorite spices you love when making the mixture for coating. The cheese makes the outside smooth and tender.

2 tablespoons olive oil
2 eggs
1 tablespoon dried mixed herbs
½ teaspoon ground black pepper

¾ cup grated Parmesan cheese
1 teaspoon paprika
1½ teaspoons garlic powder
2 pounds (907 g) zucchinis, cut into ½-inch French fry strips

1. Start by preheating the oven to 425°F (220°C). Line a baking tray with aluminum foil and grease with olive oil.
2. In a bowl, beat the eggs. Add the mixed herbs, pepper, Parmesan cheese, paprika, and garlic powder in another bowl, and stir well.
3. Dredge the zucchini fries into the beaten eggs, then dip them in the Parmesan mixture until coated evenly.
4. Arrange the coated zucchini fries on the prepared baking tray and bake for 35 minutes until golden brown.
5. Transfer to a plate lined with paper towels and serve.

STORAGE: Store in an airtight container in the fridge for up to 4 days or in the freezer for up to 1 month.
REHEAT: Microwave, covered, until the desired temperature is reached or reheat in an air fryer or instant pot, covered, on medium.
SERVE IT WITH: To make this a complete meal, serve the zucchini fries with a keto dipping sauce.
PER SERVING
calories: 262 | fat: 18.0g | total carbs: 12.9g | fiber: 4.2g | protein: 16.3g

CAULIFLOWER CASSEROLE

Macros: Fat 78% | Protein 18% | Carbs 4%
Prep time: 10 minutes | Cook time: 35 minutes | Serves 2

Easy Cauliflower Keto Casserole is a delicious recipe ideal for a family meal. It will make every member happy.

½ head cauliflower, cut into florets
½ cup heavy cream
¼ teaspoon salt

¼ teaspoon freshly ground black pepper
1 cup Cheddar cheese, shredded

1. Start by preheating the oven to 400°F (205°C).
2. Salt a large pot of water and bring to a boil over medium heat. Add and cook the cauliflower for about 10 minutes until lightly softened. Remove the cauliflower from the pot and pat dry. Set aside on a plate.
3. In a large bowl, combine salt, pepper, cream, and Cheddar cheese. In a casserole dish, put the cauliflower and pour the cheese mixture on top.
4. Arrange the casserole dish in the oven and bake for about 25 minutes, or until the cheese is melted.
5. When ready, let it cool for about 20 minutes, then serve.

STORAGE: Store in an airtight container in the fridge for up to 2 days. It is not recommended to freeze.
REHEAT: Microwave, covered, until the desired temperature is reached or reheat in a frying pan or air fryer / instant pot, covered, on medium.
SERVE IT WITH: To make this recipe complete meal, serve with veggie salad.
PER SERVING
calories: 388 | fat: 33.6g | total carbs: 5.0g | fiber: 1.3g | protein: 17.8g

SPINACH CASSEROLE

Macros: Fat 68% | Protein 16% | Carbs 16%
Prep time: 10 minutes | Cook time: 25 minutes | Serves 4

This casserole is savory and creamy. It is a perfect for holiday or a family dinner on a Sunday. Besides, spinach is one of the popular veggies to bring abundant nutrients for the people.

2 tablespoons olive oil, for greasing
1 (1-ounce / 28-g) package dry onion soup mix
2 cups sour cream

2 (10-ounce / 284-g) packages frozen chopped spinach, cooked and drained
½ cup Cheddar cheese, shredded

1. Start by preheating an oven to 350°F (180°C) and then grease a casserole dish with the olive oil.
2. Combine the soup mix, sour cream and spinach together in a medium mixing bowl. Pour the mixture into the casserole dish and then scatter with the shredded cheese.
3. Bake in the preheated oven for 25 minutes, or until cooked through and the cheese melts.
4. Cool for 5 minutes and then serve.

STORAGE: Store in an airtight container in the fridge for up to 3 days. It is not recommended to freeze.
REHEAT: Microwave, covered, until the desired temperature is reached or reheat in a frying pan or air fryer / instant pot, covered, on medium.
SERVE IT WITH: To make this a complete meal, serve it with the fried fish.
PER SERVING
calories: 339 | fat: 25.6g | total carbs: 18.7g | fiber: 4.9g | protein: 13.3g

CHEESY CAULIFLOWER BAKE

Macros: Fat 82% | Protein 13% | Carbs 5%
Prep time: 15 minutes | Cook time: 25 minutes | Serves 4

This recipe is creamy, cheesy and very yummy! This is a great deal to enjoy as it is easy to prepare and does not take long.

1 head cauliflower, cut into florets
1 teaspoon mixed herbs
½ teaspoon black pepper, ground
1 teaspoon salt
3 tablespoons olive oil

1 tablespoon butter
½ cup heavy whipping cream
1 pinch nutmeg, ground
1 cup Cheddar cheese, shredded
3 tablespoons Parmesan cheese, grated

1. Preheat the oven to 450°F (235°C) and then line an aluminum foil in a baking sheet.
2. Put the cauliflower florets in the baking sheet, then sprinkle with mixed herbs, pepper, salt, and olive oil. Toss to coat well.
3. Place the baking sheet in the preheated oven. Bake for 10 to 15 minutes until crunchy.
4. Meanwhile, heat the butter, heavy whipping cream, nutmeg and Cheddar cheese in a saucepan over medium heat. Bring them to a simmer for 5 minutes, or until they are foamy. Keep stirring during the cooking.
5. Pour the mixture over the cauliflower and scatter with Parmesan cheese, then bake in the oven for another 10 minutes or until golden brown.
6. Remove from the oven and cool for 5 minutes before serving.

STORAGE: Store in an airtight container in the fridge for up to 3 days. It is not recommended to freeze.
REHEAT: Microwave, covered, until the desired temperature is reached or reheat in a frying pan or air fryer / instant pot covered, on medium.
SERVE IT WITH: To make this a complete meal, serve with baked shrimp scampi.
PER SERVING
calories: 329 | fat: 30.1g | total carbs: 5.3g | fiber: 1.6g | protein: 10.7g

SYRIAN-STYLE GREEN BEANS

Macros: Fat 86% | Protein 4% | Carbs 10%
Prep time: 5 minutes | Cook time: 25 minutes | Serves 4

Prepare this awesome green bean enriched with nutrients and share with family and friends. They are easy and quick to prepare, and can be served for dinner or lunch.

1 (1-pound / 454-g) package frozen cut green beans
Salt, to taste

¼ cup extra virgin olive oil
1 minced garlic clove
¼ cup chopped fresh cilantro

1. Heat the oil in a large pot on medium-high heat, then add the green beans and sprinkle the salt to season.
2. Sauté for about 5 to 7 minutes, stirring occasionally, or until the beans are just tender.
3. Add the garlic and cilantro, then cook until the cilantro begins to wilt.
4. Remove from the heat and serve warm on a plate.

STORAGE: Store in an airtight container in the fridge for up to 4 days. It is not recommended to freeze.
REHEAT: Microwave, covered, until the desired temperature is reached or reheat in a frying pan or instant pot, covered, on medium.
SERVE IT WITH: To make this a complete meal, serve the green beans with a bowl of cauliflower rice.
PER SERVING
calories: 172 | fat: 16.0g | total carbs: 7.3g | fiber: 3.3g | protein: 1.7g

EASY ASPARAGUS F1RY

Macros: Fat 79% | Protein 13% | Carbs 8%
Prep time: 5 minutes | Cook time: 15 minutes | Serves 4

The fried asparagus is full on nutrients and creates tender stalks that are crispy and tasty. You will surely enjoy the resulting crunchy stalks.

¼ cup butter	2 tablespoons olive oil
¼ teaspoon ground black pepper	3 cloves garlic, minced
1 teaspoon coarse salt	1 pound (454 g) fresh asparagus spears, trimmed

1. In a skillet over medium-high heat, melt the butter. Add pepper, salt, and olive oil. Stir to combine well. Add the garlic and cook for 1 minute or until aromatic.
2. Add the asparagus and cook for about 10 minutes or until tender. Flip the asparagus during the cooking to make sure it cooked evenly.
3. Remove from the heat and serve in a big platter.

STORAGE: Store in an airtight container in the fridge for up to 3 days. It is not recommended to freeze.
REHEAT: Microwave, covered, until the desired temperature is reached or reheat in a frying pan or air fryer / instant pot, covered, on medium.
SERVE IT WITH: To make this a complete meal, serve with cooked eggs and shredded Parmesan.
PER SERVING
calories: 85 | fat: 7.4g | total carbs: 5.3g | fiber: 2.5g | protein: 2.7g

EASY BAKED CABBAGE

Macros: Fat: 88% | Protein: 4% | Carb: 8%
Prep time: 10 minutes | Cook time: 20 minutes | Serves 4

The baked cabbage is a keto-friendly side dish. It is easy to digest and won't upset your stomach. I don't use any artificial flavors or spices to make it hot and appealing to the taste buds. Any garden-fresh vegetable has its advantage in frozen products. Spread diced onion over it and bake along with the cabbage for a delicious experience. The baked cabbage is all set to win your heart because of the freshness it carries.

6 ounces (170 g) butter, melted	¼ teaspoon ground black pepper
2 pounds (907 g) fresh cabbage, cored and sliced into wedges	1 teaspoon salt

1. Preheat the oven to 400°F (205°C). Line the oven with a baking sheet.
2. Place the wedges on the baking sheet without overlapping.
3. Sprinkle the ground pepper and salt on the wedges for seasoning, and pour the melted butter over it.
4. Bake in the preheated oven for about 20 minutes or until wilted and roasted.
5. Remove the cabbage from the oven and serve warm.

STORAGE: Store in an airtight container in the fridge for up to 4 to 5 days or in the freezer for up to 1 month.
REHEAT: The dish can reheat and use it as a fresh salad. Microwave it as per the instruction or reheat in a frying pan or air fryer or instant pot under moderate heat.
SERVE IT WITH: Serve it as a side dish along with roasted meat, chicken, or fish. Sprinkle spices of your choice for unique taste other than ground pepper.
PER SERVING
calories: 366 | fat: 35.3g | total carbs: 8.0g | fiber: 6.0g | protein: 3.0g

GUACAMOLE

Macros: Fat: 86% | Protein: 6% | Carb: 8%
Prep time: 15 minutes | Cook time: 0 minutes | Serves 4

Enjoy the mashed delicacy of avocadoes, combined with grated onion, lime juice, and spices. The salad is quick to make and easy to make some alteration. Consider adding salsa and sour cream along with the ingredients to augment the taste. The calorie content justifies its ketogenic effect.

2 ripe avocados	cilantro, finely chopped
½ lime, juice extracted	1 clove garlic, finely grated
½ white onion, finely grated	2 tablespoons virgin olive oil
1 tomato, diced	¼ teaspoon ground pepper
4 tablespoons garden-fresh	¼ teaspoon salt

1. Peel the avocados and mash it in a medium bowl using a fork.
2. Combine it with lime juice, grated onion, tomato, cilantro, minced garlic, and olive oil.
3. Add pepper and salt as per your taste and combine well before serving.

STORAGE: Store in an airtight container in the fridge for 4 to 5 days.
SERVE IT WITH: Combine well with fried fish, roasted chicken, and meat.
PER SERVING
calories: 238 | fat: 22.4g | total carbs: 5.1g | fiber: 3.2g | protein: 3.4g

OVEN-BAKED KETO ZUCCHINI

Marcos: Fat: 80% | Protein: 10% | Carb: 10%
Prep time: 5 minutes | Cook time: 30 minutes | Serves 4

Salads are an ideal side dish, and they can get along with any main meals. Fresh salads are much better than frozen ones, and if you have time for making, try to make and refrigerate it for later use. A neatly prepared salad can make for 4 to 5 days if you can freeze it in an airtight container. So, people like me, who lead a hectic schedule, can plan to make the salad using for an extended period! No more waste of food!

1 large zucchini	cheese
1 tablespoon finely chopped garlic	1 (8-ounce / 227-g) package softened cream cheese
1 cup sour cream	Ground paprika, to taste
¼ cup shredded Parmesan	

1. Preheat the oven to 350°F (180°C).
2. Boil water in a large pot and put the zucchini. Cook it for 15 minutes or until lightly softened. Drain the water, and allow it to cool. Cut the zucchini into half and into lengthwise, and then scoop out the seeds.
3. In a medium bowl, blend the garlic, sour cream, Parmesan cheese, and cream cheese. Fill the mixture into zucchini halves and sprinkle the paprika on top.
4. Place the stuffed zucchini in a lightly greased baking pan. Put the pan in the oven and bake for 10 to 15 minutes or until cooked through.
5. Remove the zucchini from the oven and serve warm.

STORAGE: Store in an airtight container in the fridge for up to 4 days or in the freezer for up to 1 month.
REHEAT IT: Microwave, covered, until the desired temperature is reached or reheat in a frying pan or instant pot, covered, on medium.
SERVE IT WITH: To make this a complete meal, serve it with baked or roasted chicken.
PER SERVING
calories: 313 | fat: 27.8g | total carbs: 8.3g | fiber: 0.2g | protein: 7.5g

CAULIFLOWER, AND MUSHROOM CASSEROLE

Macros: Fat 74% | Protein 13% | Carbs 13%
Prep time: 2 minutes | Cook time: 45 minutes | Serves 8

This recipe is amazingly delicious and filled with very nice flavor. It is creamy and very nutritious. You will love every bit of it.

2 tablespoons olive oil, divided
2 onions, chopped

1 large head cauliflower, cut into florets
½ cup mayonnaise, keto-friendly
1 clove garlic, minced
½ cup sour cream
¼ teaspoon ground black

pepper
½ teaspoon salt
6 tablespoons fresh chives, chopped and divided
2 cups shredded Parmesan cheese, divided
1 (8-ounce / 227-g) package cremini mushrooms, chopped coarsely

1. Start by preheating the oven to 425°F (220°C). Grease a baking dish with 1 tablespoon oil.
2. Heat 1 tablespoon olive oil in a nonstick skillet over medium heat for 2 minutes. Add onions and fry for 2 minutes or until translucent.
3. Put a steamer insert in a saucepan, then pour into the water so that it almost reaches the steamer and bring to a boil. Add the cauliflower florets, cover and steam for 15 to 20 minutes or until tender.
4. Meanwhile, in a large bowl, combine mayonnaise, garlic, sour cream, black pepper, and salt; add cauliflower florets, 3 tablespoons chives, 1 cup Parmesan cheese, and mushroom and mix.
5. Pour the mixture into the greased baking dish, then scatter with the remaining crumbled bacon and Parmesan cheese.
6. Place in the preheated oven and bake for 20 minutes, or until it is foamy and the cheese melts.
7. Remove from the oven and top the casserole with the remaining chives before serving.

STORAGE: Store in an airtight container in the fridge for up to 2 days.
REHEAT: Microwave, covered, until the desired temperature is reached or reheat in a frying pan or air fryer/ instant pot, covered, on medium.
PER SERVING
calories: 362 | fat: 30.0g | total carbs: 13.4g | fiber: 1.8g | protein: 11.7g

BROCCOLI AND MUSHROOM SOUP CASSEROLE

Macros: Fat 82% | Protein 13% | Carbs 5%
Prep time: 15 minutes | Cook time: 1 hour | Serves 8

This recipe is yummy and very comforting. It is made with fresh broccoli with plenty of nutrients. It is also a very easy recipe to prepare. You cannot fail to love it.

1 tablespoon olive oil
¼ cup onions, chopped
1 egg, beaten
1 (10.75-ounce / 305-g) can condensed cream of mushroom soup
1 cup mayonnaise, keto-friendly

3 (10-ounce / 284-g) packages frozen broccoli, chopped
8 ounces (227 g) Cheddar cheese, shredded
¼ teaspoon pepper
¼ teaspoon salt
¼ teaspoon paprika

1. Start by preheating the oven to 350°F (180°C). Grease a baking dish with olive oil.

2. Mix together the onions, egg, condensed soup, and mayo in a medium bowl.
3. In a separate bowl, put the frozen broccoli and break it. Scoop the egg-soup mixture over the broccoli and combine. Add the cheese and combine.
4. Transfer the mixture to the greased baking dish and spread with a spatula to make the mixture smooth. Add the paprika, pepper, and salt to season.
5. Bake in the preheated oven for at least 45 minutes or until cooked through.
6. Remove the baking dish from the oven. Cool for about 20 minutes and serve.

STORAGE: Store in an airtight container in the fridge for up to 3 days. It is not recommended to freeze.
REHEAT: Microwave, covered, until the desired temperature is reached or reheat in a frying pan or air fryer / instant pot, covered, on medium.
SERVE IT WITH: To make this a complete meal, serve with cooked bacon.
PER SERVING
calories: 383 | fat: 35.0g | total carbs: 8.6g | fiber:3.4g | protein: 11.9g

RITZY RATATOUILLE

Macros: Fat 83% | Protein 8% | Carbs 9%
Prep time: 20 minutes | Cook time: 1 hour | Serves 5

Ratatouille (p.s: not the American movie, but the French recipe) can bring you the European taste, flavor, and inspiration. You can make this dish with your families and share them with your experience the first time you messed up with this recipe.

1 cup tomatoes, crushed
¼ teaspoon apple cider vinegar
4 tablespoons extra-virgin olive oil, plus more for greasing and spraying
1 teaspoon herbs de Provence
¼ teaspoon chili powder
1 teaspoon garlic, minced

1 tablespoon fresh basil, chopped
¼ teaspoon salt
¼ teaspoon freshly ground black pepper
1 large Japanese eggplant, sliced
2 large zucchinis, sliced
1 red onion, sliced
3 large fresh tomatoes, sliced

1. Preheat the oven to 350°F (180°C).
2. Combine the crushed tomatoes, vinegar, and olive oil in a bowl, then mix in the herbs de Provence, chili powder, garlic, basil, salt, and ground black pepper.
3. Pour the mixture in a lightly greased baking dish. Use a spatula to spread the mixture so it covers the bottom evenly.
4. Arrange the eggplant slices, zucchini slices, onion slices, and tomato slices alternatively on top of the tomato mixture in rows. Spray them with olive oil.
5. Place the baking dish in the preheated oven and bake for 1 hour or until the vegetables are soft and the sauce is foamy.
6. Remove them from the oven and serve warm.

STORAGE: Store in an airtight container in the fridge for up to 5 days.
REHEAT: Microwave, covered, until the desired temperature is reached or reheat in a frying pan or instant pot, covered, on medium.
SERVE IT WITH: To make this dish complete, you can serve it with steak or chicken thighs.
PER SERVING
calories: 262 | fat: 24.0g | total carbs: 11.3g | fiber: 5.2g | protein: 5.3g

CRUSTED ZUCCHINI STICKS

Macros: Fat: 59% | Protein: 28% | Carb: 13%
Prep time: 30 minutes | Cook time: 25 minutes | Serves 6

3o minutes preparation might be a prolonged exercise, and you will find it difficult to squeeze time. But zucchini sticks can be refrigerated and used for an extended period. Baking with Parmesan cheese adds up the flavor and seasoning with Italian herbs making it a delicious side dish.

2 zucchinis, cut into nine 3-inch-long sticks
Salt, to taste
2 eggs
½ cup shredded Parmesan
cheese
½ cup ground almonds
½ teaspoon dried Italian herbs, for seasoning

1. Preheat the oven to 425°F (220°C). Line the oven with a baking sheet.
2. Put the zucchini sticks in a sieve and sprinkle salt over it. Allow it to drain for 1 hour.
3. In a medium shallow bowl, beat the eggs. Combine the grated Parmesan cheese, ground almonds, and Italian seasoning in another medium bowl. Rinse the zucchini sticks and pat dry with paper towels.
4. Dredge the zucchini sticks in the beaten egg. Shake to remove excess egg liquid and dredge in the cheese mixture. Place the well-coated zucchini sticks on the baking sheet.
5. Bake the zucchini sticks for about 25 minutes, flipping sides in between throughout the process, or until the coating becomes crisp and brown.
6. Remove from the oven and serve warm.

STORAGE: Store in an airtight container in the fridge for up to 4 to 5 days or in the freezer for up to 1 month.
REHEAT: Refrigerated zucchini can use by microwaving as per the instructions or reheating on moderate heat using a frying pan, instant pot, or air fryer.
SERVE IT WITH: Best served as a side dish along with fried or roasted chicken, meat, or fish.
PER SERVING
calories: 92 | fat: 6.0g | total carbs: 4.1g | fiber: 1.1g | protein: 6.4g

ZUCCHINI AND WALNUT SALAD

Macros: Fat: 92% | Protein: 7% | Carb: 1%
Prep time: 20 minutes | Cook time: 15 minutes | Serves 4

Dressings are the key ingredients that make any salad delicious. Design the dressing menu as the way you wish and give a surprise to your guests. I have divided the zucchini and walnut salad into two sections, starting with the salad and followed by the dressing. You will fall in love with the crunchy and nutty taste of roasted zucchinis.

FOR DRESSING:
¾ cup keto-friendly mayonnaise
2 tablespoons virgin olive oil
2 teaspoons lemon juice
1 tablespoon minced clove garlic
¼ teaspoon chili powder
¼ teaspoon salt

FOR SALAD:
4 ounces (113 g) arugula lettuce
¼ cup sliced fresh chives
1 head Romaine lettuce
2 zucchinis
1 tablespoon virgin olive oil
¼ teaspoon salt
½ teaspoon ground pepper
3½ ounces (99 g) chopped walnuts

1. Make the dressing: In a medium bowl, combine all the dressing ingredients. Set aside..

2. Make the salad: Trim the ends of the vegetables if required and cut them into uniform size. In a large bowl, combine the sliced arugula, chives, and Romaine lettuce.
3. Cut the zucchini in lengthwise and remove the seeds. Then cut the zucchini splits into halves making it into half-inch pieces.
4. In a large frying pan, pour olive oil and bring to medium heat. When the oil becomes hot, put zucchini into the pan, sprinkle salt and pepper to season. Sauté until the zucchini pieces become brown but remain firm.
5. Transfer the cooked zucchini pieces into the salad bowl and combine them gently.
6. Roast the nuts in the frying pan for 7 minutes or until browned evenly. Sprinkle with pepper and salt. Transfer the nuts onto the salad and mix.
7. Pour the dressing over the salad and combine gently before serving.

STORAGE: Ideally, you can keep the salad refrigerated for 5 days in an airtight container. Scoop out only what you want to serve 15 minutes before serving.
SERVE IT WITH: The salad goes well with roasted or grilled chicken, fish, and meat. There is no limit for experimenting, as long it can make you confident.
PER SERVING
calories: 565 | fat: 58.1g | total carbs: 8.4g | fiber: 6.9g | protein: 9.3g

MILKY MUSHROOM SOUP

Macros: Fat 78% | Protein 11% | Carbs 11%
Prep time: 10 minutes | Cook time: 30 minutes | Serves 4

Soup is another way to build your vegetable recipe island. Compared with the land of grilled vegetables, roasted vegetables, and sautéed vegetables, vegetable soup is the sea of the gourmet. So it has a huge space for us to discover.

3 tablespoons olive oil, plus more for greasing and drizzling
1½ pounds (680 g) mushrooms, trimmed
2 red onions, chopped
4 cups vegetable stock
2 cups coconut milk
1 tablespoon fresh thyme
1 clove garlic, minced
A sprig of thyme
⅛ teaspoon sea salt
⅛ teaspoon freshly ground black pepper

1. Preheat the grill to medium heat and grease the grill grates with olive oil.
2. Grill the mushrooms on the grill grates for 5 minutes, or until soft and deep browned. Flip constantly and drizzle with olive oil during the grilling.
3. Pour 3 tablespoons olive oil in a saucepan and heat over medium heat. Add the red onion and sauté for about 2 minutes or until translucent, then mix in the vegetable stock and cook for no more than 10 minutes.
4. Put the cooked red onion and grilled half of the mushrooms in a food processor. Process until they are smooth, then add coconut milk, thyme, and garlic. Process to make them creamy.
5. Pour the soup back to the saucepan, and sprinkle with thyme sprig, salt, and ground black pepper. Bring them to a simmer for at least 20 minutes, stirring occasionally.
6. Transfer to a large soup bowl, and scatter the remaining mushrooms on top to serve.

STORAGE: Store in an airtight container in the fridge for 3 to 4 days.
REHEAT: Microwave, covered, until the desired temperature is reached or reheat in a frying pan or instant pot, covered, on medium.
SERVE IT WITH: To make this dish complete, you can serve it with roasted pork chops and asparagus salad.
PER SERVING
calories: 335 | fat: 29.2g | net carbs: 15.1g | fiber: 5.8g | protein: 8.8g

CAULIFLOWER HASH WITH POBLANO PEPPERS AND EGGS

Macros: Fat: 88% | Protein: 8% | Carb: 4%
Prep time: 10 minutes | Cook time: 15 minutes | Serves 4

The dish gives you a variety of options to have some makeover. Try any other dairy products of your choice to make it special. Serving crumbled feta along with the baked peppers will be a fantastic option to make the dish tasty. If you want to make the salad more colorful, go for different colored peppers, and maintain the spiciness as per your preference.

½ cup keto-friendly mayonnaise
1 teaspoon garlic powder
1 pound (454 g) shredded cauliflower
3 ounces (85 g) butter, melted

Salt and freshly ground black pepper, to taste
1 teaspoon virgin olive oil
3 ounces (85 g) poblano peppers
4 eggs

1. In a small bowl, combine the mayonnaise and garlic powder and set aside.
2. In a food processor, grate the cauliflower with the stem.
3. In a large skillet, fry the grated cauliflower in melted butter. Sprinkle pepper and salt to taste. Transfer to a plate. Set aside until ready to serve.
4. Apply the olive oil on the poblano peppers and fry in the skillet until blistered. Remove from the skillet and set aside.
5. Break the eggs in the skillet and fry.for 2 minutes on each side Season with pepper and salt.
6. Serve the fried eggs with cauliflower hash and fried poblanos.

STORAGE: Store in an airtight container in the fridge for up to 3 days.
SERVE IT WITH: It can use as a breakfast or brunch. Alternatively, it can serve as a ketogenic side dish.
PER SERVING
calories: 450 | fat: 43.9g | total carbs: 4.7g | fiber: 3.0g | protein: 8.7g

ASPARAGUS AND PORK BAKE

Macros: Fat 87% | Protein 10% | Carbs 3%
Prep time: 5 minutes | Cook time: 20 minutes | Serves 4

In a casserole dish, you can always find rich and substantial flavor hidden inside. The combination of pork and asparagus is quite good and nutrients for everyone. So why not give it a try, maybe this dish will enlighten you.

1 pound (454 g) asparagus, tough ends removed
½ cup roughly ground pork

rinds
1 cup ranch dressing
Pinch of sea salt

1. Preheat the oven to 375°F (190°C).
2. Arrange the asparagus spears in a casserole dish. Spread the pork rinds and ranch dressing over the asparagus, then season with sea salt.
3. Place the casserole dish in the preheated oven and bake for 18 minutes or until lightly browned.
4. Transfer them onto a platter and serve warm.

STORAGE: Store in an airtight container in the fridge for no more than 3 days.
REHEAT: Microwave, covered, until the desired temperature is reached or reheat in a frying pan or instant pot, covered, on medium.
SERVE IT WITH: To make this dish complete, you can top with fresh parsley and serve it with roasted chicken thighs.
PER SERVING
calories: 303 | fat: 29.4g | total carbs: 7.8g | fiber: 2.4g | protein: 7.3g

EASY BROCCOLI AND DILL SALAD

Macros: Fat: 94% | Protein: 4% | Carb: 2%
Prep time: 5 minutes | Cook time: 5 minutes | Serves 4

Think about a yummy salad that can make within moments. The salad made out of garden-fresh broccoli and dill shall remain in your heart as a staple side dish. You can easily make some variation, that can satisfy your imagination. Try using cauliflower and Brussels sprouts instead of broccoli or use a mix of all these ingredients proportionately.

1 pound (454 g) broccoli, cut into florets and stems
¾ cup fresh dill

1 cup keto-friendly mayonnaise
½ teaspoon ground pepper
½ teaspoon salt

1. Boil the broccoli florets and stems in a pot of lightly salted water for about 5 minutes, or until it becomes fork-tender but firm and greenish.
2. Using a colander, drain the broccoli then put it in a medium bowl. Add the fresh dill, mayonnaise and mix gently. Lightly season with pepper and salt before serving.

STORAGE: For a long day of usage, refrigerate the salad in a tight container. You can use it for 4 to 5 days if you freeze it properly. Scoop out only the required portion 10 minutes before serving.
SERVE WITH: It is delicious if served along with baked chicken, meat, or fish.
PER SERVING
calories: 406 | fat: 42.4g | total carbs: 4.9g | fiber: 3.1g | protein: 4.3g

LEMONY COLESLAW

Macros: Fat: 92% | Protein: 2% | Carb: 6%
Prep time: 5 minutes | Cook time: 10 minutes | Serves 4

Coleslaw is a yummy side dish, and here I am, presenting a ketogenic coleslaw that will go easy with health-conscious people. It is ideal for serving along with a BBQ dish or a family get together. The low-calorie dish is easy to make, and in about 10 minutes, you are ready with the dish. The process simply matches the restaurant type coleslaw makes your friend awestruck. I recommend people to use mayonnaise to meet the keto restrictions. Make some experiments to change the traditional taste. You can roast the fennel seeds and mix with the coleslaw for having an improved taste.

8 ounces (227 g) fresh cabbage, cored
½ lemon juice extract
1 teaspoon salt
⅛ teaspoon ground black

pepper
½ cup keto-friendly mayonnaise
1 tablespoon Dijon mustard
⅛ teaspoon fennel seeds

1. Grate the cabbage in a food processor. Put the grated cabbage in a medium bowl. Drizzle with the lemon juice, and sprinkle salt and pepper over it.
2. Toss the cabbage to coat well. Let it sit for about 10 minutes until it becomes soft. Drain out excess liquid.
3. Add the mayonnaise and mustard and combine it well.
4. Sprinkle with fennel seeds and serve.

STORAGE: Refrigerate the coleslaw in a tight container for later use. It can ideally use for 3 to 4 days if stored well.
SERVE IT WITH: It is an ideal choice if served along with BBQ, roasted / baked chicken, meat, or fish.
PER SERVING
calories: 209 | fat: 21.7g | total carbs: 3.1g | fiber: 2.4g | protein: 1.3g

SPIRALIZED ZUCCHINI WITH AVOCADO SAUCE

Macros: Fat 86% | Protein 8% | Carbs 6%
Prep time: 30 minutes | Cook time: 0 minutes | Serves 1

This recipe is the early form of the usage of zoodles. The creation of zoodles makes us have chance to enjoy the texture of the noodles, and, in the same way, stay in a keto diet. Besides, the avocado sauce will increase the flavor of the zucchini.

1 large zucchini, spiralized   ½ teaspoon salt

AVOCADO SAUCE:
1 avocado, chopped   ¼ teaspoon ground pepper
2 tablespoons melted butter   ½ teaspoon fresh lemon juice

1. Put the spiralized zucchini in a bowl, and season with salt. Let it sit for 20 minutes under room temperature.
2. Meanwhile, make the avocado sauce: Put the remaining ingredients in a food processor, and pulse until creamy and smooth.
3. Dry the spiralized zucchini with paper towels and transfer to another bowl.
4. Pour the avocado mixture in the bowl to coat the zucchini, and serve.

STORAGE: Store in an airtight container in the fridge for up to 5 days.
REHEAT: Microwave, covered, until the desired temperature is reached or reheat in a frying pan or instant pot, covered, on medium.
SERVE IT WITH: To make this dish complete, you can serve it with grilled chicken breasts and Mozzarella bites.
PER SERVING
calories: 416 | fat: 39.9g | total carbs: 23.8g | fiber: 17.2g | protein: 7.7g

CHEESY CAULIFLOWER AND BROCCOLI BAKE

Macros: Fat 74% | Protein 14% | Carbs 12%
Prep time: 22 minutes | Cook time: 20 minutes | Serves 3

The forms and nutritional facts of cauliflower and broccoli have something in common. Whereas cauliflower is born in northeast Mediterranean, and the broccoli is born in Italy, different areas in European, and different cooking ways in the old time. But now we make them a group to let you enjoy the charms of these two old vegetables.

1 cup cauliflower, cut into florets   Salt and freshly ground black
1 cup broccoli, cut into florets   pepper, to taste
¼ cup butter, melted   ½ cup Parmesan cheese, grated

1. Preheat the oven to 375°F (190°C).
2. Combine the cauliflower, broccoli, butter, salt, and ground black pepper in a bowl until the vegetables are coated well.
3. Pour the mixture into a lightly greased baking pan. Scatter with grated Parmesan cheese.
4. Place the pan in the preheated oven and bake for 20 minutes or until the vegetables are tender and the cheese melts.
5. Remove them from the oven and serve warm.

STORAGE: Store in an airtight container in the fridge for no more than 5 days.
REHEAT: Microwave, covered, until the desired temperature is reached or reheat in a frying pan or instant pot, covered, on medium.
SERVE IT WITH: To make this dish complete, you can serve with beef rib steak.
PER SERVING
calories: 182 | fat: 15.1g | total carbs: 6.1g | fiber: 1.5g | protein: 6.9g

RICED BROCCOLI WITH ALMONDS

Macros: Fat 86% | Protein 6% | Carbs 8%
Prep time: 10 minutes | Cook time: 5 minutes | Serves 4

The broccoli rice is an extraordinary replacement for the ordinary rice, and can also satisfy your eagerness of the rice product because it can be served with main courses and shows vibrant support to the keto recipes.

1 tablespoon avocado oil   pepper, to taste
2 heads broccoli, riced in a food   ½-inch ginger, grated
processor   Juice from ¼ lemon
1 tablespoon garlic, minced   ½ cup almonds, chopped
2 teaspoons sesame oil   2 tablespoons parsley, chopped
1 tablespoon coconut aminos   ¼ cup green onions, chopped
Sea salt and freshly ground black

1. In a nonstick skillet, heat the avocado oil over medium-high heat.
2. Put the riced broccoli and garlic in the skillet. Stir to combine and sauté for 1 minute. Mix in the sesame oil, coconut aminos, salt and pepper, and sauté for 2 minutes more until tender.
3. Turn off the heat. Sprinkle the ginger and lemon juice on top of the broccoli. Add the almonds, parsley, and green onions. Stir to mix well.
4. Remove them from the skillet to a large platter and serve warm.

STORAGE: Store in an airtight container in the fridge for no more than 3 days.
REHEAT: Microwave, covered, until the desired temperature is reached or reheat in a frying pan or instant pot, covered, on medium.
SERVE IT WITH: To make this dish complete, you can squeeze the lemon wedges over the broccoli and serve with beef steak.
PER SERVING
calories: 191 | fat: 18.1g | total carbs: 10.0g | fiber: 3.1g | protein: 3.1g

EASY ASPARAGUS WITH WALNUTS

Prep time: 10 minutes | Cook time: 5 minutes | Serves 4
Macros: Fat 81% | Protein 9% | Carbs 10%

The walnut itself has plenty of necessary nutrients for the human body. The group of asparagus and walnuts is relatively a simple but different combination. So you can always find some chance to try it with your idea.

12 ounces (340 g) asparagus,   1½ tablespoons olive oil
woody ends trimmed   Sea salt and freshly ground
¼ cup chopped walnuts   pepper, to taste

1. Heat the olive oil in a nonstick skillet over medium-high heat.
2. Add the asparagus and sauté for 5 minutes or until soft, then sprinkle with salt, and ground black pepper.
3. Turn the heat off. Add the walnuts and sauté to combine well.
4. Serve warm on a platter.

STORAGE: Store in an airtight container in the fridge for at least days or in the freezer for up to two weeks.
REHEAT: Microwave, covered, until the desired temperature is reached or reheat in a frying pan or instant pot, covered, on medium.
SERVE IT WITH: You can top the asparagus with blue cheese on the last minute of cooking time and cook until the cheese melts. It would increase the flavor of the asparagus.
PER SERVING
calories: 126 | fat: 12.2g | total carbs: 4.0g | fiber: 2.1g | protein: 1.3g

VEGETABLES TRICOLOR

Macros: Fat: 88% | Protein: 9% | Carb: 3%
Prep time: 10 minutes | Cook time: 20 minutes | Serves 6

The colorful salad is something special everybody loves to have. It is a low-carb keto diet with a focus on the delicacy quotient. With a quick preparation, you can complete the cooking within 20 minutes in a flavor-rich aroma. For maintaining tricolor, the salad uses fresh Brussels sprouts, cherry tomatoes, and mushrooms. The grilled salad will be a trendsetter and relishing side dish delicacy.

1 pound (454 g) Brussels sprouts	½ cup olive oil
8 ounces (227 g) mushrooms	1 teaspoon salt
8 ounces (227 g) cherry tomatoes	½ teaspoon ground pepper
	1 teaspoon dried thyme

1. Preheat the oven to 400°F (205°C).
2. Rinse and chop all the vegetables in equal size. Put the chopped vegetables in a medium bowl. Add olive oil, salt, pepper, dried thyme, and mix well.
3. Line a parchment paper in a baking dish and spread the vegetable in it.
4. Roast the vegetable in the preheated oven for about 20 minutes or until the vegetable becomes soft, and the color looks good.
5. Remove them from the oven and serve.

STORAGE: After settling the heat, the dish can refrigerate in a tight container for an extended shelve life. In normal condition, you will have a shelve life of 5 days, if refrigerated properly.
SERVE IT WITH: It is an ideal dish to serve along with a dipping sauce. You can add any vegetable of choice and spices to give a personal touch. It is a perfect side dish for fried chicken, fish, and meat.
PER SERVING
calories: 188 | fat: 18.3g | total carbs: 6.1g | fiber: 4.3g | protein: 4.4g

LEMONY BRUSSELS SPROUT SALAD WITH SPICY ALMOND AND SEED MIX

Macros: Fat: 90% | Protein: 9% | Carb: 1%
Prep time: 10 minutes | Cook time: 10 minutes | Serves 4

Quick and easy making roasted keto Brussels sprout salad flavored with lemon can be your all-time favorite side dish. To add up its delicacy, a combination of different seeds roasted under moderate temperature and spiced in chili paste make all the differences. Try to toss with dried cranberries for a different flavor. No doubt, it is a holiday salad.

FOR SPICY ALMOND AND SEED MIX:

1 tablespoon olive oil or refined coconut oil	1 ounce (28 g) sunflower seeds
1 teaspoon chili paste	½ teaspoon crushed fennel seeds or ground cumin
2 ounces (57 g) almond	¼ teaspoon salt
1 ounce (28 g) pumpkin seeds	

FOR BRUSSELS SPROUT SALAD:

1 pound (454 g) Brussels sprouts, trimmed and rinsed	½ cup virgin olive oil
2 tablespoons lemon juice and zest	¼ teaspoon pepper
	¼ teaspoon salt

MAKE SPICY ALMOND AND SEED MIX:
1. In a large frying pan, pour the oil of your preference and bring to low-medium heat. When the oil becomes hot, add chili and sauté for 1 minute, then mix in the almond and all the seeds, and continue stirring.

2. Add salt and sauté for 10 minutes or until the fragrant starts to emanate. Make sure not to burn the almonds and seeds.
3. Set aside until ready to serve.

MAKE BRUSSELS SPROUT SALAD:
1. Finely grate the Brussels sprouts with a food processor and reserve in a medium salad bowl.
2. In a small bowl, combine lemon juice, lemon zest, olive oil, pepper, and salt. Pour them over the grated Brussels sprouts and gently mix.
3. Wrap the bowl in plastic and refrigerate marinate for 10 minutes.
4. Serve the Brussels sprouts salad with spicy almond and seed mix on top.

STORAGE: The salad can refrigerate in a tight container for an extended shelve life. You can use it for 4 to 5 days if refrigerated properly. Take out only the required quantity at least 10 minutes before you are ready to serve.
SERVE IT WITH: It is an ideal side dish along with roasted / baked fish, meat, or chicken.
PER SERVING
calories: 457 | fat: 45.2g | total carbs: 9.1g | fiber: 7.9g | protein: 10.8g

FOCACCIA

Macros: Fat 89% | Protein 9% | Carbs 2%
Prep time: 15 minutes | Cook time: 25 minutes | Serves 18

For making this recipe, there are various ways. You can choose the traditional one to leave the olive and tomato away, or you can find something more suitable to make a focaccia. Besides, this dish is very suitable for a large group of people to enjoy, like have a party or a big family dinner.

1 tablespoon baking powder	½ cup water
1 tablespoon Italian seasoning	12 grape tomatoes, halved lengthwise
2 cups roughly ground flaxseeds	10 pitted olives, halved lengthwise
1 teaspoon finely ground gray sea salt	18 tablespoons keto-friendly mayonnaise
5 large eggs	
⅓ cup refined avocado oil	

1. Arrange a rack in the oven, and preheat the oven to 350°F (180°C). Line the parchment paper in a baking pan.
2. Combine the baking powder, Italian seasoning, flaxseeds, and salt in a bowl.
3. Break the eggs into a blender, and add the avocado oil and water. Pulse the blender for 30 seconds or until the egg mixture is bubbly.
4. Make the focaccia: Pour the egg mixture in the bowl of mixture, and stir to combine well. Let sit for 3 minutes.
5. Spread the mixture in the baking pan with a spatula to coat the bottom of the pan evenly. Press them into the mixture until they are flush with the mixture.
6. Arrange the pan in the preheated oven and bake for 25 minutes or until the edges of the pan is lightly browned.
7. Remove the focaccia from the pan and parchment paper carefully to a cooling rack, and allow to cool for 1 hour.
8. Serve each focaccia with 1 tablespoon of mayo on top.

STORAGE: Store in an airtight container in the fridge for up to 3 days or in the freezer for up to 1 month.
REHEAT: Microwave, covered, until the desired temperature is reached or reheat in a frying pan or instant pot, covered, on medium.
SERVE IT WITH: To make this a complete meal, you can serve this dish with zoodles and roasted Brussels sprouts.
PER SERVING
calories: 207 | fat: 20.5g | total carbs: 5.1g | fiber: 4.0g | protein: 4.6g

MUSHROOM PIZZAS WITH TOMATO SLICES

Macros: Fat 71% | Protein 19% | Carbs 10%
Prep time: 15 minutes | Cook time: 5 minutes | Serves 4

The small pizza set on every mushroom is a neat method to bring the inspirations together when making a thoughtful dish. You can try to change the ingredients of making such kind of pizzas, the holders can be different, and the stuffs can be different.

4 large portobello mushrooms, stems removed	2 teaspoons chopped fresh basil
¼ cup olive oil	1 teaspoon minced garlic
1 medium tomato, cut into 4 slices	1 cup shredded Mozzarella cheese

1. Preheat the oven to 450°F (235°C).
2. Arrange the mushrooms in an aluminum foil-lined baking sheet, gill side down, then brush with olive oil on all sides gently.
3. Place the baking sheet in the preheated oven and broil the mushrooms for 2 minutes or until soft, then flip and broil for another 1 minute.
4. Make the mushroom pizza: Top each mushroom with a tomato slice, basil, minced garlic, and shredded cheese. Place the sheet back to the oven and broil for 1 minute more or until the cheese melts.
5. Remove the mushroom pizzas from the oven and serve warm.

STORAGE: Store in an airtight container in the fridge for up to 10 days or in the freezer for up to 1 month.
REHEAT: Microwave, covered, until the desired temperature is reached or reheat in a frying pan or air fryer / instant pot, covered, on medium.
SERVE IT WITH: To make this a complete meal, you can serve this dish with roasted asparagus or roasted Brussels sprouts.
PER SERVING
calories: 252 | fat: 20.1g | total carbs: 7.1g | fiber: 3.2g | protein: 14.1g

STIR-FRIED ZUCCHINI WITH GREEN BEANS

Macros: Fat 90% | Protein 4% | Carbs 6%
Prep time: 5 minutes | Cook time: 10 minutes | Serves 2

The usage of the skillet provides us many possibilities to combine different ingredients together, and a spatula is a noble tool for everyone to create a brilliant dish. The characteristics of this recipe is not only green, but also the strong crispness and flavor of this combination.

3 tablespoons olive oil	Sea salt, to taste
½ small zucchini, thinly sliced	2 tablespoons scallions, chopped
½ cup green beans, cut into small pieces	2 tablespoons lemon juice

1. Heat the olive oil in a nonstick skillet over medium heat.
2. Add and stir fry the zucchini, green beans, and salt for 9 minutes or until soft and crisp.
3. Remove them from the skillet to a plate. Garnish with chopped scallion and serve drizzled with lemon juice.

STORAGE: Store in an airtight container in the fridge for up to 3 to 5 days.
REHEAT: Microwave, covered, until the desired temperature is reached or reheat in a frying pan or instant pot, covered, on medium.
SERVE IT WITH: To make this dish complete, you can serve it with pork chops or beef meatloaf.
PER SERVING
calories: 137 | fat: 13.7g | total carbs: 3.4g | fiber: 1.3g | protein: 1.2g

ZUCCHINI LASAGNA

Macros: Fat 63% | Protein 30% | Carbs 7%
Prep time: 20 minutes | Cook time: 1 hour 5 minutes | Serves 6

This low-carb zucchini lasagna lets you enjoy the same lasagna flavors without the use of lasagna pasta. Zucchini is super-rich and nutritious; that is why it makes a perfect combination with other healthy ingredients in the recipe.

1½ large zucchinis, thinly sliced lengthwise	pepper
2 tablespoons olive oil, divided	1 (8-ounce / 227-g) container ricotta cheese
1 pound (454 g) ground beef	1 egg, whisked
1½ cups low-carb marinara sauce	½ teaspoon ground nutmeg
2 teaspoons salt, divided	2 cups shredded Mozzarella cheese, divided
1 teaspoon dried oregano	¼ cup grated Parmesan cheese
½ teaspoon ground black	1 teaspoon olive oil

1. Preheat your oven to 375°F (190°C). Coat a baking dish with 1 tablespoon olive oil and set aside.
2. Use a paper towel to pat dry all the zucchini slices to remove their excess moisture. Set aside.
3. Add the remaining olive oil in a saucepan and place it over medium-high heat.
4. Stir in the ground beef and sauté for 5 to 8 minutes, or until it is browned.
5. Add the 1 teaspoon salt, marinara sauce, oregano, and black pepper; then let it simmer for 10 minutes.
6. Meanwhile, add the remaining salt, whisked egg, ricotta cheese, and nutmeg in a bowl. Mix well.
7. Spread 1 layer of zucchini slices in the greased baking dish. Then cover this layer with ½ of the sauce.
8. Spread another layer of zucchini slice on top of the sauce and then top it with ricotta cheese mixture.
9. Drizzle 1 cup Mozzarella cheese on top then spread another layer of a zucchini slice.
10. Pour over the remaining sauce and sprinkle 1 cup Mozzarella cheese and Parmesan cheese on top. Cover this baking dish with aluminum foil for baking.
11. Bake the prepared zucchini lasagna in the preheated oven for 30 minutes.
12. Remove the aluminum foil from top and bake for 15 minutes more until golden brown.
13. Cool for 5 minutes before slicing to serve.

STORAGE: Store the leftover in an airtight container in the fridge for up to 3 to 4 days or in the freezer for 1 month.
REHEAT: Microwave, covered, until the desired temperature is reached or reheat in a frying pan or instant pot, covered, on medium.
SERVE IT WITH: To make this a complete meal, serve the zucchini lasagna with fresh lettuce broccoli salad.
PER SERVING
calories: 512 | fat: 36.1g | total carbs: 10.9g | fiber: 2.1g | protein: 38.0g

ODD TASTE VEGAN PANCAKE

Macros: Fat 97% | Protein 5% | Carbs 2%
Prep time: 10 minutes | **Cook time:** 16 minutes | **Serves** 4

Under general impression, pancakes are sweet ones in most situations. So when we try to make this recipe, we are taking risks. But I'm sure after you finish this dish, you will love the amazing magic of food making and human creation.

¼ cup coconut flour	1 teaspoon salt
¼ cup almond flour	1 serrano pepper, minced
1 cup coconut milk	½ red onion, chopped
½ teaspoon chili powder	1 handful cilantro, chopped
¼ teaspoon turmeric powder	½-inch ginger, grated
¼ teaspoon black pepper	4 tablespoons coconut oil

1. Mix the coconut flour, almond flour, coconut milk, chili powder, turmeric powder, black pepper, and salt in a bowl, then fold in the serrano pepper, red onion, cilantro and ginger. Stir to combine well.
2. Make the pancake: In a frying pan, heat 1 tablespoon of the coconut oil over medium-low heat, then pour ¼ cup of the mixture in the pan. Use a spatula to spread the mixture evenly.
3. Cook for 4 minutes per side, or until lightly browned around the edges. Repeat with the remaining mixture and coconut oil.
4. Transfer the pancakes onto a platter and serve warm.

STORAGE: Store in an airtight container in the fridge for no more than 5 days or in the freezer for up to two months.
REHEAT: Microwave, covered, until the desired temperature is reached or reheat in a frying pan or instant pot, covered, on medium.
SERVE IT WITH: To make this dish complete, you can serve with a dollop of plain Greek yogurt or berries.
PER SERVING
calories: 327 | fat: 33.7g | total carbs: 7.1g | fiber: 3.4g | protein: 4.2g

SHICHIMI COLLARD GREENS WITH RED ONION

Macros: Fat 81% | Protein 10% | Carbs 9%
Prep time: 15 minutes | **Cook time:** 15 minutes | **Serves** 4

The greens are always friendly not only to the keto diet, but also for all creatures' health, and I believe after you know about the collards, you can find more possibilities to make the trials for more vegan foods or combinations with the meats.

¼ cup refined avocado oil	1 tablespoon Shichimi seasoning
½ red onion, sliced thin	2 tablespoons coconut aminos
2 bunches collard greens (18 ounces / 510 g), stems removed, roughly chopped	¼ green bell pepper, sliced thin
1 teaspoon apple cider vinegar	Finely ground gray sea salt, to taste

1. Heat the avocado oil in a frying pan over medium heat, then add the sliced red onion and cook over medium-low heat for 10 minutes or until golden brown.
2. Add the collards, vinegar, Shichimi seasoning, and coconut aminos. Put the lid on and cook for another 5 minutes or until the collards are wilted, then top with the bell pepper and gray sea salt.
3. Separate the cooked collards into 4 bowls and serve warm.

STORAGE: Store in an airtight container in the fridge for no more than 3 days.
REHEAT: Microwave, covered, until the desired temperature is reached or reheat in a frying pan or instant pot, covered, on medium.
SERVE IT WITH: To make this dish complete, you can top the collards with sesame seeds and serve it with roasted chicken thighs.
PER SERVING
calories: 160 | fat: 14.4g | total carbs: 8.8g | fiber: 5.2g | protein: 3.9g

ZUCCHINI MANICOTTI

Macros: Fat 76% | Protein 20% | Carbs 4%
Prep time: 15 minutes | **Cook time:** 30 minutes | **Serves** 4

In this recipe, we use the zucchini wrappers to replace the traditional ones in the the old recipes making the manicotti. The point is, that you can make it by using various ingredients, under this circumstance, this recipe is more than a vegetable recipe, it could be a meat recipe, or even a soup recipe.

Olive oil cooking spray	⅛-inch-thick slices
4 zucchinis, cut lengthwise into	

FILLING:

2 tablespoons olive oil	oregano
½ onion, minced	Sea salt, to taste
2 teaspoons minced garlic	Freshly ground black pepper, to taste
1 red bell pepper, diced	
1 cup shredded Mozzarella cheese	2 cups low-carb marinara sauce, divided
1 cup goat cheese	
1 tablespoon chopped fresh	½ cup grated Parmesan cheese

1. Preheat the oven to 375°F (190°C). Spritz a baking dish with olive oil cooking spray and set aside.
2. Make the filling: Heat the olive oil over medium-high heat in a nonstick skillet. Add and sauté the onion, garlic, and red bell pepper for 4 minutes or until the onion is translucent, stirring occasionally.
3. Transfer them to a large bowl, then mix in the Mozzarella cheese, goat cheese, and oregano. Sprinkle with salt and pepper.
4. Make the manicotti: Pour 1 cup of marinara sauce in the baking dish, tilting the dish so the sauce spreads the bottom evenly. Put a slice of zucchini on a work surface, then spoon a few tablespoons of the filling onto one end. Roll up and arrange on the baking dish, seam-side down. Repeat with the remaining zucchini slices and filling.
5. Scatter the Parmesan cheese on top of each manicotti. Place the baking dish in the preheated oven and bake for 30 minutes or until the zucchini is soft.
6. Remove them from the oven to a platter. Serve drizzled with the remaining marinara sauce.

STORAGE: Store in an airtight container in the fridge for 3 to 5 days.
REHEAT: Microwave, covered, until the desired temperature is reached or reheat in a frying pan or instant pot, covered, on medium.
SERVE IT WITH: To make this dish complete, you can serve it with a crispy salad on the side.
PER SERVING
calories: 358 | fat: 30.2g | total carbs: 5.0g | fiber: 1.2g | protein: 17.8g

SPINACH, ARTICHOKE AND CAULIFLOWER STUFFED RED BELL PEPPERS

Macros: Fat 76% | Protein 15% | Carbs 9%
Prep time: 10 minutes | Cook time: 20 minutes | Serves 4

Stuff the bell pepper with other vegetables is a success trial in cuisine, besides, you can try to use tomatoes or butternut squash as the holder if you want to try another flavor of vegetable.

4 red bell peppers, halved and seeded	Sea salt and freshly ground black pepper, to taste
1 tablespoon olive oil	

FILLING:

10 ounces (284 g) chopped fresh spinach	cheese, divided
2 cups chopped marinated artichoke hearts	1 cup cream cheese, softened
2 cups finely chopped cauliflower	½ cup sour cream
1½ cups shredded Mozzarella	2 teaspoons minced garlic
	2 tablespoons keto-friendly mayonnaise

1. Preheat the oven to 400°F (205°C). Line a baking sheet with parchment paper.
2. Arrange the red bell peppers on the baking sheet, cut side up. Brush the peppers with olive oil on all sides. Sprinkle with salt and ground black pepper. Set aside.
3. Make the filling: Combine the spinach, artichoke hearts, cauliflower, ¾ cup of the Mozzarella cheese, cream cheese, sour cream, garlic, and mayo in a large bowl. Stir well with a fork until combined.
4. Spoon the filling into the bell peppers, and scatter with the remaining Mozzarella cheese. Place the baking sheet in the preheated oven and bake for 20 minutes or until the cheese and bell peppers are lightly browned.
5. Remove the stuffed peppers from the oven and serve warm.

STORAGE: Store in an airtight container in the fridge for 4 to 5 days.
REHEAT: Microwave, covered, until the desired temperature is reached or reheat in a frying pan or air fryer / instant pot, covered, on medium.
SERVE IT WITH: To make this dish complete, you can serve it with roasted chicken breasts or grilled salmon.
PER SERVING
calories: 511 | fat: 43.0g | total carbs: 19.0g | fiber: 7.0g | protein: 19.0g

PECAN AND VEGGIES IN COLLARD WRAPS

Macros: Fat 88% | Protein 6% | Carbs 6%
Prep time: 20 minutes | Cook time: 0 minutes | Serves 4

The freshness and crispness of the collard warps combined with the texture of the pecans and other veggies create the fancy and charm of this recipe. Embraced with dips of lemon juice, this recipe will definitely bring you brightness.

1 lemon, cut into wedges
4 collard leaves, trimmed and rinsed

FILLING:

1 cup raw pecans	1 tablespoon extra-virgin olive oil
1 teaspoon cumin	1 ripe avocado, sliced
½ teaspoon grated ginger	⅓ cup alfalfa sprouts
1 tablespoon tamari	1 red pepper, sliced

1. Squeeze juice from half of the lemon wedges into a pot of warm water. Soak the collard leaves in the water for 10 minutes.
2. Remove the collard from the pot and dry with paper towels.
3. Cut off the central stem of the leaves to make them easy to roll. Set aside on a plate.
4. Put the pecans, cumin, ginger, tamari, and olive oil in a food processor. Process until all ingredients are fully combined.
5. Unfold the collard leaves on a clean work surface. Divide and spoon the pecan mixture onto the leaves, then top the leaves with avocado slices, alfalfa sprouts, red pepper slices. Squeeze the remaining lemon juice over them.
6. Fold the corners of the leaves over to cover the filling and roll, then slice the wrap in half before serving.

STORAGE: Store in an airtight container in the fridge for up to 1 day.
SERVE IT WITH: To make this dish complete, you can serve it with roasted salmon fillets.
PER SERVING
calories: 293 | fat: 28.8g | total carbs: 10.5g | fiber: 6.4g | protein: 4.4g

GREEDY KETO VEGETABLE MIX

Macros: Fat 74% | Protein 7% | Carbs 19%
Prep time: 10 minutes | Cook time: 15 minutes | Serves 4

This is a recipe absorbed the flavor of shallot, mushrooms, asparagus, broccoli, and tomatoes. You can never say this is a greedy choice to put so many vegetables together right? All right, I admit it, this is a greedy recipe, but also tasty.

2 tablespoons coconut oil	1 bunch asparagus, sliced into 3-inch pieces
1 large shallot, sliced	
1 tablespoon garlic, minced	1 cup broccoli, cut into florets
1 cup mushrooms, sliced	1 cup cherry tomatoes, halved
1 cup artichoke hearts, chopped	½ teaspoon sea salt

VINAIGRETTE:

1 teaspoon ground oregano	6 tablespoons extra-virgin olive oil
¼ cup fresh parsley, chopped	
3 tablespoons white wine vinegar	½ teaspoon sea salt

1. Preheat the air fryer to 400°F (205°C).
2. In a nonstick skillet, heat the coconut oil over medium heat. Add the shallot and garlic, and sauté for 2 minutes or until translucent.
3. Add the mushrooms and sauté for another 3 minutes or until lightly browned. Add the artichokes, asparagus, and broccoli and sauté for 3 minutes more, stirring occasionally.
4. Transfer the cooked vegetables into the air fryer basket. Add the cherry tomatoes and sprinkle them with salt. Cook for at least 5 minutes or until the veggies are cooked through.
5. Meanwhile, make the vinaigrette: Combine the oregano, parsley, vinegar, olive oil, and salt in a bowl.
6. Transfer the cooked vegetables to a plate. Top them with the vinaigrette before serving.

STORAGE: Store in an airtight container in the fridge for no more than 3 days.
REHEAT: Microwave the vegetables, covered, until the desired temperature is reached or reheat in a frying pan or air fryer/instant pot, covered, on medium.
SERVE IT WITH: To make this dish complete, you can serve it with roasted salmon fillets.
PER SERVING
calories: 195 | fat: 16.1g | total carbs: 13.6g | fiber: 4.4g | protein: 3.4g

FLAXSEED WITH OLIVE AND TOMATO FOCACCIA

Macros: Fat 89% | Protein 9% | Carbs 2%
Prep time: 15 minutes | Cook time: 25 minutes | Serves 18

For making this recipe, there are various ways. You can choose the traditional one to leave the olive and tomato away, or you can find something more suitable to make a focaccia. Besides, this dish is very suitable for a large group of people to enjoy, like have a party or a big family dinner.

1 tablespoon baking powder
1 tablespoon Italian seasoning
2 cups roughly ground flaxseeds
1 teaspoon finely ground gray sea salt
5 large eggs
⅓ cup refined avocado oil

½ cup water
12 grape tomatoes, halved lengthwise
10 pitted olives, halved lengthwise
18 tablespoons keto-friendly mayonnaise

1. Arrange a rack in the oven, and preheat the oven to 350°F (180°C). Line the parchment paper in a baking pan.
2. Combine the baking powder, Italian seasoning, flaxseeds, and salt in a bowl.
3. Break the eggs into a blender, and add the avocado oil and water. Pulse the blender for 30 seconds or until the egg mixture is bubbly.
4. Make the focaccia: Pour the egg mixture in the bowl of mixture, and stir to combine well. Let sit for 3 minutes.
5. Spread the mixture in the baking pan with a spatula to coat the bottom of the pan evenly. Press them into the mixture until they are flush with the mixture.
6. Arrange the pan in the preheated oven and bake for 25 minutes or until the edges of the pan is lightly browned.
7. Remove the focaccia from the pan and parchment paper carefully to a cooling rack, and allow to cool for 1 hour.
8. Serve each focaccia with 1 tablespoon of mayo on top.

STORAGE: Store in an airtight container in the fridge for up to 3 days or in the freezer for up to 1 month.
REHEAT: Microwave, covered, until the desired temperature is reached or reheat in a frying pan or instant pot, covered, on medium.
SERVE IT WITH: To make this a complete meal, you can serve this dish with zoodles and roasted Brussels sprouts.
PER SERVING
calories: 207 | fat: 20.5g | total carbs: 5.1g | fiber: 4.0g | protein: 4.6g

SEEDS AND NUTS PARFAIT

Macros: Fat 79% | Protein 18% | Carbs 3%
Prep time: 15 minutes | Cook time: 0 minutes | Serves 4

In the family of nuts, we must distinguish the keto-friendly ones and the not keto-friendly ones, for example, the cashew nut is not the friendly one. So our nut brothers abandoned him and gathered together to build an absolutely keto parfait. Just as the French meaning of parfait: perfect.

SEEDS AND NUTS M1EAL:
¼ cup flaxseeds
¼ cup chia seeds
1 cup raw almonds

1 cup raw walnuts
½ cup pumpkin seeds

PINE NUT CREAM:
1 cup pine nuts
1 teaspoon maple syrup
½ teaspoon vanilla
¼ teaspoon cinnamon

¼ teaspoon salt
⅓ cup water
1 cup blackberries and strawberries, sliced in half

1. Make the seeds and nuts meal: Combine the flaxseeds, chia seeds, almonds, walnuts, and pumpkin seeds in a food processor. Pulse until they are coarse meal and well combined.
2. Make the pine nut cream: Put the pine nuts, maple syrup, vanilla, cinnamon, salt, and water in a blender. Process until the mixture has a mousse-like consistency.
3. Put the berries on the bottom layer of a serving glass, then sprinkle with ¾ of the seeds and nuts meal, and then top all of them with the pine nut cream.
4. Sprinkle with remaining seeds and nuts meal and refrigerate for 1 hour before serving.

STORAGE: Store in an airtight container in the fridge for no more than 3 days.
SERVE IT WITH: To make this dish complete, you can serve parfait with berry cookies made by almond flour and unsweetened coconut milk.
PER SERVING
calories: 524 | fat: 46.2g | total carbs: 11.8g | fiber: 8.6g | protein: 23.4g

RICED CAULIFLOWER AND LEEK RISOTTO

Macros: Fat 80% | Protein 10% | Carbs 10%
Prep time: 5 minutes | Cook time: 25 minutes | Serves 4

Risotto is a kind of Italian flavor rice, and at this point, we use the riced cauliflower to replace the rice, this keto-unfriendly food, and the choice of mushrooms can be varied. Hope the granuliform of this recipe will comfort your desire for the carb foods.

4 cups vegetable broth
2 tablespoons olive oil
8 ounces (227 g) sliced cremini mushrooms
Salt and freshly ground black pepper, to taste

¾ cup thinly sliced leeks
1 cup riced cauliflower
¼ cup dry white wine
¼ cup vegan Parmesan cheese
1 tablespoon vegan butter
Fresh chopped parsley

1. Pour the vegetable broth in a saucepan over medium heat, then bring to a simmer. Lower the heat and leave the broth in the saucepan to keep warm.
2. In the meantime, heat 1 tablespoon of olive oil in a nonstick skillet over medium heat until shimmering. Add and sauté the mushrooms for 4 minutes or until tender, then sprinkle with salt and ground black pepper. Remove the mushrooms from the skillet to a plate and set aside.
3. Heat the remaining olive oil in the skillet over medium heat. Add and sauté the leeks for 2 minutes or until lightly browned, then add the riced cauliflower and cook for 1 minute more. Pour into the dry white wine and cook for another 2 minutes to let them infuse.
4. Make the risotto: Gently pour the vegetable broth into the skillet. Stir constantly and bring them to a simmer but not boil. Cook for 20 minutes or until the vegetables are soft.
5. Turn off the heat, and mix in ⅔ of the sautéed mushrooms, Parmesan cheese, and vegan butter to combine.
6. Transfer the risotto to a large serving bowl. Top with the remaining sautéed mushrooms and chopped parsley.

STORAGE: Store in an airtight container in the fridge for no more than 5 days. It is not recommended to freeze.
REHEAT: Microwave, covered, until the desired temperature is reached or reheat in a frying pan or instant pot, covered, on medium.
SERVE IT WITH: To make this dish complete, you can serve with ratatouille.
PER SERVING
calories: 492 | fat: 43.8g | total carbs: 15.4g | fiber: 2.6g | protein: 11.6g

ZOODLES WITH BUTTERNUT SQUASH AND SAGE

Macros: Fat 84% | Protein 2% | Carbs 14%
Prep time: 15 minutes | Cook time: 35 minutes | Serves 4

The combination between zoodles and butternut squash brilliant not only from the aspect of a keto diet, but also from a healthy and unique recipe. Hope you can enjoy this recipe and enjoy the healthy way you choose.

2 tablespoons olive oil
1 tablespoon fresh sage, finely chopped
Salt, to taste
3 cups cubed butternut squash
1 yellow onion, chopped
2 cloves garlic, finely chopped

¼ teaspoon red pepper flakes
Freshly ground black pepper, to taste
2 cups homemade vegetable broth
3 large zucchinis, spiralized or julienned into zoodles

1. Heat the olive oil in a nonstick skillet over medium heat. Add and sauté the sage until wilted. Remove the sage from the skillet to a bowl. Sprinkle with salt and set aside.
2. Add the butternut squash, onion, garlic, and red pepper flakes to the skillet and cook for 10 minutes. Sprinkle with salt and pepper.
3. Pour the vegetable broth into the skillet and bring to a boil. Allow to simmer for 20 minutes or until the butternut squash cubes are fork-tender.
4. Meanwhile, microwave the zoodles for 2 to 3 minutes until soft.
5. Turn off the heat, and remove the butternut squash from the skillet to a blender. Pulse the mixture until smooth.
6. Place the soft zoodles in the skillet over medium heat and add the butternut purée. Cook for 2 minutes or until cooked through.
7. Transfer them to a serving plate and serve topped with the sage.

STORAGE: Store in an airtight container in the fridge for up to 5 days.
REHEAT: Microwave, covered, until the desired temperature is reached or reheat in a frying pan or instant pot, covered, on medium.
SERVE IT WITH: To make this dish complete, you can serve it with grilled chicken breasts and Mozzarella bites.
PER SERVING
calories: 306 | fat: 28.5g | total carbs: 13.8g | fiber: 3.4g | protein: 1.9g

LUSCIOUS VEGETABLE QUICHE

Macros: Fat 73% | Protein 23% | Carbs 4%
Prep time: 5 minutes | Cook time: 25 minutes | Serves 4

1 tablespoon melted butter, divided
6 eggs
3 ounces (85 g) goat cheese, divided
¾ cup heavy whipping cream

1 scallion, white and green parts, chopped
½ cup mushrooms, sliced
1 cup fresh spinach, chopped
10 cherry tomatoes, cut in half

1. Preheat the oven to 350°F (180°C). Coat a pie pan with ½ teaspoon of melted butter and set aside.
2. Whisk together the eggs, 2 ounces (57 g) of goat cheese, and heavy whipping cream in a bowl until creamy and smooth, you can use a blender to make it easier. Set aside.
3. Heat the remaining butter in a nonstick skillet over medium-high heat. Add and sauté scallion and mushrooms for 2 minutes or until tender. Add and sauté the spinach for another 2 minutes or until softened.
4. Pour the vegetable mixture into the pie pan, and use a spatula to spread the mixture so it covers the bottom of the pan evenly.
5. Pour the egg mixture over the vegetable mixture. Top them with the cherry tomato halves and remaining goat cheese.
6. Place the pie pan in the preheated oven and bake for 20 minutes or until fluffy. You can check the doneness by cutting a small slit in the center, if raw eggs run into the cut, then baking for another few minutes.
7. Divide the quiche among four platters and serve warm.

STORAGE: Store in an airtight container in the fridge for 3 to 4 days or in the freezer for up to 3 to 4 months.
REHEAT: Microwave, covered, until the desired temperature is reached or reheat in a frying pan or instant pot, covered, on medium.
SERVE IT WITH: To make this dish complete, you can top it with chopped parsley and serve with roasted chicken thighs.
PER SERVING
calories: 395 | fat: 32.4g | total carbs: 4.7g | fiber: 0.7g | protein: 21.2g

SAUTÉED ZUCCHINI WITH GREENS

Macros: Fat 81% | Protein 6% | Carbs 13%
Prep time: 10 minutes | Cook time: 10 minutes | Serves 2

The cooking time of a squash is relatively long compared with other common vegetables, but the time we paid is completely worthy. For the flavor of the zucchini combined with the freshness and crispness of the greens, this recipe will definitely catch your palate.

2 tablespoons coconut oil	Sea salt and freshly ground black
1 onion, finely sliced	pepper, to taste
1 ginger, chopped	½ cup water
1 red or green chili pepper, finely	Juice of ½ lemon
chopped	1 tablespoon tamari
2 garlic cloves, peeled and	½ cup chopped leafy greens
chopped	(spinach, kale, or chard)
¼ zucchini, seeded and diced	¼ cabbage

1. Melt the coconut oil in a frying pan over medium heat. Add and sauté the onion for 4 minutes or until translucent, stirring occasionally.
2. Add and sauté the ginger, chili, and garlic for 5 minutes, then add the zucchini and sprinkle with salt. Sauté for 5 minutes, pour the water in the pan and put the lid on. Allow them to simmer for 20 minutes or until the zucchini is soft.
3. Add the lemon juice, tamari, leafy greens, cabbage, salt, and ground black pepper. Sauté for another 2 minutes or until the greens are soft.
4. Transfer the cooked vegetables to a platter and serve warm.

STORAGE: Store in an airtight container in the fridge for up to 3 to 5 days.
REHEAT: Microwave, covered, until the desired temperature is reached or reheat in a frying pan or instant pot, covered, on medium.
SERVE IT WITH: To make this dish complete, you can serve it with chicken breasts or shrimp skewers.
PER SERVING
calories: 148 | fat: 14.0g | total carbs: 5.6g | fiber: 1.6g | protein: 3.0g

SCRUMPTIOUS BRIAM

Macros: Fat 74% | Protein 13% | Carbs 13%
Prep time: 10 minutes | Cook time: 20 minutes | Serves 4

Briam is a Greek way of vegetable roasting in a casserole dish. In a traditional way, it mainly contains potatoes, zucchini, onions, and tomatoes. But for our keto-friendly recipe, we use eggplant to replace the potatoes, and add other keto vegetables to increase the flavor of this recipe.

⅓ cup olive oil, divided	oregano
1 tablespoon minced garlic	2 tablespoons chopped fresh
1 onion, thinly sliced	parsley
¾ small eggplant, diced	Sea salt and freshly ground black
2 cups chopped cauliflower	pepper, to taste
1 red bell pepper, diced	2 zucchinis, diced
2 cups diced tomatoes	1½ cups crumbled feta cheese
2 tablespoons chopped fresh	¼ cup pumpkin seeds

1. Preheat the oven to 500°F (260°C). Lightly grease a casserole dish with 1 teaspoon olive oil and set aside.
2. Heat 3 tablespoons olive oil in a nonstick skillet over medium heat. Add and sauté the garlic and onion for 3 minutes or until the onion is translucent.
3. Add and sauté the eggplant for 5 minutes, then add and sauté the tomatoes, oregano, and parsley for about 8 minutes or until the vegetables are soft, stirring occasionally. Sprinkle with salt and pepper.
4. Make the briam: Transfer the mixture in the skillet to the greased casserole dish. Spread the diced zucchini and crumbled feta cheese on top. Arrange the casserole dish in the preheated oven and broil for 4 minutes or until the cheese is lightly browned.
5. Remove the briam from the oven to four plates. Scatter the pumpkin seeds over them and serve drizzled with the remaining olive oil.

STORAGE: Store in an airtight container in the fridge for 4 to 5 days.
REHEAT: Microwave, covered, until the desired temperature is reached or reheat in a frying pan or instant pot, covered, on medium.
SERVE IT WITH: To make this dish complete, you can serve it with sliced olives on the side.
PER SERVING
calories: 340 | fat: 28.0g | total carbs: 18.0g | fiber: 7.0g | protein: 11.0g

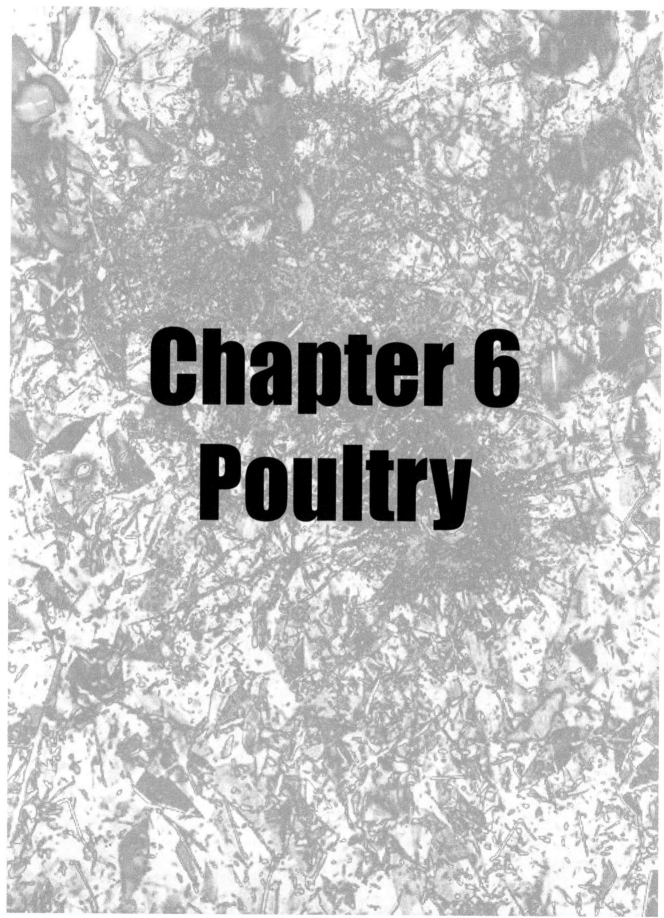

Chapter 6
Poultry

CREAMY CHICKEN AND HAM MEATBALLS

Macros: Fat: 76% | Protein: 21% | Carbs: 3%
Prep time: 30 minutes | Cook time: 15 minutes | Serves 6

Meatballs are a delicious addition to every meal. From simple dishes to complex ones, this delicious meatball dish can be served alone or can be the perfect addition to every meal. These meatballs will come out juicy and are perfect for family dinners and parties. Grab a fork and dive in.

1 pound (454 g) ground chicken	1 tablespoon butter
⅓ cup blanched almond flour	¾ cup chicken broth
½ teaspoon onion powder	1 teaspoon Dijon mustard
1 egg, lightly beaten	½ cup heavy cream
½ teaspoon salt	1 cup shredded Swiss cheese
½ teaspoon garlic powder	Freshly ground black pepper, to
6 ounces (170 g) ham steak,	taste
cubed into 20 even pieces	2 tablespoons minced fresh
1 tablespoon olive oil	parsley

1. Mix the chicken with the almond flour, onion powder, egg, salt, and garlic powder in a bowl. Roll a cube of ham into a 1½-inch ball with the chicken around it and put it on a plate. Make 20 chicken-covered ham meatballs from this mixture.
2. Heat the olive oil in a nonstick skillet over medium-high heat. Arrange the meatballs in the skillet and cook for 3 minutes or until lightly browned. Flip them and cook for another 3 to 4 minutes, then remove them from the skillet to a plate.
3. Reduce the heat to medium and add the butter to melt. Mix in the chicken broth and the mustard, then simmer for about 3 minutes.
4. Mix in the cream and Swiss cheese until it has completely melted, then put the meatballs back into the skillet. Let it cook for 3 to 4 minutes or until the sauce reduces in half.
5. Sprinkle with black pepper and parsley, then serve hot.

STORAGE: Store in an airtight container in the fridge for up to 4 days or in the freezer for up to 1 month.
REHEAT: Microwave, covered, until the desired temperature is reached or reheat in a frying pan or air fryer / instant pot, covered, on medium.
SERVE IT WITH: To make this a complete meal, serve it with mushroom and cauliflower salad.
PER SERVING
calories: 544 | fat: 45.9g | total carbs: 4.7g | fiber: 0.5g | protein: 28.4g

BUTTERY CHICKEN AND MUSHROOMS

Macros: Fat: 56% | Protein: 36% | Carbs: 8%
Prep time: 10 minutes | Cook time: 30 minutes | Serves 4

This delicious chicken and mushroom dish is a quick and easy dish to make. Whether during busy weekdays or for want of a variety, this low-carb dish is the way to go. It is perfect for parties and family gatherings.

2 boneless chicken breasts, skin-on	8 ounces (227 g) fresh mushrooms, cut into ¼-inch-thick slices
Salt and ground black pepper, to taste	½ cup of water
2 tablespoons olive oil	1 tablespoon butter

1. Start by preheating the oven to 400°F (205°C).
2. On a plate, sprinkle salt and pepper over the chicken.
3. Heat the olive oil in a frying pan over medium-high heat. Add the chicken breasts, skin side down, and cook for 5 minutes or until browned.

4. Flip the chicken and add the mushrooms. Sprinkle salt over the mushrooms and cook for 5 minutes, stirring occasionally, or until the mushrooms shrink slightly.
5. Remove the pan from the heat and put it into the oven. Bake for 15 to 20 minutes or until a meat thermometer inserted in the center of the chicken reads at least 165°F (74°C).
6. Remove the chicken from the oven and put it on a plate. Cover the plate loosely with a foil and set aside.
7. Put the pan over medium-high heat and cook the mushrooms for 5 minutes until the bottom of the pan starts to brown. Pour the water into the pan and use a spatula or a wooden spoon to scrape up the bits. Cook for 2 minutes or until the water has reduced by half.
8. Remove the pan from the heat and add any juices from the chicken to the pan. Mix in the butter until it has melted completely.
9. Season as needed with salt and pepper. Serve the chicken topped with mushroom mixture.

STORAGE: Store in an airtight container in the fridge for up to 4 days or in the freezer for up to 1 month.
REHEAT: Microwave, covered, until the desired temperature is reached or reheat in a frying pan or instant pot, covered, on medium.
SERVE IT WITH: To make this a complete meal, serve it on a bed of zucchini noodles.
PER SERVING
calories: 368 | fat: 23.2g | total carbs: 8.5g | fiber: 1.3g | protein: 31.2g

AIR-FRIED GARLIC-LEMON CHICKEN

Macros: Fat: 70% | Protein: 27% | Carbs: 3%
Prep time: 10 minutes | Cook time: 25 minutes | Serves 4

This deliciously crunchy chicken thigh dish is in a league of its own. Air fried with the best ingredients to bring out its flavor, every bite will explode in mouth-watering goodness that will overwhelm your senses and have you reaching for more.

¼ cup lemon juice	2 tablespoons olive oil
2 cloves garlic, minced	1 teaspoon Dijon mustard
¼ teaspoon salt	4 skin-on, bone-in chicken
⅛ teaspoon ground black pepper	thighs
	4 lemon wedges

1. In a bowl, mix the lemon juice, garlic, salt, black pepper, olive oil, and mustard together. Set aside.
2. Put the chicken thighs into a Ziploc bag and pour the marinade in. Make sure that the chicken thighs are well coated in the marinade, then seal the bag and put it in the refrigerator for at least 2 hours.
3. Preheat the air fryer to 375°F (190°C).
4. Remove the chicken from the marinade and dry it with paper towels.
5. Put the chicken in the air fryer basket and fry in batches for 22 to 24 minutes or until the juices are clear and a meat thermometer should read 165°F (74°C). Flip the chicken thighs halfway through the cooking time.
6. Transfer the chicken to a plate and squeeze the lemon wedges over, then serve.

STORAGE: Store in an airtight container in the fridge for up to 4 days or in the freezer for up to 1 month.
REHEAT: Microwave, covered, until the desired temperature is reached or reheat in a frying pan or air fryer / instant pot, covered, on medium.
SERVE IT WITH: To make this a complete meal, you can serve it with stir-fried zoodles.
PER SERVING
calories: 503 | fat: 39.0g | total carbs: 5.5g | fiber: 0.3g | protein: 32.3g

SOUR PEPPER CHICKEN

Macros: Fat: 46% | Protein: 51% | Carbs: 3%
Prep time: 15 minutes | Cook time: 20 minutes | Serves 6

This grilled sour pepper chicken wakes up every taste bud with its distinguishing taste. It has a crunchy, grilled skin with a perfectly-spiced, juicy, tender meat that leaves you wanting more. This dish is quick and easy to make which makes it a perfect dinner for busy weekdays.

1 teaspoon freshly ground black pepper	finely minced
½ cup lemon juice	2 tablespoons dried oregano
¼ cup olive oil	1 teaspoon red pepper flakes, to taste
1 tablespoon distilled white vinegar	6 chicken leg quarters
6 cloves garlic, crushed or very	Kosher salt, to taste
	1 lemon, cut into wedges

1. In a large bowl, whisk the black pepper, lemon juice, oil, vinegar, garlic, oregano, and red pepper flakes together.
2. Cut 2 deep slices into each chicken leg, making sure that it reaches the bone, then sprinkle generously with the kosher salt and dunk them into the bowl of mixture. Wrap the bowl in plastic and put in the refrigerator to marinate for 4 to 12 hours.
3. Preheat the grill to medium-high heat.
4. Discard the marinade and pat dry the chicken legs with paper towels.
5. Put the chicken leg on the grill, skin side down, and cook for 6 to 7 minutes on each side or until the juices run clear and no pink. Cook for another 8 minutes or until cooked through.
6. Remove the chicken legs from the grill and serve them on a plate, and squeeze the lemon wedges over.

STORAGE: Store in an airtight container in the fridge for up to 4 days or in the freezer for up to 1 month.
REHEAT: Microwave, covered, until the desired temperature is reached or reheat in a frying pan or air fryer / instant pot, covered, on medium.
SERVE IT WITH: To make this a complete meal, serve it with a glass of sparkling water.
PER SERVING
calories: 402 | fat: 20.4g | total carbs: 4.4g | fiber: 1.0g | protein: 51.3g

ITALIAN GARLIC CHICKEN KEBAB

Macros: Fat: 35% | Protein: 63% | Carbs: 2%
Prep time: 20 minutes | Cook time: 15 minutes | Serves 8

This dish is the perfect go-to for everyone. It is a crowd-pleaser in every party, gathering, brunch, or just a simple dinner. It freezes and reheats well which means that you can get your favorite dish anytime, anywhere.

¼ cup coconut aminos	1 clove garlic, crushed
¼ teaspoon onion powder	1 teaspoon grated fresh ginger root
2 tablespoons lemon juice	
4 tablespoons olive oil, divided	1 pinch ground black pepper
¾ teaspoon Italian seasoning	8 skinless, boneless chicken breasts, cut into strips
3 tablespoons dry white wine	

SPECIAL EQUIPMENT:
8 skewers, soaked for at least 30 minutes to avoid burning during grilling

1. Put the coconut aminos, onion powder, lemon juice, 2 tablespoons of olive oil, Italian seasoning, dry white wine,

garlic, ginger root, and black pepper in a Ziploc bag and mix them together. Put the chicken in the bag. Shake the bag to make sure the chicken is coated in the spices, then seal the bag and put it in the refrigerator to marinate for 3 hours.
2. Preheat an outdoor grill to medium-high heat.
3. Run each of the skewers through the chicken strips and set aside. Pour the marinade into a pan over high heat and let it boil.
4. Brush the preheated grill grates with 1 tablespoon of olive oil and place the chicken skewers on the grates to grill for 16 minutes. Brush the chicken skewers with the remaining olive oil and flip halfway through the cooking time. Cover the chicken with the sauce generously as it grills.
5. When the chicken juices run clear, remove it from the grill, and serve on a plate.

STORAGE: Store in an airtight container in the fridge for up to 4 days or in the freezer for up to 1 month.
REHEAT: Microwave, covered, until the desired temperature is reached or reheat in a frying pan or air fryer / instant pot, covered, on medium.
SERVE IT WITH: To make this a complete meal, serve it with cheesy broccoli salad.
PER SERVING
calories: 339 | fat: 13.0g | total carbs: 2.4g | fiber: 0.1g | protein: 53.2g

CHICKEN IN TOMATOES AND HERBS

Macros: Fat: 28% | Protein: 65% | Carbs: 7%
Prep time: 10 minutes | Cook time: 25 minutes | Serves 6

This herb chicken dish will become your favorite go-to recipe for every occasion. It is the perfect way to add a juicy chicken to salads, wraps, pasta, and any other dish. Perfect for kids and adults, any event with this dish will be fondly remembered.

6 skinless, boneless chicken breasts	2 tablespoons olive oil
1 teaspoon garlic salt	1 onion, thinly sliced
Freshly ground black pepper, to taste	1 (14½-ounce / 411-g) can diced tomatoes
	½ cup balsamic vinegar

HERBS:
1 teaspoon dried basil	1 teaspoon dried rosemary
1 teaspoon dried oregano	½ teaspoon dried thyme

1. Sprinkle all sides of the chicken with garlic salt and pepper.
2. Pour the olive oil into the pan over medium heat and brown the chicken breasts in the pan for 3 to 4 minutes on each side. Mix in the onions and cook for 3 o 4 minutes until it is browned.
3. Pour the tomatoes and vinegar over the chicken then season with the herbs. Cook on low heat for 15 minutes until the juices are clear.
4. Remove them from the heat and serve on a plate.

STORAGE: Store in an airtight container in the fridge for up to 4 days or in the freezer for up to 1 month.
REHEAT: Microwave, covered, until the desired temperature is reached or reheat in a frying pan or air fryer / instant pot, covered, on medium.
SERVE IT WITH: To make this a complete meal, serve it with a bowl of green salad.
PER SERVING
calories: 356 | fat: 10.9g | total carbs: 6.6g | fiber: 1.6g | protein: 53.9g

SPICY BURNT-FRIED CHICKEN

Macros: Fat: 27% | Protein: 71% | Carbs: 2%
Prep time: 10 minutes | Cook time: 20 minutes | Serves 2

You cannot deny that a slightly burnt or blackened taste gives any chicken an extra kick. This delicious burnt-fried chicken is guaranteed to leave you wanting some more. Generously coated in hot spices, it is the perfect meal to kick out the cold and delight your taste buds.

½ teaspoon cayenne pepper	1 teaspoon cumin
½ teaspoon onion powder	¼ teaspoon salt
½ teaspoon black pepper	2 (12-ounce / 340-g) skinless,
2 teaspoons paprika	boneless chicken breasts
1 teaspoon ground thyme	2 teaspoons olive oil

1. Mix the cayenne pepper, onion powder, black pepper, paprika, thyme, cumin, and salt in a bowl.
2. Rub the chicken breasts with the olive oil, then put it in the spice mixture. Make sure they are coated all around with the spices, then set aside to marinate for 5 minutes.
3. Preheat the air fryer to 375°F (190°C).
4. Put the chicken in the air fryer basket and cook for 10 minutes. Flip it over and cook for another 10 minutes.
5. Remove the chicken from the basket to a plate and let it rest for 5 minutes before serving.

STORAGE: Store in an airtight container in the fridge for up to 4 days or in the freezer for up to 1 month.
REHEAT: Microwave, covered, until the desired temperature is reached or reheat in a frying pan or air fryer / instant pot, covered, on medium.
SERVE IT WITH: To make this a complete meal, serve it with mashed cauliflower.
PER SERVING
calories: 464 | fat: 14.1g | total carbs: 3.0g | fiber: 1.4g | protein: 77.3g

CRUNCHY TACO CHICKEN WINGS

Macros: Fat: 28% | Protein: 71% | Carbs: 1%
Prep time: 5 minutes | Cook time: 15 minutes | Serves 5

Take the taste of that crunchy taco you absolutely love and put it on these chicken wings dish. This dish is a quick and easy dish that promises to take your taste buds on an amazing ride. From the crunchy, well-seasoned chicken back to the soft and spicy meat, this chicken dish will always make a reappearance on your table.

3 pounds (1.4 kg) chicken wings	2 teaspoons olive oil
1 tablespoon taco seasoning mix	

1. Put the chicken wings in a Ziploc bag, then add the taco seasoning and olive oil.
2. Seal the bag and shake well until the chicken is coated thoroughly.
3. Preheat the air fryer to 350°F (180°C).
4. Put the chicken in the air fryer basket and cook for 6 minutes on each side until crispy.
5. Remove the chicken from the basket and serve on a plate.

STORAGE: Store in an airtight container in the fridge for up to 4 days or in the freezer for up to 1 month.
REHEAT: Microwave, covered, until the desired temperature is reached or reheat in a frying pan or air fryer / instant pot, covered, on medium.
SERVE IT WITH: To make this a complete meal, serve it with a bowl of cauliflower rice and a glass of sparkling water.
PER SERVING
calories: 364 | fat: 11.4g | total carbs: 1.0g | fiber: 0.2g | protein: 59.9g

SPICY CHEESY STUFFED AVOCADOS

Macros: Fat: 63% | Protein: 24% | Carbs: 12%
Prep time: 10 minutes | Cook time: 8 minutes | Serves 8

Perfect for brunch and parties with kids and adults, this dish is a healthy, low-carb healthy alternative to unhealthy snacks. Each bite is loaded with the delicious, healthy avocado which is the perfect ingredients for every low-carb diet.

4 avocados, halved and pitted	pepper
2 cooked chicken breasts, shredded	1 pinch cayenne pepper
	¼ cup tomatoes, chopped
4 ounces (113 g) cream cheese, softened	¼ teaspoon salt
	½ cup shredded Parmesan
¼ teaspoon ground black	cheese, or more to taste

SPECIAL EQUIPMENT:
8 muffin cups, for stabilizing the avocado halves

1. Start by preheating the oven to 400°F (205°C).
2. Spoon some of the avocado flesh in a bowl. Add the chicken, cream cheese, black pepper, cayenne pepper, tomatoes, and salt to the bowl and mix well. Spoon the mixture into each of the avocado wells then top it with a layer of Parmesan cheese.
3. Put the avocado halves in muffin cups, facing up, to stabilize them.
4. Put the cups in the preheated oven to bake for 8 to 10 minutes, or until the cheese is melted.
5. Remove them from the oven and serve hot.

STORAGE: Store in an airtight container in the fridge for up to 4 days or in the freezer for up to 1 month.
REHEAT: Microwave, covered, until the desired temperature is reached or reheat in a frying pan or air fryer / instant pot, covered, on medium.
SERVE IT WITH: To make this a complete meal, serve it with jicama and daikon radish salad with a glass of sparkling water.
PER SERVING
calories: 308 | fat: 22.9g | total carbs: 10.3g | fiber: 6.8g | protein: 18.0g

CRISPY KETO WINGS WITH RICH BROCCOLI

Macros: Fat 61% | Protein 34% | Carbs 5%
Prep time:15 minutes | Cook time: 45 minutes | Serves 6

The crispness and fragrance of this tender chicken wings will catch your palate, and served with tiny broccoli florets to help balance the rich, creaminess of the dish. It's is a match made in heaven.

BAKED CHICKEN WINGS:

½ lemon, juice and zest	¼ cup olive oil
2 teaspoons ground ginger	1 teaspoon salt
¼ teaspoon cayenne pepper	3 pounds (1.4 kg) chicken wings

CREAMY BROCCOLI:

1½ pounds (680 g) broccoli, cut into florets	1 cup mayonnaise, keto-friendly
	Salt and freshly ground black
¼ cup chopped fresh dill	pepper, to taste

1. Preheat the oven to 400°F (205°C).
2. Combine the lemon juice, lemon zest, ground ginger, cayenne pepper, olive oil, and salt in a Ziploc bag, then put the chicken wings in the bag. Shake to coat well.
3. Arrange the bag in the refrigerator to marinate for at least 45 minutes.
4. Arrange the well-coated chicken wings in a lightly greased baking dish. PLace the dish in the preheated oven.

5. Bake for 45 minutes, or until no pink and the juice of the chicken wings run clear.
6. Meanwhile, blanch the broccoli in a pot of salted water for 5 minutes or until lightly softened.
7. Transfer the broccoli to a large bowl, and add the remaining ingredients. Toss to combine well.
8. Serve the baked chicken wings with creamy broccoli aside.

STORAGE: Store in an airtight container in the fridge for up to 4 days.
REHEAT: Microwave, covered, until the desired temperature is reached or reheat in a frying pan or air fryer / instant pot, covered, on medium.
SERVE IT WITH: To make this a complete meal, you can serve it with mushroom and salmon salad, and strawberry smoothie.
PER SERVING
calories: 657 | fat: 44.9g | total carbs: 8.5g | fiber: 3.1g | protein: 53.5g

KETO CHICKEN CASSEROLE

Macros: Fat 46% | Protein 46% | Carbs 8%
Prep time: 15 minutes | Cook time: 25 minutes | Serves 4

Keto chicken casserole is a recipe you have come across not once but several times. However, it is worth cooking over and over again because of its great taste and essential nutrients especially on keto diet. This recipe is perfect for dinner.

4 skinless, boneless chicken breast halves	condensed cream of mushroom soup
¼ cup butter	2 (13½-ounce / 383-g) cans
1 tablespoon Italian seasoning	drained spinach
3 teaspoons minced garlic	4 ounces (113 g) fresh sliced
½ cup grated Parmesan cheese	mushrooms
1 tablespoon lemon juice	⅔ cup bacon bits
½ cup heavy cream	2 cups shredded Mozzarella
1 (10¾-ounce / 305-g) can	cheese

1. Start by preheating the oven to 350°F (180°C), then put the chicken breast halves on a greased baking tray.
2. Bake in the preheated oven for 30 minutes until the juices are clear. Remove from the oven and put aside.
3. Increase the temperatures in the oven to 400°F (205°C).
4. Melt the butter in a medium saucepan over medium heat.
5. Add the Italian seasoning, garlic, Parmesan cheese, lemon juice, heavy cream, and mushroom soup, stirring continuously, for about 4 minutes. Set aside.
6. Place the spinach at the bottom of a baking dish.
7. Add the mushrooms then pour ½ of the mixture from the saucepan on top.
8. Place the chicken then pour the remaining sauce mixture.
9. Sprinkle the bacon bits then top with Mozzarella cheese.
10. Bake in the preheated oven for about 25 minutes until the chicken is lightly browned and the cheese is bubbly.
11. Remove form the oven and slice to serve.

STORAGE: Store in an airtight container in the fridge for up to 1 week
REHEAT: Microwave, covered, until the desired temperature is reached or reheat in an air fryer, covered, on medium.
SERVE IT WITH: To make this a complete meal, serve the chicken casserole with buttered mushrooms.
PER SERVING
calories: 717 | fat: 36.6g | total carbs: 21.3g | fiber: 6.3g | protein: 81.9g

CHICKEN BREAST WITH GUACAMOLE

Macros: Fat 69% | Protein 23% | Carbs 8%
Prep time: 20 minutes | Cook time: 20 minutes | Serves 6

This is a super delicious recipe. The taste of cheese with the flavor of the spiced chicken is balanced, and the cheese can be changed to Parmesan cheese for additional salty flavor. This is a meal with low budget to maintain a healthy body.

CHEESE STUFFED CHICKEN:

1 green bell pepper or red bell pepper, chopped	shredded
1 garlic clove, granulated	2 tablespoons pickled jalapeños, finely chopped
2 tablespoons olive oil	½ teaspoon ground cumin
1½ pounds (680 g) chicken breasts	1 ginger, minced
3 ounces (85 g) cream cheese	Salt and freshly ground black pepper, to taste
4 ounces (113 g) Cheddar cheese,	

SPECIAL EQUIPMENT:	**FOR SERVING:**
4 toothpicks, soak in water for at least 30 minutes	8 ounces (227 g) lettuce
	1 cup sour cream

GUACAMOLE:

2 ripe avocados, peeled	5 tablespoons fresh cilantro, finely chopped
½ lime, the juice	
2 garlic cloves, minced	Salt and freshly ground black pepper, to taste
1 diced tomato	
3 tablespoons olive oil	

1. Preheat the oven to 350°F (180°C).
2. Warm the olive oil in a nonstick skillet over medium heat. Add the garlic and bell pepper and sauté for about 3 minutes until the bell pepper is soft. Transfer to a bowl and allow to cool for 5 minutes.
3. Sprinkle the cheeses, jalapeños, cumin, and ginger in the bowl. Toss to combine well. Set aside.
4. Butterfly the chicken breasts by cutting them crosswise and leave a 1-inch space uncut at the end of the breasts.
5. Unfold the breasts on a clean working surface like a book, then divide and spread the cheese mixture in the breasts. Close the 'book' and secure each chicken breast with a toothpick. Sprinkle with salt and pepper.
6. Arrange the stuffed chicken breasts in a lightly greased frying pan and fry for 8 minutes or until lightly browned. Place the fried chicken in a baking dish.
7. Pour the remaining cheese mixture over the chicken breasts and bake in the preheated oven for 20 minutes or until a meat thermometer inserted in the middle of the chicken reads at least 165°F (74°C).
8. Remove the toothpicks and serve with lettuce, guacamole, and sour cream.

GUACAMOLE:
1. Mash the guacamole with a fork in a large bowl. Top with lime juice and minced garlic.
2. Add tomato, olive oil and finely chopped cilantro. Season with salt and pepper, and blend well.

STORAGE: Chicken breast filled cheese with guacamole can be stored covered in the fridge for 2 up to 3 days, you can even freeze it in a freezer-safe container for up to 1 month.
REHEAT: Microwave, until it reaches the desired temperature.
SERVE IT WITH: To make it a complete meal, you can serve it with a mushroom and salmon salad and berry smoothie.
PER SERVING
calories: 599 | fat: 47.1g | total carbs: 13.5g | fiber: 5.9g | protein: 32.8g

BUTTERY CHEESY GARLIC CHICKEN

Macros: Fat: 46% | Protein: 51% | Carbs: 3%
Prep time: 15 minutes | Cook time: 40 minutes | Serves 8

This buttery cheesy garlic chicken dish is perfectly cooked for all occasions. It is easy to make with ingredients you probably have at home. This recipe is going to be a constant request from family and friends during any parties.

½ cup butter
4 cloves garlic, minced
1½ cups shredded Cheddar cheese
¼ teaspoon dried parsley
¼ teaspoon dried oregano
¼ cup coconut flour

½ cup freshly grated Parmesan cheese
¼ teaspoon ground black pepper
⅛ teaspoon salt
8 skinless, boneless chicken breasts, pounded thin

1. Start by preheating the oven to 350°F (180°C).
2. Put the butter in a pan and melt over low heat. Add the garlic to cook for 3 minutes or until lightly browned. Transfer the garlic butter to a bowl. Set aside.
3. Mix the Cheddar cheese, parsley, oregano, coconut flour, Parmesan cheese, black pepper, and salt together in a separate bowl.
4. Dredge each chicken breast into the garlic butter, then coat it with the cheese mixture.
5. Place the chicken breasts on a baking dish and pour the remaining garlic butter and cheese mixture over them, then put the baking dish in the preheated oven.
6. Bake for 30 minutes until an instant-read thermometer inserted in the center of the chicken register at least 165°F (74°C).
7. Remove the chicken from the oven and serve warm.

STORAGE: Store in an airtight container in the fridge for up to 4 days or in the freezer for up to 1 month.
REHEAT: Microwave, covered, until the desired temperature is reached or reheat in a frying pan or air fryer / instant pot, covered, on medium.
SERVE IT WITH: To make this a complete meal, serve it with a bowl of green salad.
PER SERVING
calories: 506 | fat: 26.3g | total carbs: 2.9g | fiber: 0.1g | protein: 61.3g

PAN-FRIED CREAMY CHICKEN WITH TARRAGON

Macros: Fat: 41% | Protein: 58% | Carbs: 1%
Prep time: 15 minutes | Cook time: 30 minutes | Serves 4

This pan-fried chicken dish is creamy and delicious. Made with mustard and fresh tarragon, this low-carb dish will hit you with a hint of spice and flavor with the buttery juiciness of the chicken.

1 tablespoon butter
1 tablespoon olive oil
4 skinless, boneless chicken breasts
Salt and freshly ground black

pepper, to taste
½ cup heavy cream
1 tablespoon Dijon mustard
2 teaspoons chopped fresh tarragon

1. Melt the butter in a pan over medium-high heat, then add the olive oil.
2. Season the chicken with salt and pepper then put it in the pan to fry for 15 minutes on both sides until the juices are clear. Remove them from the pan and set aside.
3. Pour the heavy cream in the pan and use a wooden spoon to scrape the parts stuck to the pan, then add the mustard and the

tarragon. Mix well and let it simmer for 5 minutes.
4. Put the chicken back into the pan and cover it with the creamy sauce.
5. Serve the chicken drizzled with the sauce on a plate.

STORAGE: Store in an airtight container in the fridge for up to 4 days or in the freezer for up to 1 month.
REHEAT: Microwave, covered, until the desired temperature is reached or reheat in a frying pan or air fryer / instant pot, covered, on medium.
SERVE IT WITH: To make this a complete meal, serve it with a bowl of green salad.
PER SERVING
calories: 395 | fat: 18.2g | total carbs: 1.2g | fiber: 0.3g | protein: 53.7g

CHEESY LOW-CARB CHICKEN

Macros: Fat: 41% | Protein: 54% | Carbs: 5%
Prep time: 10 minutes | Cook time: 1 hour | Serves 4

This cheesy chicken dish is seasoned with oregano and topped with cheese to make a delicious low-carb meal that is perfect for the healthy eaters and kids. It is a family-friendly meal that is perfect for any night of the week.

1 (2- to 3-pound / 0.9- to 1.4-kg) whole chicken, cut into uniform pieces
⅛ cup extra virgin olive oil
1 cup chicken stock
1 clove garlic, crushed

1 teaspoon dried oregano
Salt and freshly ground black pepper, to taste
¼ cup grated Romano cheese
3 tablespoons balsamic vinegar

1. Start by preheating the oven to 450°F (235°C).
2. Put the chicken in a baking dish, then pour the olive oil and chicken stock over it. Sprinkle with the garlic. Season with oregano, salt, and pepper, then scatter the cheese over the chicken.
3. Put the baking dish in the preheated oven to bake for 45 to 60 minutes until cooked through.
4. Remove from the oven and serve the chicken drizzled with the vinegar on a plate.

STORAGE: Store in an airtight container in the fridge for up to 4 days or in the freezer for up to 1 month.
REHEAT: Microwave, covered, until the desired temperature is reached or reheat in a frying pan or air fryer / instant pot, covered, on medium.
SERVE IT WITH: To make this a complete meal, serve it with a bowl of green salad.
PER SERVING
calories: 389 | fat: 17.7g | total carbs: 5.1g | fiber: 0.1g | protein: 52.3g

SOUR AND SPICY CHICKEN BREAST

Macros: Fat: 45% | Protein: 54% | Carbs: 1%
Prep time: 10 minutes | Cook time: 10 minutes | Serves 4

This delicious chicken breast brings the perfect tangy and spicy combination to any chicken dish. Marinated and grilled, it is perfectly crispy on the outside and juicy on the inside, making it a lip-smacking experience for every tongue.

4 skinless, boneless chicken breast halves

⅛ cup extra virgin olive oil
1 lemon, juiced

2 teaspoons crushed garlic ⅓ teaspoon paprika
1 teaspoon salt 2 tablespoons olive oil, divided
1½ teaspoons black pepper

1. Combine the olive oil, lemon, garlic, salt, pepper, and paprika in a bowl, then set aside.
2. Cut 3 slits into the chicken breasts to allow the marinade to soak in. Put the chicken in a separate bowl and pour the marinade over it.
3. Cover the bowl with plastic wrap and put in the refrigerator to marinate overnight.
4. Preheat the grill to medium heat and brush the grill grates with 1 tablespoon of olive oil.
5. Remove the chicken from the marinade and place it on the grill to cook for about 5 minutes until the juices are clear. Flip the chicken over and brush with the remaining olive oil. Grill for 3 minutes more.
6. Remove the chicken from the grill and serve on plates.

STORAGE: Store in an airtight container in the fridge for up to 4 days or in the freezer for up to 1 month.
REHEAT: Microwave, covered, until the desired temperature is reached or reheat in a frying pan or air fryer / instant pot, covered, on medium.
SERVE IT WITH: To make this a complete meal, serve it with cheesy baked asparagus or creamy cucumber salad.
PER SERVING
calories: 399 | fat: 19.8g | total carbs: 2.1g | fiber: 0.4g | protein: 53.4g

BAKED CHICKEN THIGHS WITH LEMON BUTTER CAPER SAUCE

Marcos: Fat 71% | Protein 26% | Carbs 3%
Prep time: 15 minutes | Cook time: 30 minutes | Serves 4

Sometimes, we are hungry for a tasty meal, but never have the time for it, or do we? That's right my dear hungry friend. These delicious chicken thighs alongside with lemon butter caper sauce could be prepared in less than an hour. So get your ingredients ready and prepare yourself for an exquisite meal packed with flavor.

1 teaspoon sea salt chicken thighs, skin-on
½ teaspoon ground black 2 tablespoons olive oil
pepper 3 tablespoons butter
1 tablespoon Italian seasoning 2 tablespoons lemon juice
1 tablespoon garlic powder 1 lemon, divided into wheels
2 pounds (907 g) bone-in

SERVING:
2 ounces (57 g) leafy vegetables

1. Preheat the oven to 400°F (205°C).
2. Use salt, pepper, Italian seasoning and garlic powder to season the thighs on both sides.
3. Heat the olive oil in a large skillet over medium heat. Add the chicken thighs, skin side down, and cook for about 5 minutes until the skin turns crispy and nice.
4. Flip the chicken thighs over and put the skillet into the preheated oven. Bake for 15 to 20 minutes until the chicken is cooked through.
5. Remove the chicken from the oven to a plate and set aside.
6. Add the butter and lemon juice to the same skillet over medium-high for 2 to 3 minutes, and keep stirring until the sauce gets thickened. Scarp any leftover bits stuck to the bottom of the skillet with a spatula.
7. Pour the sauce over the chicken and garnish with lemon wheels, then serve with leafy vegetables.

STORAGE: Store in a sealed airtight container in the fridge for up to 5 days or in your freezer for about 1 month.
REHEAT: Microwave, covered, until the desired temperature is reached or reheat in a frying pan or instant pot, covered, on medium.
SERVE IT WITH: It could be served with the vegan kale salad.
PER SERVING
calories: 635 | fat: 50.3g | total carbs: 5.5g | fiber: 0.8g | protein:38.6g

SPICY OVEN-BAKED CHICKEN

Macros: Fat: 21% | Protein: 74% | Carbs: 5%
Prep time: 10 minutes | Cook time: 20 minutes | Serves 8

This spicy oven-baked chicken is the perfect highlight of every gathering. It is a juicy dish that is perfect for salads, wraps, pasta, and any sandwiches of your choice. It has a delicious crispy skin with soft and juicy meat that makes each bite a pleasure.

1 teaspoon dried thyme ½ teaspoon black pepper
1 teaspoon white pepper ½ teaspoon garlic powder
½ teaspoon cayenne pepper 2 onions, quartered
4 teaspoons salt 2 (4-pound / 1.8-kg) whole
2 teaspoons paprika chickens, giblets removed,
1 teaspoon onion powder rinsed and drained

1. Mix the thyme, white pepper, cayenne, salt, paprika, onion powder, black pepper, and garlic powder in a bowl.
2. Coat the inside of the chicken and the outer part with the spice mixture, then put 1 onion inside the chicken.
3. Put the chicken in a Ziploc bag and seal it. Place the chicken in a refrigerator for 4 to 6 hours, preferably overnight.
4. Preheat the oven to 400°F (205°C).
5. Remove the chicken from the bag and put it in a roasting pan. Put the pan in the oven to bake for about 20 minutes, or until an instant-read thermometer inserted into the thickest part registers at least 165°F (74°C).
6. Remove the chicken from the oven. Let it rest for 10 minutes before slicing to serve.

STORAGE: Store in an airtight container in the fridge for up to 4 days or in the freezer for up to 1 month.
REHEAT: Microwave, covered, until the desired temperature is reached or reheat in a frying pan or air fryer / instant pot, covered, on medium.
SERVE IT WITH: To make this a complete meal, serve it with a bowl of green salad.
PER SERVING
calories: 268 | fat: 6.3g | total carbs: 3.7g | fiber: 0.9g | protein: 46.6g

GRILLED SPICED CHICKEN

Macros: Fat: 78% | Protein: 21% | Carbs: 1%
Prep time: 15 minutes | Cook time: 20 minutes | Serves 10

A grill and a generous heart are all you need to make this dish a reality, don't forget the ingredients too! This grilled spiced chicken dish is a quick and easy dish to cook because it uses ingredients that you already have at home. Perfect for busy weekdays with the added value of being keto-friendly, this dish is the best bet for you.

1 teaspoon garlic powder ½ cup apple cider vinegar
1 teaspoon ground paprika 1 tablespoon salt
1 teaspoon poultry seasoning 1 teaspoon black pepper
1 cup of olive oil 10 skinless chicken thighs

1. Pour the garlic powder, paprika, poultry seasoning, oil, vinegar, salt, and black pepper into a jar with a lid, cover the jar and shake it well to combine.
2. Put the chicken thighs on a baking dish and pour three-quarters of the powder mixture over them. Cover the dish with plastic wrap and put it in the refrigerator to marinate for 8 hours, preferably overnight.
3. Preheat the grill to high heat.
4. Place the chicken on the grill to cook for 10 minutes on each side.
5. Transfer the chicken to a plate and brush with the remaining powder mixture, then serve.

STORAGE: Store in an airtight container in the fridge for up to 4 days or in the freezer for up to 1 month.
REHEAT: Microwave, covered, until the desired temperature is reached or reheat in a frying pan or air fryer / instant pot, covered, on medium.
SERVE IT WITH: To make this a complete meal, serve it with a bowl of green salad.
PER SERVING
calories: 615 | fat: 53.7g | total carbs: 1.2g | fiber: 0.2g | protein: 32.0g

SPICY GARLIC CHICKEN KEBABS

Macros: Fat: 50% | Protein: 44% | Carbs: 6%
Prep time: 15 minutes | Cook time: 12 minutes | Serves 6

Chicken kebabs has always been a party pleaser but this spicy variation will kick your party up a notch. It can be stored and reheated which makes it a suitable leftover meal and can replace carb-laden snacks.

1 cup plain Greek yogurt
2 tablespoons freshly squeezed lemon juice, or more to taste
1 tablespoon kosher salt
1½ teaspoons ground cumin
1 teaspoon freshly ground black pepper

⅛ teaspoon ground cinnamon
2 tablespoons olive oil, divided
6 cloves garlic, minced
1 tablespoon red pepper flakes
1 teaspoon paprika
2½ pounds (1.1 kg) boneless, skinless chicken thighs, halved

SPECIAL EQUIPMENT:
4 long metal skewers

1. Mix the yogurt, lemon juice, kosher salt, cumin, black pepper, cinnamon, 1 tablespoon olive oil, garlic, red pepper flakes, and paprika together in a bowl.
2. Put the chicken in the marinade to coat, then cover the bowl with plastic wrap and refrigerate to marinate for 2 to 8 hours.
3. Preheat the grill to medium-high heat and brush the grill grates with the remaining olive oil.
4. Make the kebabs: Thread half of the chicken on two skewers and shape it into a thick log.
5. Put the kebabs on the grill and cook for 4 to 5 minutes. Flip the kebabs over and cook the for about 6 minutes more, or until cooked through and a meat thermometer inserted in the center registers 165°F (74°C).
6. Remove the kebabs from the grill and serve on a plate.

STORAGE: Store in an airtight container in the fridge for up to 4 days or in the freezer for up to 1 month.
REHEAT: Microwave, covered, until the desired temperature is reached or reheat in a frying pan or air fryer / instant pot, covered, on medium.
SERVE IT WITH: To make this a complete meal, serve it with a bowl of green salad.
PER SERVING
calories: 512 | fat: 28.5g | total carbs: 11.7g | fiber: 4.1g | protein: 56.3g

CHICKEN AND HERB BUTTER WITH KETO ZUCCHINI ROLL-UPS

Macros: Fat 83% | Protein 13% | Carbs 4%
Prep time: 15 minutes | Cook time: 40 minutes | Serves 4

Chicken and herb butter with keto zucchini is the best recipe for a family gathering at dinner, where you find vitamins, protein, and calcium in one dish your child will enjoy a healthy and delicious meal as the family warms up.

ZUCCHINI ROLL-UPS:
1½ pounds (680 g) zucchini
½ teaspoon salt
3 ounces (85 g) butter
6 ounces (170 g) mushrooms, finely chopped
6 ounces (170 g) cream cheese
6 ounces (170 g) shredded Cheddar cheese
½ green bell pepper, chopped

2 ounces (57 g) air-dried chorizo, chopped
1 egg
1 teaspoon onion powder
2 tablespoons fresh parsley, chopped
½ teaspoon salt
¼ teaspoon pepper

CHICKEN:
4 (6-ounce / 170-g) chicken breasts
Salt and freshly ground pepper,

to taste
1 ounce (28 g) butter, for frying

HERB BUTTER:
4 ounces (113 g) butter, at room temperature
1 garlic clove
½ teaspoon garlic powder

1 tablespoon fresh parsley, finely chopped
1 teaspoon lemon juice
½ teaspoon salt

1. Preheat the oven to 350°F (180°C). Cut the zucchini lengthwise into equal slices, half an inch, Pat dry with paper towels or a clean kitchen towel.and place it on a baking tray lined with parchment paper. Sprinkle salt on the zucchini and let stand for 10 minutes.
2. Bake for 20 minutes in the oven, or until the zucchini is tender. Transfer to a cooling rack from the oven, Dry more if needed.
3. Put the butter in the saucepan over medium heat, cut the mushrooms and put it in and stir fry well, let cool.
4. Add the remaining ingredients for the zucchini roll-ups to a bowl, except a third of the shredded cheese. Add the mushrooms and blend well.
5. Place a large amount of cheese on top of each zucchini slice.
6. Roll up and put it inside the baking dish with seams down, Sprinkle on top the remainder of the cheese.
7. Raise the temperature to 400°F (205°C). Bake for 20 minutes, or until the cheese turns bubbly and golden.
8. In the meantime, season your chicken and fry it over medium heat in butter until it is crispy on the outside and cooked through.

HERB BUTTER:
1. To prepare Herb butter mix the butter, garlic, garlic powder, fresh parsley, lemon juice, and salt. thoroughly in a small bowl.
2. Let sit for 30 minutes and serve on top of the chicken and zucchini roll-ups.

STORAGE: Store in an airtight container in the fridge for up to 5 days or in the freezer for up to 2 weeks.
REHEAT: Microwave, covered, until the desired temperature is reached or reheat in a frying pan.
SERVE IT WITH: Serve with a herb butter or keto-friendly mayonnaise and a green salad.
PER SERVING
calories: 913 | fat: 84.0g | total carbs: 10.0g | fiber: 3.0g | protein: 30.0g

CHEESY CHICKEN DISH WITH SPINACH AND TOMATOES

Macros: Fat: 54% | Protein: 40% | Carbs: 6%
Prep time: 10 minutes | Cook time: 15 minutes | Serves 4

This mouth-watering cheesy chicken dish with spinach and tomatoes is just bursting with flavorful deliciousness. It is a family favorite dish and can bring any boring dish to life. Dip your fork into this cheesy deliciousness and you certainly won't regret it.

2 tablespoons olive oil
1½ pounds (680 g) skinless, boneless chicken breast, thinly sliced
1 cup heavy cream
1 teaspoon garlic powder

1 teaspoon Italian seasoning
½ cup chicken broth
½ cup Parmesan cheese, grated
1 cup spinach, chopped
½ cup sun-dried tomatoes, chopped

1. Heat the olive oil in a large skillet over medium-high heat.
2. Add the chicken to the skillet and cook for 3 to 5 minutes on each side or until lightly browned. Transfer the chicken to a plate and set aside.
3. Pour the heavy cream in the skillet and add the garlic powder, Italian seasoning, chicken broth, and Parmesan cheese, then whisk well for 5 minutes or until the sauce starts to thicken.
4. Mix in the spinach and the tomatoes and cook on low heat for 1 minute. Put the chicken back into the skillet and cook for 2 to 3 minutes. Keep stirring during the cooking.
5. Remove from the heat and serve on plates.

STORAGE: Store in an airtight container in the fridge for up to 4 days or in the freezer for up to 1 month.
REHEAT: Microwave, covered, until the desired temperature is reached or reheat in a frying pan or instant pot, covered, on medium.
SERVE IT WITH: To make this a complete meal, serve it with Greek salad or coleslaw.
PER SERVING
calories: 437 | fat: 26.1g | total carbs: 7.7g | fiber: 1.2g | protein: 44.0g

DELICIOUS PARMESAN CHICKEN

Macros: Fat 75% | Protein 23% | Carbs 2%
Prep time: 20 minutes | Cook time: 8 minutes | Serves 4

The kids will enjoy this delicious Parmesan chicken especially for dinner. The chicken is enriched with essential nutrients from the cream, pork rinds, eggs, and Parmesan cheese. It is a fulfilling recipe for keto diet.

1 (8-ounce / 227-g) skinless, boneless chicken breast
1 tablespoon heavy whipping cream
1 egg
½ teaspoon salt
½ teaspoon red pepper flakes
1 ounce (28 g) grated Parmesan cheese

1½ ounces (43 g) crushed pork rinds
½ teaspoon ground black pepper
½ teaspoon garlic powder
½ teaspoon Italian seasoning
1 tablespoon butter
¼ cup shredded Mozzarella cheese

1. Start by preheating the oven's broiler and put the oven rack about 6 inches from the heat source.
2. On a flat work surface, slice the chicken breast horizontally through the middle, Pound the chicken to ½-inch thickness with a meat mallet.
3. In a bowl, beat the cream and the egg until smooth. Set aside.
4. In another bowl, combine the salt, red pepper flakes, Parmesan cheese, pork rinds, black pepper, garlic powder, and Italian seasoning. Transfer the breading mixture to a plate.
5. Dip the chicken into the egg mixture, then press the chicken into the breading mixture to coat thickly on both sides.
6. Melt the butter in a skillet over medium-high heat.
7. Cook the chicken for about 3 minutes per side, or until it is no longer pink and juices are clear.
8. Put the cooked chicken in a baking tray then top up with Mozzarella cheese.
9. Broil in the preheated oven for about 2 minutes until the cheese is barely brown and bubbly.

STORAGE: Store in an airtight container in the fridge for up to 1 week.
REHEAT: Microwave, covered, until the desired temperature is reached or reheat in a frying pan or air fryer, covered, on medium.
SERVE IT WITH: To make this a complete meal, serve the Parmesan chicken with zucchini noodles.
PER SERVING
calories: 492 | fat: 41.2g | total carbs: 2.5g | fiber: 0.4g | protein:28.1g

ALMOND CHICKEN CORDON BLEU

Macros: Fat 46% | Protein 52% | Carbs 2%
Prep time: 10 minutes | Cook time: 35 minutes | Serves 4

If you want to surprise your family with a unique and tasty chicken recipe, then go for almond chicken cordon bleu. The almond flavor gives the chicken a tasty approach that will leave you craving for more. For best results, use a chicken breast without bones.

2 tablespoons olive oil
4 skinless, boneless chicken breast halves
⅛ teaspoon ground black pepper

¼ teaspoon salt
6 slices Swiss cheese
4 slices cooked ham
½ cup almond meal

SPECIAL EQUIPMENT:
Toothpicks, soaked for at least 30 minutes

1. Start by preheating the oven to 350℉ (180℃) then grease a baking sheet with olive oil.
2. On a flat work surface, using a meat mallet to pound the chicken until it is ¼-inch thickness.
3. Sprinkle the pepper and salt on each piece of the chicken evenly.
4. Put 1 slice of ham and 1 slice of cheese on each breast.
5. Roll each breast and tightly secure with a toothpick.
6. Arrange them on the prepared baking sheet and evenly sprinkle with the almond meal.
7. Bake in the preheated oven until cooked through, for about 35 minutes
8. Remove from the oven and top each breast with ½ cheese slice.
9. Return to the oven and bake for 5 minutes more, until the cheese is bubbly.
10. Remove from the oven and serve on plates.

STORAGE: Store in an airtight container in the fridge for up to 1 week
REHEAT: Microwave, covered, until the desired temperature is reached or reheat in an air fryer, covered, on medium.
SERVE IT WITH: To make this a complete meal, serve the almond chicken cordon bleu with saucy chili-garlic cucumber noodles
PER SERVING
calories: 532 | fat: 27.1g | total carbs: 3.4g | fiber: 0.4g | protein: 69.1g

GRILLED CHICKEN BREAST

Macros: Fat 34% | Protein 65% | Carbs 1%
Prep time: 15 minutes | Cook time: 20 minutes | Serves 4

If you are craving for some juicy grilled chicken while on keto diet then this grilled chicken breast is the best option. You can prepare this recipe for lunch or dinner and enjoy with your family.

1 tablespoon olive oil
1 teaspoon steak sauce
2 tablespoons keto-friendly mayonnaise

⅓ teaspoon liquid stevia
⅓ cup Dijon mustard
4 skinless, boneless chicken breast halves

1. Start by preheating the grill on medium heat and lightly grease the grill grate with olive oil.
2. Mix together the steak sauce, mayonnaise, stevia, and mustard in a bowl. Reserve some mustard sauce for basting in another bowl, then coat the chicken with the remaining sauce.
3. Grill the chicken for about 20 minutes until the juices are clear, flipping occasionally and basting frequently with the reserved sauce.
4. Remove from the grill and serve hot.

STORAGE: Store in an airtight container in the fridge for up to 1 week
REHEAT: Microwave, covered, until the desired temperature is reached or reheat in a frying pan or air fryer / instant pot, covered, on medium.
SERVE IT WITH: To make this a complete meal, serve the grilled chicken with creamy spinach dill.
PER SERVING
calories: 333 | fat: 12.6g | total carbs: 1.5g | fiber: 0.9g | protein: 54.3g

GARLIC CHICKEN LOW-CARB

Macros: Fat 66% | Protein 31% | Carbs 3%
Prep time: 15 minutes | Cook time: 45 minutes | Serves 4

For those who look for simplicity, strong taste, and few calories, this recipe offers you great taste, distinct flavor, and simplicity of preparation.

2 ounces (57 g) butter
2 pounds (907 g) chicken drumsticks
Salt and freshly ground black pepper, to taste

2 tablespoons olive oil
1 lemon, the juice
7 garlic cloves, sliced
½ cup fresh parsley, finely chopped

1. Start by preheating the oven to 450°F (235°C).
2. Grease the baking pan with butter and put the chicken drumsticks, season with salt and pepper generously.
3. Drizzle the olive oil and lemon juice over the chicken pieces. Sprinkle the garlic and parsley on top.
4. Bake the chicken for 30 to 40 minutes or until the garlic slices become golden and chicken pieces turn brown and roasted, the baking time may be longer if your drumsticks are on the large size. Lower the temperature considerably towards the end.

STORAGE: Low-carb garlic chicken can be stored covered in the fridge for 1 up to 4 days, it can even be kept in the freezer for 15 days.
REHEAT: Microwave, covered, until the desired temperature is reached or reheat in a frying pan or air fryer / instant pot, covered, on medium.
SERVE IT WITH: This wonderful recipe is served cold or hot, can be Serve with aioli and a hearty salad and toast with garlic. Some people favor it with a delectable cauliflower mash.
PER SERVING
calories: 542 | fat: 40.0g | total carbs: 4.0g | fiber: 1.0g | protein: 42.0g

CHICKEN NUGGETS WITH FRIED GREEN BEAN AND BBQ-MAYO

Marcos: Fat 71% | Protein 24% | Carbs 5%
Prep time: 20 minutes | Cook time:25 minutes | Serves 6

Looking for another yummy scrummy keto meal? The Chicken nuggets with fried green bean is what you are looking for. As a young boy I used to eat nuggets all the time, and at that time I thought they were the best thing ever, so if you like normal nuggets as I do then surely these nuggets with BBQ-mayo and fried beans will blow your mind my friend. Chicken nuggets are not only for kids to enjoy, so make yourself this delicious meal and enjoy it regardless of your age.
There is no problem if you want to use chicken fingers instead of the nuggets.

CHICKEN NUGGETS:
1½ pounds (680 g) boneless chicken thighs, cut into bite size pieces
4 ounces (113 g) shredded Parmesan cheese
1 tablespoon onion powder

¼ tablespoon salt
¼ tablespoon ground black pepper
1 egg
1 tablespoon coconut oil

GREEN BEAN FRIES:
8 ounces (227 g) fresh green beans, trimmed
1 tablespoon coconut oil
¾ cup mayonnaise, keto-friendly

½ tablespoon smoked chili powder
1 tablespoon garlic powder
Salt and freshly ground black pepper, to taste

1. Put the Parmesan, onion powder, salt and pepper in a medium bowl and stir them till they are mixed very well
2. In another bowl, add the egg and whisk until it gets frothy.
3. Start Dipping the chicken pieces in the egg, and make sure to cover them entirely.
4. Coat the chicken nuggets in the Parmesan mixture by dipping them and shake off any excess.
5. Melt the coconut oil in a large skillet over medium heat, then fry the chicken nuggets on each side for 5 minutes until they become golden brown and cooked through.
6. Heat up coconut oil in a large skillet to medium-high, then put the trimmed beans and fry them for a couple of minutes. They should be crispy. Season the beans with salt before serving.
7. Now for the BBQ-mayo sauce, you should prepare a medium bowl and mix the mayonnaise, smoked chili powder, garlic powder, and a little bit of salt and pepper together, then stir very well and refrigerate for 30 minutes before serving.

STORAGE: Nuggets unfortunately last only for a day or two in the refrigerator. To maximize the quality of the nuggets. Wrap them with aluminum foil, or put them in a shallow airtight container.
REHEAT: It heats well in the microwave, but if you wanted them to be a bit tough then place the nuggets on a parchment paper lined cookie sheet, and make sure you preheat the oven to 350℉ (180°C), keeping them in there for 10 minutes will be enough to get them tasty and crunchy again.
SERVE IT WITH: There are a lot of things that could go along with this dish. Such as broccoli rice. The choices are not limited to certain things.
PER SERVING
calories: 644 | fat: 51.0g | total carbs: 8.5g | fiber: 1.7g | protein: 37.7g

CHICKEN FAJITAS BAKE

Macros: Fat 74% | Protein 21% | Carbs 5%
Prep time: 10 minutes | Cook time: 15 minutes | Serves 4 to 6

This keto chicken casserole is the perfect low-carb meal for the whole family. It has all of your favorite fajita flavors all in one skillet. It is super simple, with only 7 main ingredients, and can be made in about 20 minutes. This would be a great weeknight family-friendly keto recipe. It's an easy keto recipe for beginners, too!

⅓ cup mayonnaise, keto-friendly
1 yellow onion, chopped
1 red bell pepper, chopped
1 rotisserie chicken breast, shred into bite-sized pieces
2 tablespoons Tex-Mex seasoning

2 tablespoons olive oil
5⅓ ounces (150 g) lettuce
7 ounces (198 g) cream cheese
Salt and freshly ground black pepper, to taste
7 ounces (198 g) shredded Cheddar cheese, divided

1. Preheat the oven to 400°F (205°C).
2. Add all the ingredients except for a third of the cheese to a lightly greased casserole dish. Stir to combine well.
3. Top the mixture with remaining cheese, then arrange the casserole dish in the preheated oven. Bake for 15 minutes or until lightly browned.
4. Remove the casserole dish from the oven and serve warm.

STORAGE: Store in an airtight container in the fridge for up to 4 days.
REHEAT: Microwave, covered, until the desired temperature is reached or reheat in a frying pan or air fryer / instant pot, covered, on medium.
SERVE IT WITH: To make this a complete meal, you can serve this casserole dish with leafy greens dressed in olive oil.
PER SERVING
calories: 526 | fat: 43.1g | total carbs: 7.0g | fiber: 1.5g | protein: 27.7g

PIE KETO CHICKEN CURRY

Macros: Fat 84% | Protein 14% | Carbs 2%
Prep time:25 minutes | Cook time:40 minutes | Serves 4

Pie keto chicken curry is a popular recipe for children and adults, as it has a high nutritional value, this recipe is especially suitable for keto to preserve health and have i mentioned its distinctive taste? It is very suitable for family trips, too.

PIE CRUST:
¾ cup almond flour
4 tablespoons sesame seeds
4 tablespoons coconut flour
1 tablespoon ground psyllium husk powder
1 tablespoon baking powder

1 pinch salt
3 tablespoons olive oil or coconut oil
1 egg
4 tablespoons water

FILLING:
⅔ pound (302 g) cooked chicken
1 cup mayonnaise, keto-friendly
3 eggs
½ green bell pepper, finely chopped
1 teaspoon curry powder
½ teaspoon paprika powder

½ teaspoon onion powder
¼ teaspoon ground black pepper
4 ounces (113 g) cream cheese
5 ounces (142 g) shredded cheese

SPECIAL EQUIPMENT:
A 10-inch (25-cm) springform pan

1. Start by Preheating the oven to 350°F (180°C).

2. Place all the ingredients for the pie crust in a food processor for a couple of minutes until the dough firms into a ball. You can also mix the dough with a fork If you don't have a food processor.
3. Bring a springform pan with a diameter of no more than 10 inches (25 cm) (the spring form pan makes it easier to remove the pie when it is done). Attach a piece of parchment to the pan and grease the sides and bottom of the pan.
4. Spread the dough into the saucepan. Using your fingers or an oiled spatula. Pre-bake the crust for 10 to 15 minutes.
5. Mix together the other filling ingredients, and fill the pie crust. Bake for 35 to 40 minutes or until a good, golden brown has turned on the cookie.

STORAGE: The pie can be kept in the fridge for 2 days and in the freezer for a period not exceeding 3 months.
REHEAT: Microwave, covered, until the desired temperature is reached or reheat in a frying pan or air fryer / instant pot, covered, on medium.
SERVE IT WITH: The pie can be cut in medium size and served with hot sauce and vegetable salad for a great and delicious taste.
PER SERVING
calories: 1130 | fat: 105.0g | total carbs: 8.0g | fiber: 7.0g | protein: 39.0g

ROTISSERIE-STYLE ROAST CHICKEN

Macros: Fat 64% | Protein 35% | Carbs 1%
Prep time:10minutes | Cook time: 5 hours | Serves 8

With minimal preparation and about 5 hours' cooking time,you can get that restaurant-style rotisserie chicken at home as you ever wish. It is super simple to make. No special skills are required. It is delicious and the leftovers are just as good the next day!

1 teaspoon onion powder
1 teaspoon white pepper
1 teaspoon dried thyme
½ teaspoon garlic powder
½ teaspoon cayenne pepper
1 teaspoons paprika

2 teaspoons salt
½ teaspoon black pepper
1 (4-pound / 1.8-kg) whole chickens, giblets removed, rinsed and pat dry
1 onion, quartered

1. Combine the onion powder, white pepper, thyme, garlic powder, cayenne pepper, paprika, salt, and black pepper in a bowl.
2. Rub the whole chicken with the powder mixture on all sides. Arrange the onion quarters into the cavity of the chicken.
3. Wrap the chicken with two layers of plastic and refrigerate for at least 4 hours.
4. Preheat the oven to 250°F (120°C).
5. Arrange the chicken in a baking pan and bake in the preheated oven for 5 hours or until a meat thermometer inserted in the center of the chicken reads at least 180°F (82°C).
6. Remove the chicken from the oven. Allow to cool for 10 minutes and slice to serve.

STORAGE: Store in an airtight container in the fridge for up to 4 days or in the freezer for up to 1 month.
REHEAT: Microwave, covered, until the desired temperature is reached or reheat in a frying pan or air fryer / instant pot, covered, on medium.
SERVE IT WITH: Easy lemon-ginger spinach is a perfect match for this dish, or you can have it with oven-roasted frozen broccoli cooked in the left juices. It will burst the flavors inside your mouth.
PER SERVING
calories: 484 | fat: 34.2g | total carbs: 2.2g | fiber: 0.6g | protein: 42.5g

LEMON HERB CHICKEN BREASTS

Macros: Fat 35% | Protein 63% | Carbs 2%
**Prep time:10 minutes | Cook time: 25 to 30 minutes |
Serves 2**

If you're looking for an easy, simple, and drop-dead-delicious way to cook chicken breasts quickly, you've found it! It's guaranteed to win the hearts of friends and family!

2 skinless, boneless chicken breast halves	1 tablespoon extra virgin olive oil
1 lemon, cut in half	1 pinch dried oregano
Salt and freshly ground black pepper, to taste	2 sprigs fresh parsley, for garnish

1. Squeeze the juice from ½ lemon to a large bowl, then add the chicken breast, salt and pepper. Toss well.
2. Meanwhile, heat the olive oil in a skillet over medium-low heat. Add the seasoned chicken breast, oregano, pepper, and juice from remaining lemon. Sauté for 6 to 10 minutes per side until the chicken is cooked through.
3. Remove from the heat and garnish with fresh parsley.

STORAGE: Fried chicken left in the refrigerator is good only for 3 to 4 days.
REHEAT: To reheat, let it in the room temperature for an hour then place the chicken in an oven-safe dish, pour a cup of chicken broth in the bottom of the dish, and cover everything with foil. Place it in the oven, at 350°F (180°C), for about 25 minutes.
You can also set it on a plate covered and microwave it on medium for 2 to 5 minutes.
PER SERVING
calories: 337 | fat: 13.0g | total carbs: 2.0g | fiber: 0.3g | protein: 53.3g

COLESLAW WITH CRUNCHY CHICKEN THIGHS

Macros: Fat 79% | Protein 19% | Carbs 2%
Prep time: 15 minutes | Cook time: 40 minutes | Serves 8

Who doesn't like coleslaw with crunchy keto chicken thighs? this recipe was really amazing, the marinade was very easy to make. It's one of my favorite keto dishes, it is so flavorful and all the ingredients are natural.

CHICKEN THIGHS:

1 teaspoon salt	2 pounds (907 g) chicken thighs
½ cup sour cream	5 ounces (142 g) pork rinds
2 tablespoons jerk seasoning (cinnamon, paprika, tumeric, ginger, saffron and cumin)	3 ounces (85 g) unsweetened shredded coconut
	3 tablespoons olive oil

COLESLAW:

1 pound (454 g) green cabbage	Salt and freshly ground black pepper, to taste
1 cup mayonnaise, keto-friendly	

SPECIAL EQUIPMENT:
2 big plastic bags

1. Preheat the oven to 350°F (180°C).
2. Mix together a marinade of jerk seasoning, salt and sour cream. And pour in a big plastic bag with the drumsticks, please keep the skin on the drumsticks.
3. Thoroughly shake and allow to marinate for 15 minutes.
4. Take the drumsticks out, and into a new, clean bag.
5. Put the pork rinds into a food processor and blend into fine crumbs, add in coconut flakes and blend a few more seconds.

6. Pour the pork mixture into the bag with the marinated chicken and shake.
7. Grease a baking dish, and put the chicken into it, drizzle with olive oil and bake for 40 to 50 minutes, or until the chicken is cooked through. Turn the drumsticks halfway through, if the breading has already turned a desirable golden brown color, lower the heat.
8. In the meantime, cut the cabbage finely with a sharp knife or with a mandolin or even a food processor. Put the coleslaw into a bowl, season with salt and pepper, and add mayonnaise, mix well and let sit for 10 minutes.

STORAGE: Store in an airtight container in the fridge for up to 5 days. You can freeze the chicken for 1 to 2 months, but can't freeze the coleslaw.
REHEAT: Microwave, covered or reheated in a frying pan until the desired temperature is reached.
SERVE IT WITH: To make this a complete meal, Serve the thighs chicken and the coleslaw with a glass of orange juice, enjoy!
PER SERVING
calories: 586 | fat: 51.2g | total carbs: 6.4g | fiber: 2.4g | protein: 27.2g

BACON-WRAPPED CHICKEN BREASTS STUFFED WITH SPINACH

Macros: Fat 59% | Protein 39% | Carbs 2%
Prep time: 25 minutes | Cook time: 1 hour | Serves 4

Trust me, this easy bacon-wrapped chicken breasts stuffed with spinach will become your family favorite! The flavor of the cheeses will bring you and your families tons of flavor. And the choice of spinach for this recipe will also increase the nutritional value of the meal.

1 (10-ounce / 284-g) package frozen chopped spinach, thawed and drained	½ cup feta cheese, shredded
	2 cloves garlic, chopped
½ cup mayonnaise, keto-friendly	4 skinless, boneless chicken breasts
	4 slices bacon

1. Preheat the oven to 375°F (190°C).
2. Combine the spinach, mayo, feta cheese, and garlic in a bowl, then set aside.
3. Cut the chicken crosswise to butterfly the chicken breasts, (butterfly cutting technique: not to cut the chicken breast through, leave a 1-inch space uncut at the end of the chicken. So when flipping open the halved chicken breast, it resembles a butterfly.)
4. Unfold the chicken breasts like a book. Divide and arrange the spinach mixture over each breast, then wrap each breast with a slice of bacon and secure with a toothpick.
5. Arrange them in a baking dish, and cover a piece of aluminum foil. Place the dish in the preheated oven and bake for 1 hour or until the bacon is crispy and the juice of chicken breasts run clear.
6. Remove the baking dish from the oven and serve warm.

STORAGE: Store in an airtight container in the fridge for up to 4 days or in the freezer for up to 1 month.
REHEAT: Microwave, covered, until the desired temperature is reached or reheat in a frying pan or air fryer / instant pot, covered, on medium.
SERVE IT WITH: To make this a complete meal, serve them on a bed of greens or serve with a cherry tomato and zucchini salad.
PER SERVING
calories: 626 | fat: 41.3g | total carbs: 3.7g | fiber: 1.4g | protein: 61.2g

MICHIGANDER-STYLE TURKEY

Macros: Fat 40% | Protein 59% | Carbs 1%
Prep time: 10 minutes | Cook time: 4 hours | Serves 16

Wondering what to prepare your entire family for dinner? Michigander-style turkey will sort out all your worries. During the last minutes of cooking, remember to remove the foil so that the turkey browns nicely.

1 (12-pound / 5.4-kg) whole turkey	2 tablespoons dried onion, minced
6 tablespoons butter, divided	2 tablespoons dried parsley
3 tablespoons chicken broth	2 tablespoons seasoning salt
4 cups warm water	

1. Start by preheating the oven to 350°F (180°C).
2. Rinse the turkey and pat dry with paper towels.
3. Put the turkey on a roasting pan, then separate the skin over the breast to make pockets.
4. Put 3 tablespoons of butter into each pocket.
5. Mix the broth and water in a medium bowl.
6. Add the minced onion and parsley, then pour over the turkey. Sprinkle some salt on the turkey then cover with aluminum foil.
7. Bake in the preheated oven until the internal temperatures of the turkey reads 180°F (80°C), for about 4 hours.
8. When 45 minutes are remaining, remove the foil so that the turkey browns well.
9. Remove from the oven and serve warm.

STORAGE: Store in an airtight container in the fridge for up to 1 week
REHEAT: Microwave, covered, until the desired temperature is reached or reheat in an air fryer covered, on medium.
SERVE IT WITH: To make this a complete meal, serve the turkey with sautéed garlic kale and lemon.
PER SERVING
calories: 497 | fat: 22.1g | total carbs: 0.6g | fiber: 0g | protein: 73.8g

SAVOURY AND STICKY BAKED CHICKEN WINGS

Macros: Fat 37% | Protein 62% | Carbs 1%
Prep time: 5 minutes | Cook time: 45 minutes | Serves 4

These wings are great. There is a heat to them, but non-spice lovers enjoy them too because of the sweetness. They have a sweet, spicy, smoky flavor that will make you do a happy dance for sure! Made with a keto-friendly homemade marinade you can ensure there's no nasty preservatives or refined sugars in these bad boys!

2 pounds (907 g) chicken wings	1 teaspoon sea salt

SAUCE:

¾ cup coconut aminos	¼ teaspoon onion powder
¼ teaspoon garlic powder	¼ teaspoon ground ginger
¼ teaspoon red pepper flakes	

1. Preheat oven to 450°F (235°C).
2. Arrange the chicken wings in a baking pan, skin side down. Make sure to keep a little distance between wings.
3. Sprinkle salt to season the wings, then bake in the preheated oven for 45 minutes or until crispy and cooked through.
4. Meanwhile, make the sauce: Warm a nonstick skillet over medium heat, then add the coconut aminos, garlic powder, red pepper flakes, onion powder, and ginger powder. Bring them to a simmer.
5. Reduce the heat to low and keep simmering. Stir the mixture constantly to combine well until the sauce is lightly thickened.
6. Arrange the chicken wings on a large serving dish. Pour the sauce over to coat the chicken wings and serve warm.

STORAGE: Store in an airtight container in the fridge for up to 4 days.
REHEAT: Microwave, covered, until the desired temperature is reached or reheat in a frying pan or air fryer / instant pot, covered, on medium.
SERVE IT WITH: Serve them with roasted Brussels sprout and rich cod fish soup.
PER SERVING
calories: 450 | fat: 18.5g | total carbs: 9.4g | fiber: 0.1g | protein: 69.2g

LOW-CARB CHICKEN WITH TRICOLORE ROASTED VEGGIES

Macros: Fat 71% | Protein 21% | Carbs 8%
Prep time: 15 minutes | Cook time: 30 minutes | Serves 8

It really is a beautiful and most colorful dish. So easy-to-make with lots of good flavor, and you can choose to cook it with either a whole chicken or chicken breasts.

TRICOLORE ROASTED VEGGIES:

8 ounces (227 g) mushrooms	1 teaspoon sea salt
1 pound (454 g) Brussels sprouts	½ teaspoon ground black pepper
8 ounces (227 g) cherry tomatoes	½ cup olive oil
1 teaspoon dried rosemary	

FRIED CHICKEN:

4 chicken breasts	pepper, to taste
1 ounce (28 g) butter, for frying	4 ounces (113 g) herb butter, for serving
Salt and freshly ground black	

1. Preheat the oven to 400°F (205°C).
2. Arrange the mushrooms, Brussels sprouts, and cherry tomatoes in a baking pan.
3. Sprinkle with rosemary, salt, and ground black pepper. Pour the olive oil over. Stir to coat the veggies well.
4. Arrange the baking pan in the preheated oven and bake for about 20 minutes or until the Brussels spouts are wilted and the veggies are soft.
5. In the meantime, melt the butter in a nonstick skillet over medium heat, then place the chicken breasts in the pan. Sprinkle with salt and pepper.
6. Fry the chicken in the skillet for 8 to 10 minutes or until there is no pink on the chicken and the juices run clear.
7. Remove the baked veggies from the oven and serve with the fried chicken.

STORAGE: Roasted vegetables can be stored in the refrigerator for 3 to 4 days. Store any leftover chicken in the fridge. This will store for up to three days.
REHEAT: Heat roasted vegetables again in a hot oven to keep them firm and crisp. A microwave will just turn them to mush. Spread the vegetables out on a baking sheet, drizzle them with olive oil, and bake at 450°F (235°C) for 4 or 5 minutes.
SERVE IT WITH: To make this a complete meal, you can serve it with with roasted Brussels sprout and rich sea white fish soup.
PER SERVING
calories: 390 | fat: 30.8g | total carbs: 10.4g | fiber: 3.1g | protein: 20.9g

BUFFALO DRUMSTICKS WITH CHILI AIOLI

Macros: Fat 68% | Protein 30% | Carbs 2%
Prep time:10 minutes | Cook time:40 minutes | Serves 4

For those who love chicken with spices, peppers, and olive oil in an easy and simple way, and for those who work all day and want to enjoy a delicious meal, keto buffalo drumsticks with chili aioli and garlic is the best choice for fun and health. It's take 40 minutes to get ready. Cook it and enjoy the taste.

2 pounds (907 g) chicken drumsticks or chicken wings

CHILI AIOLI:

⅓ cup mayonnaise, keto-friendly	2 tablespoons white wine vinegar
1 tablespoon smoked paprika powder or smoked chili powder	1 teaspoon salt
1 garlic clove, minced	1 teaspoon paprika powder
2 tablespoons olive oil, and more for greasing the baking dish	1 tablespoon tabasco

1. Preheat the oven to 450°F (235°C).
2. Make the chili aioli: Combine the mayonnaise, smoked paprika powder, garlic clove, olive oil white wine vinegar, salt, paprika powder and tabasco for the marinade in a small bowl,
3. Put the drumsticks in a plastic bag, and pour the chili aioli into the plastic bag. Shake the bag thoroughly and let marinate for 10 minutes at room temperature.
4. Coat a baking dish with olive oil. Place the drumsticks in the baking dish and let bake in the preheated oven for 30 to 40 minutes or until they are done and have turned a nice color.
5. Remove the chicken wings from the oven and serve warm.

STORAGE: Store in an airtight container in the fridge for up to 3 days or in the freezer for week up to 1 month.
REHEAT: The chicken drumsticks or chicken wings with chili aioli, Can be heated with a frying pan, a microwave or grill easily.
SERVE IT WITH: serve with mayonnaise sauce, yogurt, and vegetable salad for a great and delicious taste.To make this a complete meal, serve the soup with crisp salad or roasted vegetables.
PER SERVING
calories: 570 | fat: 43.0g | total carbs: 3.0g | fiber: 1.0g | protein: 43.0g

CHUBBY AND JUICY ROASTED CHICKEN

Macros: Fat 64% | Protein 34% | Carbs 2%
Prep time: 15 minutes | Cook time: 45 minutes | Serves 4

Thinking of the perfect dish for your special occasion or a simple dinner with the family, palmy roasted chicken is always a crowd-pleaser. Butter, garlic, and lemon give the chicken a rich flavor, while it's cooked away with healthy, aromatic butter or olive oil. Lemon and garlic are just such a wonderful combination!

1 teaspoon olive oil	Sea salt and freshly ground black pepper, to taste
1 lemon, zested and cut in half	
½ tablespoon ground cinnamon	1 (3-pound / 1.4-kg) whole chicken
½ tablespoon ground ginger	
3 sprigs fresh thyme, chopped	4 whole garlic cloves
2 sprigs fresh rosemary, chopped	¾ cup water
2 cloves garlic, minced	

1. Preheat the oven to 400°F (205°C).
2. In a bowl, mix together the olive oil, lemon zest, cinnamon, ginger, rosemary, thyme, and minced garlic. To taste, add a pinch salt and pepper.
3. Rub ⅔ of the mixture over the meat under the skin of the chicken. Stuff the cavity with half of the lemon along with the 4 garlic cloves. This will render the chicken a delicious flavor.
4. Rub the remaining mixture over the outside of the chicken and season with salt and pepper.
5. Arrange the chicken in a roasting pan and pour ¾ cup of water into the pan, Squeeze the juice from the remaining lemon half and rub evenly over the chicken.
6. Place the chicken in the preheated oven for 45 minutes until completely cooked through and an instant-read thermometer inserted into the thickest part of the thigh, near the bone registers at least 165°F (74°C).
7. Remove from the oven and cover the pan with a doubled sheet of aluminum foil. Let rest for 5 to 10 minutes before serving.

STORAGE: Store in an airtight container in the fridge for up to 4 days or in the freezer for up to 1 month.
REHEAT: Microwave, covered, until the desired temperature is reached or reheat in a frying pan or air fryer / instant pot, covered, on medium.
SERVE IT WITH: To make this a complete meal, it's best served with Mashed Cauliflower with Parmesan and Chives or Roasted Asparagus with Browned Butter.
PER SERVING
calories: 745 | fat: 52.7g | total carbs: 5.3g | fiber: 1.8g | protein: 64.1g

OVEN-BAKED CHICKEN IN GARLIC

Macros: Fat 56% | Protein 43% | Carbs 0%
Prep time: 10 minutes | Cook time: 55 minutes | Serves 4

Looking for a one-pan meal with your family? Or maybe you're just looking for a meal with easy preparation? This oven-baked keto chicken in garlic just needs a big baking dish. It is beautifully flavorful and fragrant. Who knew that a chicken dish would fit into a diet so well?

3 pounds (1.4 kg) chicken	pepper
2 teaspoons sea salt	2 garlic cloves, minced
½ teaspoon ground black	6 ounces (170 g) butter

1. Preheat the oven to 400°F (205°C). Season the chicken with salt and pepper, both inside and out.
2. Place chicken breast up in a baking dish.
3. Combine the garlic and butter in a small saucepan over medium heat. The butter should not turn brown, just melt.
4. Let the butter cool for a couple of minutes.
5. Pour the garlic butter over and inside the chicken. Bake on lower oven rack for 1-1 ½ hours, or until internal temperature reaches 180°F (82°C). Baste with the juices from the bottom of the pan every 20 minutes.
6. Serve with the juices and a side dish of your choice.

STORAGE: Keeping foods separate and well covered helps to combat potential cross-contamination. store it in a plastic container in the fridge for up to 3 to 4 days or in the freezer for up to 3 weeks
REHEAT: Microwave, covered, or reheated in a frying pan or instant pot, covered, on medium until the desired temperature is reached. Don't reheat leftovers more than once. This is because the more times you cool and reheat food, the higher the risk of food poisoning.
SERVE IT WITH: Serve with salad or steamed low-carb vegetables and a glass of fresh juice.
PER SERVING
calories: 686 | fat: 43.7g | total carbs: 0.8g | fiber: 0.1g | protein: 69.7g

KETO CHICKEN WITH HERB BUTTER

Macros: Fat 82% | Protein 17% | Carbs 1%
Prep time: 10 minutes | Cook time: 10 minutes | Serves 8

There is truly nothing better than a quick, delicious keto chicken with herb butter recipe that gets the dinner on the table in no time. Recipes for fast chicken breasts help me get the dinner on the table fast during the hectic weekends.

This 10-minute keto chicken with herb butter is a true gem and will become a family favorite.

HERB BUTTER:

6 ounces (170 g) herb butter, at room temperature	¼ cup fresh parsley, finely chopped
1 garlic clove, minced	1 teaspoon lemon juice
½ teaspoon garlic powder	½ teaspoon salt

FRIED CHICKEN:

3 tablespoons butter	Salt and freshly ground black pepper, to taste
4 chicken breasts	

SERVING:

8 ounces (227 g) leafy greens (such as baby spinach)

1. Start with the herb butter. Mix the garlic, parsley, lemon juice and a pinch of salt thoroughly in a small bowl and let sit until it's time to serve.
2. Cut in half horizontally to make two thin chicken breasts so they cook evenly and quickly. Season the chicken with Italian seasoning, salt, pepper, and crushed red pepper.
3. Melt the butter over medium heat, in a large frying pan. Put in the chicken and fry in butter until the fillets are cooked through, or a meat thermometer inserted and registers 165°F (75°C). To prevent dry chicken fillets, lower the temperature toward the end.
4. Serve the chicken on a leafy greens bed and put a generous amount of herb butter over it.

STORAGE: Keep it in the fridge for up to 4 days or in the freezer for up to 1 month.
REHEAT: Reheat it until piping hot throughout. If you're using a microwave, be aware they do not heat evenly throughout, so take your food out halfway through cooking time and give it a stir.
SERVE IT WITH: To make this a complete meal, you can serve it with a side of pasta, veggies, or cauliflower rice.
PER SERVING
calories: 772 | fat: 70.3g | total carbs: 1.5g | fiber: 0.7g | protein: 34.1g

CHICKEN WITH MUSHROOMS AND PARMESAN

Macros: Fat 63% | Protein 33% | Carbs 4%
Prep time: 10 minutes | Cook time: 30 minutes | Serves 4

Chicken is always a favorite at week-night. This simple chicken with mushroom and Parmesan cheese features a creamy, cheesy mushroom sauce. It is a quick keto meal, ideal for busy evenings because it can be cooked and prepared in less than 30 minutes.

If you think you don't like mushrooms, think again, because this recipe is about to change the way you feel about mushrooms forever! And if you're already a fan of mushrooms like me and are looking for a way to uplift your game of mushroom-lovin dinner, this recipe has your name all over it.

2 tablespoons avocado oil	8 ounces (227 g) cremini mushrooms, sliced
1½ pounds (680 g) boneless chicken thighs	1½ cups heavy whipping cream
Salt and freshly ground black pepper, to taste	2 ounces (57 g) Parmesan cheese, grated
4 garlic cloves, minced	1 teaspoon fresh parsley

1. Heat the avocado oil in a large skillet over medium heat. Season the chicken thighs with salt and pepper. Fry in the skillet until browned or cooked; remove the chicken to a slotted spoon plate, conserve the juices in the pan.
2. Add garlic to the frying pan and stir-fry until soft; add mushrooms and sauté for around 5 to 7 minutes, until softened.
3. Put heavy cream on low heat, and stir well. Stirring frequently for about 10 minutes, allow to simmer, incorporate Parmesan cheese to melt. Add salt and chili pepper to taste.
4. Return the chicken to the skillet and garnish with sauce. Serve with parsley.

STORAGE: Keep a stash of lidded containers so that you have something to store your leftovers in. Use freezer bags if you don't have space to store a lot of containers. Keep it in the fridge for up to 2 to 3 days or in the freezer for up to 3 weeks.
REHEAT: Microwave, covered, or reheated in a frying pan or instant pot, covered, on medium until the desired temperature is reached.
SERVE IT WITH: Serve with a fresh side salad or steamed low-carb vegetables like broccoli, spinach, or asparagus.
PER SERVING
calories: 584 | fat: 41.0g | total carbs: 6.0g | fiber: 0.6g | protein: 48.4g

KETO FRIED CHICKEN WITH BROCCOLI

Marcos: Fat 85% | Protein 12% | Carbs 3%
Prep time: 5 minutes | Cook time: 15 minutes | Serves 3

Not many things could be done in 20 minutes, right? Well, you might want to reconsider that opinion because this luscious dish of broccoli and fried chicken takes only 20 minutes to prepare. I remember the first time I made this dish. It tastes like something that I would order from a Chinese restaurant but even better. It saves me through many days when I was busy, and it's delicious at the same time, so what are you waiting for? Prepare the ingredients and get yourself ready for an enjoyable journey.

9 ounces (255 g) broccoli	Salt and freshly ground black pepper, to taste
3½ ounces (99 g) butter	
10 ounces (284 g) boneless chicken thighs	½ cup keto-friendly mayonnaise

1. Wash and cut the broccoli and the stem into small pieces.
2. Heat up a good amount of butter in a big frying pan where you will be able to fit both the broccoli and the chicken.
3. Season the chicken with salt and pepper, then fry over medium heat for 5 minutes on each side, or until it turns golden brown and cooked through. You can check by using a cooking thermometer in the thickest part, it gets fully cooked when it reaches 180°F (82°C)
4. Add a bit more butter and place the broccoli in the frying pan, and fry for another 2 minutes.
5. Season to taste with salt and pepper, and pour the remained butter on top, then serve.

STORAGE: place the leftovers in an air tight container and put it in the fridge. It lasts up to 3 days in the fridge. It lasts for about 1 month in the freezer in a freezer-safe container.
REHEAT: You could reheat it in the microwave with no problem, or in the oven at 350°F (180°C) for 15 minutes.
SERVE IT WITH: You could serve it with a keto salad of your choice such as the grilled vegetable salad with pesto.
PER SERVING
calories: 653 | fat: 61.7g | total carbs: 6.2g | fiber: 2.3g | protein: 19.5g

CHICKEN WITH COCONUT CURRY

Macros: Fat 71% | Protein 22% | Carbs 7%
Prep time: 20 minutes | Cook time: 30 minutes | Serves 6

This flavorful chicken with keto coconut curry recipe is EASY, with a secret trick! You are only 9 ingredients away from low-carbon coconut curry, and 30 minutes away. The easy chicken curry will be a family-wide dinner winner. Plus, it is gluten-free and keto-friendly.

2 stalks of lemongrass	pepper, to taste
1½ pounds (680 g) boneless chicken thighs	1 leek
2 tablespoons coconut oil	2 garlic cloves
1 tablespoon curry powder	1 small red bell pepper, sliced
1 thumb-sized piece of fresh ginger	½ red chili pepper, finely chopped
Salt and freshly ground black	14 ounces (397 g) coconut cream
	1 lemon, zest

1. Crush the rough part of the lemongrass with the broad side of a knife or a pestle.
2. Cut the chicken into coarse pieces.
3. Gently heat the coconut oil in a wok or a large frying pan.
4. Grate the ginger and fry together with the lemongrass and curry.
5. Add half of the chicken and sauté over medium heat until the strips are golden. Salt and pepper to taste.
6. Set aside and fry the rest of the chicken in the same way, perhaps add a little more curry for the second batch. The lemon grass can remain in the pan.
7. Slice the leek into pieces and sauté them in the same pan together with the other vegetables and the finely chopped garlic. The vegetables should turn golden, but retain their crispiness.
8. Add the coconut cream and chicken and let simmer for 5 to 10 minutes until everything is warm.
9. Remove the lemon grass and sprinkle over the lime zest.

STORAGE: Keep your leftovers well sealed and separate. Keeping foods separate and well covered helps to combat potential cross-contamination. store it in a glass or plastic container or to save room for 4 days in the fridge and for 1 month in the freezer, put it into a freezer bag and lay it flat so that it freezes flat.
REHEAT: Microwave, covered, or reheated in a frying pan or instant pot, covered, on medium until the desired temperature is reached. Don't reheat leftovers more than once. This is because the more times you cool and reheat food, the higher the risk of food poisoning.
SERVE IT WITH: Serve with keto eggplant salad with capsicum and a glass of fresh juice.
PER SERVING
calories: 578 | fat: 46.6g | total carbs: 10.8g | fiber: 2.8g | protein: 32.6g

SIMPLE CHICKEN TONNATO

Macros: Fat 71% | Protein 28% | Carbs 1%
Prep time: 10 minutes | Cook time: 20 minutes | Serves 4

Get your keto on with this amazing and simple chicken tonnato keto dish! Fall in love with fresh basil and rich tuna and enveloping savory chicken. It doesn't get much more keto-taste than this!

TONNATO SAUCE:

4 ounces (113 g) tuna	friendly
2 garlic cloves	¼ cup olive oil
¼ cup fresh basil, chopped	½ teaspoon salt
1 teaspoon dried parsley	¼ teaspoon ground black pepper
2 tablespoons lemon juice	
½ cup mayonnaise, keto-	

CHICKEN:

1½ pounds (680g) chicken breasts	Water, as needed
Salt, to taste	7 ounces (198 g) leafy green

1. Mix all of the sauce ingredients in an immersion blender or in a food processor. Reserve the Tonnato sauce to allow the aromas to grow.
2. In a pot, put the chicken breasts with only enough lightly salted water to cover them. Bring to a boil.
3. Let simmer for around 15 minutes over medium heat, or until the chicken is completely cooked through. When you are using a meat thermometer, when finished, it will say 165℉ (74℃).
4. Enable the breasts of chicken to rest, at least 10 minutes before slicing.
5. Place the leafy greens on the serving plates, and top with the sliced chicken. Pour the sauce over the chicken and serve with a slice of fresh lemon and extra capers.

STORAGE: store it in a glass or plastic container in the fridge for up to 3 to 4 days or in the freezer for up to 1 month.
REHEAT: Grill, skillet, or reheated in frying pan or air fryer / instant pot.
SERVE IT WITH: Serve with beef stock and cauliflower rice.
PER SERVING
calories: 652 | fat: 51.3g | total carbs: 2.8g | fiber: 0.8g | protein: 43.2g

CHICKEN WITH TOMATO CREAM

Macros: Fat 69% | Protein 24% | Carbs 7%
Prep time: 10 minutes | Cook time: 1 hour 30 minutes | Serves 4

This mushrooms and chicken with tomato cream is full of flavor and ready in less than 90 minutes. Elegant enough for a date night, fast enough and easy enough for a week-end dinner. It's sure to be a family favorite! I love this Chicken with Mushroom and Tomato cream! It's just so delicious. It is super-fast and simple

7 ounces (198 g) skinless, boneless chicken breasts	sliced
1 tablespoon olive oil	1 cup heavy whipping cream
Ground black pepper and sea salt, to taste	3 ounces (85 g) Parmesan cheese, finely grated
2 tablespoons salted butter	4 ounces (113 g) fresh tomatoes, diced
3 garlic cloves, minced	Fresh basil, for garnish
6 cremini mushrooms, thinly	

1. Season the chicken breasts generously with salt and pepper on both sides.
2. Heat up the olive oil over medium to high heat in a large skillet. Pan-sear the chicken breasts until each side is golden brown and caramelized, about 4 to 5 minutes. Take off the pan and cover to keep warm.
3. Add the butter, garlic and mushrooms to the same pan, reduce the heat to medium-low, and sauté until the garlic is fragrant and the mushrooms have released their liquid.
4. In the pan add the heavy cream, Parmesan and diced tomatoes. To thicken, mix in and let simmer, about 10 minutes.
5. Add the chicken back to the saucepan and cook until completely cooked. Taste, and if necessary, add more salt and pepper.
6. Plate and top with fresh basil.

STORAGE: store it in a glass or plastic container in the fridge for up to 3 days or in the freezer for up to 2 weeks.
REHEAT: Microwave, grill, covered, or reheated in frying pan or air fryer / instant pot.
SERVE IT WITH: Serve with Loaded Cauliflower Salad.
PER SERVING
calories: 326 | fat: 25.6g | total carbs: 5.8g | fiber: 0.4g | protein: 18.5g

LEMON-ROSEMARY ROASTED CORNISH HENS

Macros: Fat 66% | Protein 30% | Carbs 4%
Prep time: 10 minutes | Cook time: 55 minutes | Serves 4

If you are only ever going to really master a single recipe, let it be this one! It's really simple. If you can cook chicken, you can cook cornish game hen.
This Cornish Game Hen Recipe is perfect for any occasion! The bright flavors of the lemon and rosemary will have everyone on the planet go crazy for having it and still wanting more.

4 Cornish game hen	2 teaspoons paprika
Salt and freshly ground black pepper, to taste	1 lemon, quartered
3 tablespoons olive oil	24 cloves garlic
4 sprigs fresh rosemary, plus 4 more sprigs for garnish	⅓ cup low-sodium chicken broth
	⅓ cup dry white wine

1. Preheat the oven to 450°F (235°C).
2. Make the marinade: In a small bowl, stir together the salt, pepper, 2 tablespoons of olive oil, rosemary, and paprika. Set aside.
3. Clean and dry each hen. Squeeze the lemon juice inside the cavity and on the surface of each hen. Place 1 sprig of rosemary and 1 lemon wedge inside each hen. Evenly rub each hen with the marinade until well coated.
4. Place hens in a large roasting dish (at least an inch apart) and arrange garlic cloves around hens. (A bit of space between each hen leads to even browning and crispy skin.)
5. Place the roasting dish in the preheated oven and roast for about 25 minutes.
6. Reduce the oven temperature to 350°F (180°C).
7. Combine the remaining olive oil, chicken broth, and wine in a mixing bowl. Pour the mixture over hens and continue roasting for 25 minutes, or until hens are a deep golden color and reach at least 165°F (74°C) on a meat thermometer.
8. Remove the hens from the oven to a plate. Pour any remaining juices and garlic cloves to a medium saucepan. Cover the hens with aluminum foil to keep warm.
9. Boil the left juices and garlic cloves in the saucepan for 6 minutes until the liquid thickens to a sauce consistency.
10. Cut each hen half lengthwise into slices and place on serving plates. Pour the sauce and garlic cloves over them. Garnish with rosemary sprigs on top before serving.

STORAGE: Store in an airtight container in the fridge for up to 4 days or in the freezer for up to 1 month.
REHEAT: Microwave, covered, until the desired temperature is reached or reheat in a frying pan or air fryer / instant pot, covered, on medium.
SERVE IT WITH: To make this a complete meal, serve these hens alongside some mushrooms cooked in the hen juices.
PER SERVING
calories: 796 | fat: 58.3g | total carbs: 10.5g | fiber: 2.5g | protein: 59.8g

ROAST CHICKEN WITH BROCCOLI AND GARLIC

Macros: Fat 68% | Protein 23% | Carbs 9%
Prep time: 10 minutes | Cook time: 45 minutes | Serves 4

Roast Chicken with broccoli and garlic -yum! It's a quick, savory, nutritious, cheap keto meal. Works well as a short dinner, or a balanced lunch box. It'll become a favorite go-to. Cooked chicken and broccoli in 45 minutes in a garlic butter sauce, all in one oven!

CHICKEN LEGS:

4 (5-ounce / 140-g) chicken legs	½ teaspoon salt (if not have salt in the Italian seasoning)
1 teaspoon garlic powder	Freshly ground black pepper, to taste
2 tablespoons olive oil	
1 tablespoon Italian seasoning	

GARLIC BUTTER:

4 tablespoons unsalted butter, softened	chopped
2 garlic cloves, pressed	Salt and freshly ground black pepper, to taste
1 tablespoon fresh parsley, finely	

BROCCOLI:

20 ounces (567 g) broccoli	Salt, to taste

1. Preheat oven to 400°F (205°C).
2. Season both sides of chicken legs with salt, garlic powder, black pepper, and Italian seasoning.
3. Heat 1 tablespoon olive oil in a large skillet or cast iron pan over medium-high heat. Cook chicken breasts 4 to 5 minutes per side or until browned and cooked through and reaches 165°F (74°C).
4. Cut the broccoli into florets when the chicken is in the skillet, and slice the stem. In a saucepan, boil in light salted water for 5 minutes. Drain and put the water on the lid to keep it warm.
5. In a bowl, mix all the ingredients for the garlic butter. And serve with chicken legs and broccoli.

STORAGE: store it in a glass or plastic container in the fridge for up to 3 to 4 days or in the freezer for up to 3 weeks.
REHEAT: Microwave, grill, covered, or reheated in frying pan or air fryer / instant pot. Don't reheat leftovers more than once.
SERVE IT WITH: Serve with broccoli and garlic butter on the chicken.
PER SERVING
calories: 494 | fat: 37.6g | total carbs: 12.1g | fiber: 4.1g | protein: 28.0g

GRILLED TANDORI CHICKEN THIGHS

Macros: Fat 68% | Protein 30% | Carbs 2%
Prep time:15 minutes | Cook time: 30 to 45 minutes | Serves 16

The flood of fat in chicken thighs is coming for you. We coat the thighs with great flavor of tandoori and the grilling will keep the thighs juicy. Without the bone, you can enjoy the chicken thighs entirely free.

2 (6-ounce / 170-g) containers plain Greek yogurt	4 teaspoons paprika
2 tablespoons freshly grated ginger	3 cloves garlic, minced
½ teaspoon ground cloves	2 teaspoons ground cinnamon
2 teaspoons kosher salt	2 teaspoons ground cumin
1 teaspoon black pepper	2 teaspoons ground coriander
	16 chicken thighs
	1 tablespoon olive oil

1. Mix together the yogurt, ginger, cloves, salt and pepper in a medium bowl. Add the paprika, garlic, cinnamon, cumin, and coriander. Stir well and set the marinade aside.
2. Rinse and pat dry the chicken thighs. Cut 4 to 5 slits in each thigh, then place in a plastic zip-top bag.
3. Pour the marinade over chicken, seal the bag and shake until it is coated completely. (Don't forget to press air out of it.). Put the bag in the refrigerator to marinate about 8 hours or overnight for the best results.
4. Preheat a grill to medium heat and lightly grease the grill grate with olive oil.
5. Get chicken out of the bag, and discard the marinade. Rub out the excess marinade with towel papers. Spray the chicken thighs with olive oil spray.
6. Grill the thighs about 2 minutes per side until nicely caramelized, then cook approximately 35 to 40 minutes until the internal temperature reaches at least 165°F (74°C) on an instant-read thermometer.

STORAGE: Store in an airtight container in the fridge for up to 4 days or in the freezer for up to 1 month.
REHEAT: Microwave, covered, until the desired temperature is reached or reheat in a frying pan or air fryer / instant pot, covered, on medium.
SERVE IT WITH: To make this a complete meal, it's best served with a whipped cucumber raita with plain Greek yogurt, crushed garlic, and a dash of salt.
PER SERVING
calories: 445 | fat: 33.8g | total carbs: 2.7g | fiber: 0.5g | protein: 32.9g

DELICIOUS FRIED CHICKEN WITH BROCCOLI

Marcos: Fat 72% | Protcin 22% | Carbs 6%
Prep time: 10 minutes | Cook time: 25 minutes | Serves 4

There are too many recipes that could be done with chicken thighs, and for that every time I try a new one. Sometimes they are yummy sometimes not, so let me say this clearly. This fried thigh with broccoli and butter is one of the best recipes that I have discovered. If you are looking for a simple, basic, and flavorful approach to cook chicken. You have discovered it! These chicken thighs with broccoli and butter have become a regular in my household since they are so exquisite.

5 ounces (142 g) separated butter	pepper, to taste
1½ pounds (680 g) chicken thighs, boneless	1 pound (454 g) broccoli
Salt and freshly ground black	½ leek
	1 tablespoon garlic, powder

1. Put half of the butter over medium high heat in a large frying pan to melt it.
2. Add salt and pepper to the chicken for seasoning, and then place it on pan. Keep flipping the chicken for 20 to 25 minutes (depends on the thighs size) until it turns brown on both of the sides, then remove them it from the pan, but keep it warm by covering it with aluminum foil or in the oven on over low heat.
3. While the thighs are in the oven, wash the broccoli including the stem and trim it. Slice it into small pieces. Rinse and wash the leek, but be careful to remove any sandy deposits between the layers. chop the leek into big pieces.
4. In a different skillet, melt the rest of the butter on medium heat, then add in the salt and pepper, and the garlic powder. Put the leek to them, and start stirring slowly until it starts to get softer, then put the broccoli. Cook it for about 5 minutes, until it becomes tender.
5. Serve the vegetables and chicken with an extra amount melted butter on top.

STORAGE: The chicken thighs could be stored in the refrigerator and will last for up to 4 days in the, and for 2 months in the freezer, but make sure you keep it in freezer-safe container.
REHEAT: It heats perfectly in the microwave, but you can also heat it in the oven. Heat your oven in advance to 350°F (180°C). Place the chicken wings on a baking sheet in a single layer. Put the wings in the preheated oven for about 15 to 20 minutes.
SERVE IT WITH: It could be served with keto salads of your choice such as the classic Greek salad.
PER SERVING
calories: 602 | fat: 48.3g | total carbs: 10.3g | fiber: 3.2g | protein: 32.8g

ROTISSERIE CHICKEN AND KETO CHILI-FLAVORED BÉARNAISE SAUCE

Marcos: Fat 69% | Protein 30% | Carbs 1%
Prep time: 10 minutes | Cook time: 15 minutes | Serves 6

To Rotisserie or not to Rotisserie, that is the question! Well, it's definitely one of the most delicious dishes to me. I have tried Rotisserie chicken in many places, but it never tastes as good as the homemade one. I realized that I don't need a cook to make me Rotisserie chicken because the world's best Rotisserie chicken could come out of your own kitchen. What do you need in order to make that happen? All you need is chicken, few spices, an oven, and love.

2 rotisserie chickens	red chili pepper
4 egg yolks	10 ounces (284 g) butter
2 tablespoons white wine vinegar	Salt and freshly ground black pepper, to taste
½ tablespoon onion powder	3 ounces (85 g) leafy vegetables
1 finely chopped and deseeded	

1. Split the chicken into two pieces, and make a fresh leafy salad or basically another side dish of your choice.
2. Crack the eggs and take only egg yolks, then put them into a heat-resistant bowl. Mix the wine vinegar, chili and onion powder in a mug, then put the butter in a saucepan and melt it.
3. Slowly beat the egg yolks and add the butter one drop at a time into the yolk while whisking. Increase the pace as the sauce thickens. Continue to whisk until you are done with all the butter. You'll see that white milk protein has accumulated at the pan's bottom; however, it should be removed.
4. Put the vinegar in, then stir together with salt and pepper to add taste. Make sure to keep the sauce warm.
5. Serve it with green salad and a fried chicken or any other side dish of your choice, personally I prefer the green salad because it adds variation to the taste.

STORAGE: It lasts for up to 4 days in the refrigerator, and for 2 months in the freezer, but make sure you keep it in freezer-safe container.
REHEAT: To heat Rotisserie chicken you'll need to place it in an oven-safe dish, and roast in the oven for 25 minutes at 350°F (180°C).
SERVE IT WITH: You can serve it with any kind of green salad, two of my favorites are caprese zoodles and classic Greek salad.
PER SERVING
calories: 505 | fat: 38.9g | total carbs: 2.1g | fiber: 0.4g | protein: 37.5g

CHICKEN WINGS AND BLUE CHEESE DIP

Macros: Fat 58% | Protein 39% | Carbs 3%
Prep time: 1 hour | Cook time: 25 minutes | Serves 4

Something I learned in my early ages is that you simply cannot enjoy chicken wings without the blue cheese dressing. To me it feels like a rule that should be taught in school, and the equation should be that chicken wings plus blue cheese dip equals happiness. If you have never tried the blue cheese dip with chicken wings then what are you waiting for? Let your tongue enjoy the creaminess of the cheese with the mouth-watering wings.
You could have any other dip of your choice such as the curry sauce or the traditional hot sauce.

⅓ cup mayonnaise, keto-friendly	2 tablespoons olive oil
¼ cup sour cream	¼ tablespoon garlic powder
3 tablespoons lemon juice	1 garlic clove, minced
¼ tablespoon garlic powder	1 teaspoon salt
¼ tablespoon salt	¼ tablespoon ground black pepper
¼ cup heavy whipping cream	2 ounces (57 g) Parmesan cheese, grated
3 ounces (85 g) blue cheese, crumbled	
2 pounds (907 g) chicken wings	

1. Put the mayonnaise, sour cream, lemon juice, garlic powder, salt, and cream in a large bowl, and whisk to combine. Add the blue cheese crumbles in and mix well.
2. Let it chill for about 45 minutes before you serve it. You can use this dressing over salads or as I recommend as a dip for the wings or vegetables.
3. Prepare the chicken wings: place the wings in large bowl. Add the olive oil, garlic powder, minced garlic, salt, and black pepper. Start stirring slowly in order to coat the chicken. Let it marinate in the fridge for 30 minutes.
4. Preheat the oven to 425°F (220°C).
5. Grill or bake in the preheated oven for about 25 minutes, or until brown and tender; the skin should be crispy.
6. Carefully take out the wings and place them in a large bowl, then add the Parmesan cheese. Finally, put the wings in the cheese until they are coated, and Serve warm.

REHEAT: Preheat your oven to 350°F (180°C). Place the chicken wings on a baking sheet in a single layer. Put the wings in the preheated oven for about 15 to 20 minutes.
STORAGE: The chicken wings could last for four days in the refrigerator, and make sure that you wrap the cheese dip in parchment or wax paper and keep it in the refrigerator because otherwise it won't last for more than 2 days.
SERVE IT WITH: You could add your own choice of vegetables to go along with the wings. Or you can serve it with sliced cucumber or celery.
PER SERVING
calories: 658 | fat: 42.8g | total carbs: 6.0g | fiber: 0.3g | protein: 59.6g

LIME CHICKEN GINGER

Macros: Fat 28% | Protein 66% | Carbs 6%
Prep time: 10 minutes | Cook time: 20 minutes | Serves 4

Chicken, a perfect meat to cook for any occasion. It's incredibly versatile and takes on flavors really well! Ginger and lime in the marinade used to produce this recipe create the ideal combination of flavors. The marinade can be made forwards and is easy to toss along with lime juice, lime zest, ginger, garlic, oil, sesame, and coriander. And this lime chicken ginger is one meal that's perfect to make all year around. It is perfect to throw on the barbecue in the summer but is equally as good to grill in a pan and make a fresh salad or fajitas with any time of the year.

1½ pounds (680 g) boneless, skinless chicken breasts
¼ cup coconut aminos
2 tablespoons lime juice
2 teaspoons olive oil
1 teaspoon lime zest

1 teaspoon fresh ginger
Pinch red pepper flakes, to taste
1 teaspoon sesame seeds, toasted
1 tablespoon fresh cilantro, chopped

1. Put the breasts of chicken in a huge, shallow dish. Poke holes in the chicken using a fork. This helps the chicken to drink the marinade.
2. Fill a small bowl with the aminos coconut, lime juice, olive oil, lime zest, ginger and red pepper flakes and blend to combine. Pour the mixture over the chicken and allow to marinate in the fridge for at least 3 hours.
3. Place over medium to high heat on a large grill pan. Once the pan is hot, add the chicken to the grill pan and pour the extra marinade over the top. Cook, turning halfway through until the chicken become golden brown and caramelized outside, and cooked for about 10 to 15 minutes all the way through.
4. Before eating, sprinkle with the red pepper flakes, sesame seeds and coriander.

STORAGE: Keeping foods separate and well covered helps to combat potential cross-contamination. store it in a plastic container in the fridge for up to 3 to 4 days or in the freezer for up to 3 weeks
REHEAT: Microwave, grill, covered, or reheated in frying pan or air fryer / instant pot. Don't reheat leftovers more than once. This is because the more times you cool and reheat food, the higher the risk of food poisoning.
SERVE IT WITH: Serve with salad or steamed low-carb vegetables.
PER SERVING
calories: 232 | fat: 7.2g | total carbs: 3.8g | fiber: 0.2g | protein: 38.5g

CAESAR SALAD

Prep time: 15 minutes | Cook time: 20 minutes | Serves 4
Marcos: Fat 78% | Protein 20% | Carbs 2%

I owe my uncle a lot since he was the one that introduced me to Caesar salad. As a kid I always thought that salads were never meant to be tasty; however, I could recall the first time I tasted Caesar salad and the way I enjoyed it. The rich, and wonderful taste of the anchovy. The crustiness on each bite that makes it so exquisite. Enjoy this easy to make meal.
You could add edible flowers or even croutons, but they are totally optional

¾ pound (340 g) chicken breasts
1 tablespoon olive oil
Salt and freshly ground black pepper, to taste

3 ounces (85 g) bacon
7 ounces (198 g) Romaine lettuce
1 ounce (28 g) of freshly grated Parmesan cheese

DRESSING:
½ cup mayonnaise, keto-friendly
1 tablespoon Dijon mustard
½ lemon, juice and zest
½ ounce (14 g) grated Parmesan cheese, finely grated

2 tablespoons anchovy paste
1 garlic clove, finely chopped or pressed
Salt and freshly ground black pepper, to taste

1. Preheat the oven to 350°F (180°C).
2. Spread the chicken breasts in a greased baking dish.
3. Add salt and pepper to the chicken, then drizzle melted butter or olive oil on top of it.
4. Bake the chicken in the preheated oven for 20 minutes, or until you notice that it's fully cooked through by sticking a knife into the thickest part, and making sure that the juices are colorless and smooth. (You can also check by using a cooking thermometer in the thick part, its fully cooked when it reaches 180°F (82°C)). you could also cook the chicken by using the stovetop.
5. Fry the bacon until it gets crispy. Chop the lettuce and put it as a base on two plates, then place the crispy, crumbles bacon on top of the sliced pieces of chicken.
6. In order to make the dressing, put the ingredients in a bowl and mix them with a whisk or with an immersion blender, then set it aside in the refrigerator.
7. End it with a good dollop of dressing and a fine grating of the cheese.

STORAGE: It lasts for about 3 to 5 days in the refrigerator, but it might lose the crispiness on the second day.
REHEAT: You could heat the cold left-over sliced chicken pieces by frying them in a small amount of butter for a delicious, warm addition.
SERVE IT WITH: If you want to serve it side by side with something, then you can make the salad basically go with any type of meat of your choice.
PER SERVING
calories: 521 | fat: 44.5g | total carbs: 4.4g | fiber: 1.3g | protein: 26.0g

CHICKEN PROVENÇALE

Marcos: Fat 77% | Protein 20% | Carbs 3%
Prep time: 10 minutes | Cook time: 45 minutes | Serves 6 to 8

Do you want to have a quick trip to France in the middle of a busy week? Then you must try this chicken Provençale. I tried it the first time when I travelled to France for a week with my family, and ever since then, this meal has a special place in my heart for its unique flavor that I don't get to taste in everyday meals. The perfect balance between the ingredients in this dish takes it to a whole different level from every day to day meals, so treat yourself with an exquisite meal.

2 pounds (907 g) chicken drumsticks
8 ounces (227 g) tomatoes
2½ ounces (71 g) pitted black olives

¼ cup olive oil
5 sliced garlic cloves
1 tablespoon dried oregano
Salt and freshly ground black pepper, to taste

FOR SERVING:
7 ounces (198 g) lettuce
1 cup mayonnaise, keto-friendly
¼ lemon zest

1 tablespoon paprika powder
Salt and freshly ground black pepper, to taste

1. Start by preheating the oven to 400°F (205°C). Set the chicken's skin side up in an oven-safe baking dish. Add olives, garlic and tomatoes on top of the meat and around it.
2. Drizzle over it a good amount of olive oil, then spatter it with oregano and put salt and pepper to season.
3. Put in the oven and roast. It should take about 45 to 60 minutes, depending on the size of the pieces. You can check internal temperature with a meat thermometer. When the temperature reaches 180°F (82°C), the chicken is cooked through. However, you could check by sticking a knife into the thickest part of the chicken, and making sure that the juices run clear.
4. Serve it with a salad of your choice, mayo, lemon zest, and paprika or a mild chili and a sprinkle of salt and pepper.

STORAGE: It could last for up to 4 days in a refrigerator. Allow it to cool first then wrap very well, and make sure it's away from any raw meat. It stays in the freezer for a good 2 months.
REHEAT: It could be reheated in the oven at 350°F (180°C) for about 20 minutes, and make sure you keep stirring occasionally, or by using the microwave for about 5 minutes at medium-high.
SERVE IT WITH: It could be served with salads such as the classic Greek salad or any type of keto salads of your choice.
PER SERVING
calories: 606 | fat: 51.8g | total carbs: 5.7g | fiber: 2.1g | protein: 29.0g

GRAVY BACON AND TURKEY

Macros: Fat 45% | Protein 53% | Carbs 2%
Prep time: 15 minutes | Cook time: 3 hours | Serves 14

This gravy bacon and turkey is very simple to make given that it is made in the same way conventional turkey gravy is made. One extra step is added when making the turkey, which sets this amazing gravy recipe apart!
To my family, it's one of our favorite dishes. I will show you in detail how to make turkey with bacon gravy here.

12 pounds (5.4 kg) turkey
Sea salt and fresh ground black pepper, to taste
1 pound (454 g) cherry tomatoes
1 cup red onions, diced
2 garlic cloves, minced
1 large celery stalk, diced

4 teaspoons fresh thyme, four small sprigs
8 ounces (227 g) bacon (10 slices, diced)
8 tablespoons butter
2 lemon, the juice
⅛ teaspoon guar gum (optional)

SPECIAL EQUIPMENT:
Kitchen twine

1. Start by preheating the oven to 350°F (180°C).
2. Remove the neck and giblets from the turkey, pat the turkey dry with paper towels and season both inside and outside of the turkey with salt and pepper.
3. Insert cherry tomatoes, onions, celery, garlic and thyme into the turkey cavity. Tie the legs together with kitchen twine, and put the turkey on a large roasting pan, tuck its wings under the body.
4. Cook the bacon in a large skillet over medium heat until crisp, for 7 to 8 minutes. Transfer to paper towels to drain, reserving the drippings in the skillet.
5. Add the ghee or butter to the skillet with the drippings and stir until melted, then pour into a bowl and stir in the lemon juice. Rub mixture all over the turkey.
6. Place into oven for 30 minutes. After every 30 minutes, baste the turkey with the drippings. Roast for about 3 hours or until a thermometer inserted into the thigh registers 165°F (74°C).
7. Remove from oven onto a serving tray to rest for at least 25 minutes before serving.
8. Meanwhile, pour the drippings into a saucepan. Whisk in the guar gum to thicken, after 2 minutes of whisking, add a touch more if you want a thicker gravy. Then add the reserved bacon for one amazing gravy.

STORAGE: Store in an airtight container in the fridge for up to 5 days. You can freeze the chicken for 1 to 2 months.
REHEAT: Microwave, covered or reheated in a frying pan until the desired temperature is reached.
SERVE IT WITH: Serve the dish with Antipasto Salad and a glass of juice!
PER SERVING
calories: 693 | fat: 35.0g | total carbs: 3.7g | fiber: 0.7g | protein: 86.7g

ROASTED CHICKEN THIGHS AND CAULIFLOWER

Marcos: Fat 70% | Protein 25% | Carbs 4%
Prep time: 3 hours 15 minutes | Cook time: 35 minutes |
Serves 6

Since I'm attempting to constrain the number of carbs, I eat around evening time, I got a couple of cauliflower heads and transformed them into the smoothest, the richest purée which was the ideal backup to the succulent, flavorful chicken. What's more, the garlic! Gracious, the garlic. You folks, I could most likely live off broiled garlic. I made them alongside the chicken. At the point when cooked, the garlic turns out to be sweet and subtle, and draining them out of their papery skins is genuinely the best time you can have with your pants on.

CHICKEN THIGHS:
3 pounds (1.4 kg) chicken thighs, 2 thighs per serving, skin on and bone in
4 tablespoons olive oil
4 tablespoons lemon juice
2 tablespoons red wine vinegar
3 tablespoons finely cut fresh

oregano.
2 tablespoons finely cut fresh thyme
2 garlic diced cloves
2 teaspoons salt
1 teaspoon black pepper

CAULIFLOWER PUREE:
1 pound (454 g) cauliflower, cut into florets
3 ounces (85 g) Parmesan cheese, grated

3 tablespoons melted butter, unsalted
½ lemon, zest and juice
1 tablespoon olive oil

CHICKEN THIGHS:
1. Put the olive oil, lemon juice, red wine vinegar, oregano, thyme, diced garlic cloves, salt, and pepper in bowl or a large zip lock bag, then add the thighs and flip it on sides in the mixture to fully coat.
2. Seal or cover, and put in the fridge for 3 hours. Keep turning them every now and then for a better taste.
3. Heat the oven in advance to 400°F (205°C). Place one large baking tray, or two regular ones with parchment paper.
4. Take out the chicken thighs from the mixture, and gently put them skin-side up, on top of the tray(s).
5. Keep them in the oven for about 30 to 35 minutes, or use a cooking thermometer, and make sure that the internal temperature is 165°F (74°C), and that the skin color is golden brown. After that let it rest for 10 minutes before you serve it with the cauliflower mash.

CAULIFLOWER MASH:
1. Boil a pot of slightly salted on high heat, then add on the cauliflower to the pot and boil for 2 to 5 minutes, or until tender but remain firm. Strain all the cauliflower florets in a colander, and get rid of the water.
2. Put the cauliflower in a food processor, along with the cheese, butter, lemon zest and juice, and olive oil. Keep pulsing until they gain a creamy and smooth consistency. You have the choice of using an immersion blender.
3. Salt and pepper to taste. You could put more butter or olive oil if you wish.

STORAGE: The purée could be prepared in advance and kept in the refrigerator for up to 3 days. It lasts for a month in the freezer, but make sure to keep it in a freezer-safe container. The chicken will remain 3 to 4 days in the refrigerator in an airtight container.
REHEAT: In order to warm it up, you can place it on a dry skillet over medium heat until it gets warm enough.
SERVE IT WITH: It can be served with any keto salad of your choice. I recommend the classic Greek salad for a kind of variation.
PER SERVING
calories: 725 | fat: 57.1g | total carbs: 9.1g | fiber: 2.4g | protein: 43.5g

CHICKEN BREAST WRAPPED WITH BACON AND CAULIFLOWER PURÉE

Macros: Fat 73% | Protein 22% | Carbs 5%
Prep time: 10 minutes | Cook time: 30 minutes | Serves 4

Have you ever thought of a meal so fancy yet so easy to make? Well, you've arrived to your destination. This bacon-wrapped chicken breast is one of my favorite meals to make, everything about it is convenient. It pretty much takes no effort to make, and exquisite at the same time. I grew up in a household full of different people with different tastes, yet they almost never refused to eat the mouth-watering bacon-wrapped chicken.

CAULIFLOWER PURÉE:
4 garlic cloves
2 ounces (57 g) butter
¾ pound (340 g) cauliflower

⅓ cup heavy whipping cream
Salt and freshly ground black pepper, to taste

CHICKEN BREAST:
1 pound (454 g) chicken breast
10 ounces (284 g) bacon
2 tablespoons olive oil

Salt and freshly ground black pepper, to taste
1 pound (454 g) fresh spinach

1. Slightly mash the garlic cloves by pressing hard on them with the handle of a knife, then peel the skin off. Fry them with butter over medium heat until they turn golden. Be careful because it can go from golden to burned in a blink of an eye, and you certainly don't want a bitter taste in your food. Turn off the heat and keep the garlic in the pan while you do the rest.
2. Rinse then trim the cauliflower and divide to smaller florets. Start cooking them in lightly salted water until they are tender, then remove the florets with a strainer and keep some of the water.
3. Place the cauliflower in a food processor or in a blender. Add garlic cloves and the pan juices. The pan juices will add tasty flavor!
4. Add the cream and the purée until it turns smooth. If you wanted it thinner you could add a little bit of the reserved water to the purée. Begin with a couple of tablespoons of reserved water and keep adding more if needed, until it becomes as you desired. Season with salt and pepper to taste.
5. Wrap each chicken breast with one or two pieces of bacon. Put them gently in a pan and fry with olive oil until the bacon is crisp and chicken is cooked through. Keep the pan over low temperature or you could cook them in a hot oven (400°F / 205°C) for 15 minutes until an instant read thermometer inserted in the center of the chicken registers at least 165°F (74°C).
6. Take the chicken off the pan and keep it warm. Use the same pan to fry the spinach, then Serve immediately with the purée.

STORAGE: The purée could be prepared ahead and stored in the refrigerator for 3 days. However, It lasts up to a month in the freezer, but be sure to keep it in a freezer-safe container.
REHEAT: In order to reheat it you can place it on a dry skillet over medium heat until it gets warm enough.
SERVE IT WITH: You can serve it with salads such as Keto Broccoli salad, or Parmesan Brussels Sprouts Salad.
PER SERVING
calories: 700 | fat: 57.3g | total carbs: 10.3g | fiber: 4.3g | protein: 38.3g

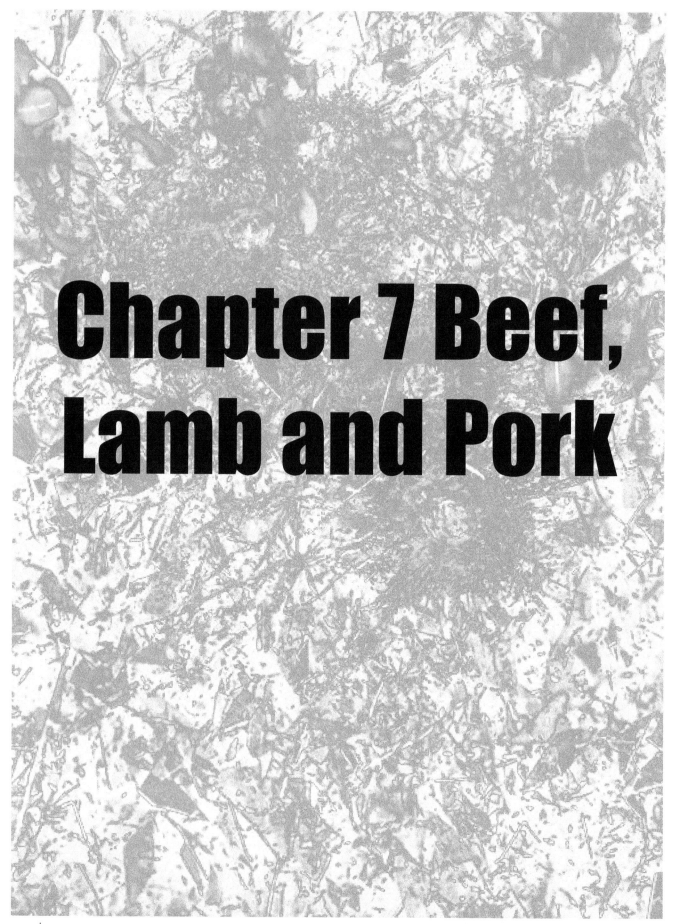

Chapter 7 Beef, Lamb and Pork

ROASTED LAMB RACK

Macros: Fat 69% | Protein 28% | Carbs 3%
Prep time: 20 minutes | Cook time: 20 minutes | Serves 4

Crispy, juicy, and soft roasted lamb rack is that perfect meal to serve on every special occasion. Whether you are on a low-carb diet or you just want to heat healthy, this lamb rack will tempt you to the core through its appealing aroma and irresistible flavors.

2 tablespoons fresh rosemary, chopped
2 tablespoons garlic, minced
¼ cup coconut flour
1 tablespoon Dijon mustard
¼ teaspoon black pepper

4 tablespoons olive oil, divided
1 teaspoon salt
1 (7 bone) rack of lamb, trimmed
Salt and freshly ground black pepper, to taste

1. Preheat the oven to 450°F (235°C).
2. Add the rosemary, garlic, flour, mustard, ¼ teaspoon black pepper, 2 tablespoons of olive oil, and 1 teaspoon of salt in a large bowl. Mix well until well combined and set aside.
3. On a flat work surface, season the lamb rack with salt and black pepper on both sides.
4. In a skillet over high heat, heat the remaining olive oil until shimmering. Sear the lamb rack for 2 minutes per side. Remove from the heat and brush the rosemary mixture over the lamb rack.
5. Wrap the lamb rack with aluminum foil and place in a baking sheet.
6. Roast in the preheated oven for about 15 minutes until the internal temperature reads 145°F (63°C) on a meat thermometer.
7. Remove from the oven and cool for 5 to 7 minutes before serving.

STORAGE: Store in a sealed airtight container in the fridge for up to 5 days or in your freezer for about 1 month.
REHEAT: Microwave, covered, until the desired temperature is reached or reheat in a frying pan or air fryer / instant pot, covered, on medium.
SERVE IT WITH: To add more flavors to this meal, serve the lamb rack with fried cauliflower rice.
PER SERVING
calories: 736 | fat: 56.2g | total carbs: 6.0g | fiber: 0.4g | protein: 51.5g

KALAMATA PARSLEY TAPENADE AND SALTED LAMP CHOPS

Macros: Fat 72% | Protein 25% | Carbs 3%
Prep time: 15 minutes | Cook time: 25 minutes | Serves 4

It is a delicious and easy to cook dish with a rich flavor. It is nutritious with a rich fat content. And the meat of the lamp is one of the best meats on lands. The secret ingredients for making a tapenade will definitely catch your heart.

TAPENADE:
1 cup pitted Kalamata olive
2 teaspoons minced garlic
2 tablespoons extra-virgin olive oil

2 tablespoons chopped fresh parsley
2 teaspoons freshly squeezed lemon juice

LAMB CHOPS:
2 (1-pound / 454-g) racks French-cut lamb chops (8 bones each)

Sea salt and ground black pepper, to taste
1 tablespoon olive oil

MAKE THE TAPENADE:
1. In a food processor, add the olives, garlic, olive oil, parsley, and lemon juice and blend well until it becomes slightly chunky purée.
2. Add the purée in a container. Cover with a plastic wrap and reserve in the refrigerator until ready to use.

MAKE THE LAMB CHOPS:
1. Preheat the oven to 450°F (235°C).
2. Sprinkle the lamb racks with salt and pepper.
3. Heat olive oil in a skillet over medium-high heat. Sear for about 5 minutes until the lamb racks are browned. Flip the lamb racks halfway through the cooking time.
4. Turn the racks and interlace the bones. Roast in the preheated oven for about 20 minutes to get medium-rare results.
5. Allow the lamb to rest for about 10 minutes, then slice into chops.
6. Serve the chops equally to 4 plates, then top with the tapenade before serving.

STORAGE: Store in an airtight container in the refrigerator for up to 4 days or in the freezer for up to 1 month.
REHEAT: Microwave the lamb chops, covered, until the desired temperature is reached or reheat in a frying pan or air fryer / instant pot, covered, on medium.
SERVE IT WITH: To make this a complete meal, serve with keto broccoli salad.
PER SERVING
calories: 347 | fat: 27.0g | total carbs: 2.0g | fiber: 1.0g | protein: 20.0g

BRAISED BEEF BRISKET

Macros: Fat 37% | Protein 62% | Carbs 1%
Prep time:15 minutes | Cook time: 5 hours and 10 minutes | Serves 10

Are you planning to serve delicious and healthy beef brisket at the dinner table? Then this basic brisket recipe is just the right fit for you. The coconut aminos dipped brisket first seared and then roasted for hours in the oven, which gives the meat a crispy texture on the outside and super soft and juicy texture on the inside.

1 (5-pound / 2.3-kg) flat-cut corned beef brisket
2 tablespoons coconut aminos, or more as needed
2 tablespoons olive oil, or more

as needed
6 garlic cloves, sliced
1 onion, sliced
2 tablespoons water

1. Preheat the oven to 275°F (135°C).
2. In a bowl, coat the beef brisket with coconut aminos generously.
3. In a large skillet over medium-high heat, heat the olive oil until it shimmers.
4. Sear this beef brisket for 5 minutes per side. Transfer to a roasting pan and then add the garlic, onion, and water.
5. Tightly cover the pan with aluminum foil. Place in the preheated oven and roast for about 5 hours until tender.
6. Let cool for about 10 minutes before slicing to serve.

STORAGE: Store in a sealed airtight container in the fridge for up to 5 days or in your freezer for about 1 month.
REHEAT: Microwave, covered, until the desired temperature is reached or reheat in a frying pan or instant pot, covered, on medium.
SERVE IT WITH: To add more flavors to this meal, serve the brisket on top of salad greens.
PER SERVING
calories: 645 | fat: 51.73g | total carbs: 1.3g | fiber: 0.1g | protein: 40.4g

BEEF CHUCK ROAST

Macros: Fat 40% | Protein 57% | Carbs 3%
Prep time:5 minutes | Cook time: 8 hours | Serves 6

No healthy meat menu is complete without a delicious beef chuck roast recipe. And here is your chance to expand your special menu and try this simple beef roast recipe. Cooked with onion soup mix for hours, this roast gets a mouth-pleasing and satisfying flavor.

1 (1-ounce / 28-g) package dry onion soup mix
⅓ cup coconut aminos
3 pounds (1.4 kg) beef chuck

roast
2 teaspoons freshly ground black pepper

1. Add the dry onion soup mix and coconut aminos to a slow cooker, then mix well. Add the beef chuck roast and pour in the water until ½ inch of the roast is covered.
2. Sprinkle with ground black pepper, then cover the lid. Cook on low heat for about 8 hours or until the meat is fork-tender.
3. Remove from the heat and cut into slices to serve.

STORAGE: Store in a sealed airtight container in the fridge for up to 5 days or in your freezer for about 1 month.
REHEAT: Microwave, covered, until the desired temperature is reached or reheat in a frying pan or instant pot, covered, on medium.
SERVE IT WITH: To add more flavors to this meal, serve the pork roast with nutty, green beans salad.
PER SERVING
calories: 436 | fat: 19.2g | total carbs: 3.7g | fiber: 0.5g | protein: 60.9g

SAUCY PERNIL PORK

Macros: Fat 42% | Protein 53% | Carbs 5%
Prep time:20 minutes | Cook time: 6 hours | Serves 6

Saucy and tangy pork makes a good serving for all the ketogenic dieters. The pork roast is cooked with peppers, garlic, dried herbs, spices, and vinegar in a slow cooker for hours to get a deep and penetrating taste.

4 garlic cloves
2 tablespoons fresh oregano, chopped
1 large onion, quartered
2 teaspoons salt
1 tablespoon ground cumin
2 teaspoons ground ancho chile pepper

2 teaspoons ground black pepper
1 tablespoon white wine vinegar
1 tablespoon olive oil, or as needed
1 (3-pound / 1.4-kg) boneless pork loin roast
1 lime, cut into wedges

1. Add the garlic, oregano, onion, salt, cumin, chile pepper, black pepper, vinegar and olive to a food processor, then process until all ingredients are fully combined.
2. Rub the mixture all over the pork loin, and transfer to a slow cooker.
3. Cover and cook on low heat for about 6 to 8 hours until cooked through.
4. When ready to serve, slice the pork loin to small chunks. Garnish with lime wedges on top before serving.

STORAGE: Store in a sealed airtight container in the fridge for up to 5 days or in your freezer for about 1 month.
REHEAT: Microwave, covered, until the desired temperature is reached or reheat in a frying pan or instant pot, covered, on medium.
SERVE IT WITH: To add more flavors to this meal, serve the pork roast with grilled zucchini steaks.
PER SERVING
calories: 485 | fat: 22.6g | total carbs: 6.7g | fiber: 1.4g | protein: 61.1g

CREAMY PORK TENDERLOIN

Macros: Fat 50% | Protein 48% | Carbs 2%
Prep time:15 minutes | Cook time:35 minutes | Serves 4

These pork tenderloin strips are cooked in a creamy sauce. If you are in a mood to enjoy a comforting gravy meal, then this recipe is just the right fit for you. The sauce is made of a rich mix of cream, broth, tomatoes, seasonings, and prosciutto.

2 tablespoons olive oil
2 tablespoons fresh sage, chopped
2 tablespoons sun-dried tomatoes, chopped
2 tablespoons fresh parsley, chopped
¼ cup onion, chopped

¼ cup prosciutto, chopped
1½ pounds (680 g) pork tenderloin, cut into ½-inch strips
½ cup heavy cream
½ cup chicken broth
¼ teaspoon salt

1. Take a suitable skillet and place it over medium-high heat. Add the oil to heat then add the sage, tomatoes, parsley, onion, and prosciutto.
2. Sauté the veggies for 5 minutes until soft, then add the pork tenderloin strips to sear for 5 minutes per side.
3. Pour in the heavy cream and broth, then add the salt. Bring the gravy to a boil, then reduce the heat to low. Cook for 20 minutes, stirring occasionally, or until the sauce thickens. Serve warm.

STORAGE: Store in a sealed airtight container in the fridge for up to 3 days or in your freezer for about 1 month.
REHEAT: Microwave, covered, until the desired temperature is reached or reheat in a frying pan or instant pot, covered, on medium.
SERVE IT WITH: To add more flavors to this meal, serve the pork tenderloin with asparagus bacon salad.
PER SERVING
calories: 330 | fat: 18.2g | total carbs: 2.8g | fiber: 0.7g | protein: 39.5g

SIMPLE SPICY BEEF BRISKET

Macros: Fat 72% | Protein 27% | Carbs 1%
Prep time: 5 minutes | Cook time: 35 minutes | Serves 4

Beef brisket is a tasty and easy dish. It has an amazing flavor and one of the best for anyone who loves beef.

1 tablespoon butter
2 minced garlic cloves
1 small sliced onion

Salt and freshly ground black pepper, to taste
2 pounds (907 g) beef brisket

1. In a large nonstick skillet, heat butter over medium heat, then add garlic and onion.
2. Sauté for 3 minutes. Add black pepper, salt, and beef briskets.
3. Put the lid on and cook for 30 minutes over medium-low heat.
4. Transfer the ready brisket to a flat surface and slice into 1-inch (2.5-cm) sizes before serving.

STORAGE: Store in an airtight container in the refrigerator for up to 4 days or in the freezer for up to 1 month.
REHEAT: Microwave, covered, until the desired temperature is reached or reheat in a frying pan or air fryer / instant pot, covered, on medium.
SERVE IT WITH: To make this a complete meal, serve with grilled chicken salad.
PER SERVING
calories: 665 | fat: 53.1g | total carbs: 2.4g | fiber: 0.3g | protein: 41.4g

ITALIAN SAUSAGE SATAY

Macros: Fat 58% | Protein 33% | Carbs 9%
Prep time: 15 minutes | **Cook time:** 25 minutes | **Serves 6**

Sausage lovers will definitely find this recipe interesting, as it is a crispy and saucy vegetable and sausage mix. A colorful mix of bell pepper with seasoned sausage mix makes a delicious every time meal. It can make your low-carb go-to meal.

6 (4-ounce / 113-g) links Italian sausage	1 green bell pepper, sliced
2 tablespoons butter	1 large red bell pepper, sliced
4 garlic cloves, minced	1 teaspoon dried oregano
½ red onion, sliced	1 teaspoon dried basil
1 yellow onion, sliced	¼ cup white wine

1. Take a large skillet and place it over medium heat. Add the sausage to the hot skillet and cook until it is browned. Transfer the sausage to a plate and cut into slices.
2. Add the butter to the same skillet and heat to melt. Toss in the garlic, red onion, and yellow onion.
3. Sauté for about 3 minutes, then add the green bell pepper, red bell pepper, oregano, basil, and white wine. Cook them until the onions are soft.
4. Return the sausage slices to the skillet and reduce the heat to low, then continue cooking covered for about 15 minutes until warmed through.
5. Remove from the heat and serve hot.

STORAGE: Store in a sealed airtight container in the fridge for up to 2 days or in your freezer for about 1 month.
REHEAT: Microwave, covered, until the desired temperature is reached or reheat in a frying pan or instant pot, covered, on medium.
SERVE IT WITH: To add more flavors to this meal, serve the satay with cheesy cauliflower mash on the side.
PER SERVING
calories: 461 | fat: 39.4g | total carbs: 9.0g | fiber: 2.0g | protein: 17.1g

SEASONED BEEF ROAST

Macros: Fat 41% | Protein 57% | Carbs 2%
Prep time: 10 minutes | **Cook time:** 50 minutes | **Serves 4**

It is a perfect dish for a Sunday lunch. It's easy to cook and you can enjoy it with friends or family. You can store it for future use if you wish. The roast beef with broth will bring you a very nice taste.

2 pounds (907 g) beef roast	Salt and freshly ground black pepper, to taste
1 cup onion soup	
1 cup beef broth	

1. Add beef roast in a pressure cooker. Add onion soup, beef broth, black pepper and salt. Cover the lid of the pressure cooker and cook for 50 minutes at high pressure.
2. Naturally release the pressure. Transfer to a serving plate to cool before serving.

STORAGE: Store in an airtight container in the refrigerator for up to 4 days.
REHEAT: Microwave, covered, until the desired temperature is reached or reheat in a frying pan or air fryer / instant pot, covered, on medium.
SERVE IT WITH: To make this a complete meal, serve with creamy cucumber salad.
PER SERVING
calories: 432 | fat: 19.2g | total carbs: 2.7g | fiber: 0.5g | protein: 61.8g

SEASONED PORK CHOPS

Macros: Fat 57% | Protein 42% | Carbs 1%
Prep time: 10 minutes | **Cook time:** 15 minutes | **Serves 8**

Let rejoice the old bay seasoning flavors by cooking some delicious pork chops seasoned with its delicious mix. The pork chops are marinated for an hour in the juicy marinade, which adds up to its taste and texture. When these marinated chops are grilled, they get this strong irresistible smoky flavor.

2 garlic cloves, minced	seasoning
Freshly ground black pepper, to taste	½ cup apple cider vinegar
1 lime, juiced	½ cup olive oil
1 tablespoon fresh basil, chopped	8 boneless pork chops, cut into ½ inch thick
1 tablespoon Old Bay seafood	

1. Add the minced garlic, black pepper, lime juice, basil, seasoning, apple cider vinegar, and olive oil to a Ziploc bag.
2. Place the pork chops in this bag and seal it. Shake it well to coat the pork and place it in the refrigerator for 6 hours. Continue flipping and shaking the bag every 1 hour.
3. Meanwhile, preheat your outdoor grill over medium-high heat.
4. Remove the pork chops from the Ziploc bag and discard its marinade.
5. Grill all the marinated pork chops for 7 minutes per side until their internal temperature reaches 145°F (63°C). Serve warm on a plate.

STORAGE: Store in a sealed airtight container in the fridge for up to 4 days.
REHEAT: Microwave, covered, until the desired temperature is reached or reheat in a frying pan or instant pot, covered, on medium.
SERVE IT WITH: To add more flavors to this meal, serve the pork chops with sautéed green beans.
PER SERVING
calories: 412 | fat: 26.4g | total carbs: 1.0g | fiber: 0.1g | protein: 40.0g

GARLICKY PORK ROAST

Macros: Fat 24% | Protein 74% | Carbs 2%
Prep time: 20 minutes | **Cook time:** 2 hours | **Serves 6**

If you are looking for a healthy and fulfilling meal to serve your family, the pork tenderloin is seasoned with basic garlic and rosemary, which turns out great when the pork is roasted well in the oven.

3 pounds (1.4 kg) pork tenderloin	1 tablespoon olive oil
2 garlic cloves, minced	3 tablespoons dried rosemary

1. Preheat the oven to 375°F (190°C).
2. Mix the garlic, olive oil, and rosemary in a bowl, then rub this mixture all over the pork tenderloin.
3. Place the pork tenderloin in a roasting pan and roast in the preheated oven for about 2 hours, or until the internal temperature reaches 145°F (63°C).
4. Once roasted, remove the tenderloin from the oven. Slice and serve warm.

STORAGE: Store in a sealed airtight container in the fridge for up to 5 days or in your freezer for about 1 month.
REHEAT: Microwave, covered, until the desired temperature is reached or reheat in a frying pan or air fryer / instant pot, covered, on medium.
SERVE IT WITH: To add more flavors to this meal, serve the Pork roast with roasted mushrooms. It also goes well with broccoli cheese salad.
PER SERVING
calories: 274 | fat: 7.4g | total carbs: 1.4g | fiber: 0.7g | protein: 47.7g

CHEESE STUFFED PORK CHOPS

Macros: Fat 68% | Protein 31% | Carbs 1%
Prep time:20 minutes | Cook time: 16 minutes | Serves 4

If crispy and spicy pork chops aren't enough to put into a better mood, then the cheese-stuffed pork chops are here to make your day. These chops are stuffed with a special gouda cheese bacon mixture. The crumbly bacon inside the chops makes a perfect combination.

¼ cup fresh parsley, chopped
4 bacon slices, cooked and crumbled
2 ounces (57 g) smoked Gouda cheese, shredded
⅛ teaspoon ground black pepper

2 (2¼-inch thick) center-cut, bone-in pork chops
1 teaspoon olive oil
¼ teaspoon salt
Freshly ground black pepper, to taste
1 tablespoon olive oil

SPECIAL EQUIPMENT:
Toothpicks, soaked for at least 30 minutes

1. Preheat the grill to medium heat.
2. In a small bowl, add the bacon, parsley, cheese, and black pepper. Mix well and set aside.
3. Place the chops on a cutting board and use a sharp knife to make a pocket into each pork chops up to the bone while holding the knife parallel to the board. Keep the sides of the chops intact.
4. Stuff the bacon cheese mixture into the pork pockets and seal the edges with a toothpick.
5. Rub the stuffed chops with 1 teaspoon of olive oil, black pepper and salt.
6. Lightly grease the grill grates with 1 tablespoon olive oil. Grill them for 8 minutes per side in the preheated grill until nicely browned.
7. Remove from the grill and serve hot.

STORAGE: Store in a sealed airtight container in the fridge for up to 4 days.
REHEAT: Microwave, covered, until the desired temperature is reached or reheat in a frying pan or instant pot, covered, on medium.
SERVE IT WITH: To add more flavors to this meal, serve the pork chops with fresh lettuce broccoli salad.
PER SERVING
calories: 310 | fat: 23.4g | total carbs: 0.8g | fiber: 0.1g | protein: 23.6g

SPICED PORK TENDERLOIN

Macros: Fat 27% | Protein 70% | Carbs 3%
Prep time: 10 minutes | Cook time: 2 hours | Serves 4

There is yet another way to enjoy pork tenderloin with a tangy twist of basic kitchen spices. Rub with a dry spice mix, the pork tenderloin cubes are baked for hours in the oven to give them a delicious crispy taste every time. Serve them warm with your favorite low-carb side meal.

2 teaspoons minced garlic
1 tablespoon fresh cilantro
1 dash ground black pepper
2½ teaspoons ground cumin

1 teaspoon salt
2 tablespoons chili powder
2 pounds (907g) pork tenderloin, cubed

1. In a bowl, add the garlic, cilantro, black pepper, cumin, salt, and chili powder. Mix these spices together.
2. Toss in the pork cubes and coat them well with the spice mixture.
3. Cover the pork cubes and refrigerate them for 45 minutes to marinate.
4. Meanwhile, preheat the oven to 225°F (107°C).
5. Arrange the spiced pork in a baking tray and roast for 2 hours, or until crispy.
6. Remove from the oven and serve on a plate.

STORAGE: Store in an airtight container in the fridge for up to 3 days or in your freezer for about 1 month.
REHEAT: Microwave, covered, until the desired temperature is reached or reheat in a frying pan or air fryer / instant pot, covered, on medium.
SERVE IT WITH: To add more flavors to this meal, serve the tenderloin with curried cauliflower florets.
PER SERVING
calories: 291 | fat: 8.9g | total carbs: 3.1g | fiber: 1.6g | protein: 47.7g

MARINATED STEAK SIRLOIN KABOBS

Macros: Fat 60% | Protein 33% | Carbs 7%
Prep time: 15 minutes | Cook time: 10 minutes | Serves 3

Do you love kabobs? It is a wonderful recipe you can prepare at home. The spices make the flavor to be unique. You won't spend much of your time in the kitchen since it takes 10 minutes to be ready. You can try the recipe and the results will amaze you.

MARINADE:
1½ teaspoons paprika
1 teaspoon ground cumin
1 tablespoon chili powder
½ teaspoon garlic powder

½ teaspoon salt
Juice of 1 lime
2 tablespoons avocado oil

KABOBS:
1 pound (454 g) boneless sirloin steak, sliced into 1-inch cubes
1 red bell pepper
1 green bell pepper

½ red onion, peeled and sliced in 1-inch pieces
Sliced jalapeños, for garnish

SPECIAL EQUIPMENT:
6 bamboo skewers (about 10 inches / 25 cm long), soaked for at least 30 minutes

1. Put the steak in a Ziploc bag, then set aside.
2. Make the marinade: In a small bowl, mix the paprika, cumin, chili, garlic, and salt, then mix well with a fork. Add the lime juice and avocado oil, then mix well. Transfer the mixture into the steak bag and seal tightly. Swing slowly to allow the pieces to coat evenly in the marinade. Transfer the bag into the refrigerator and chill for 45 minutes.
3. Preheat the grill to medium-high heat.
4. Deseed and remove membranes from the red and green bell peppers, then chop into 1-inch chunks.
5. Thread the marinated steak, onions, and peppers alternately onto the skewers.
6. Allow the kabobs to grill for 10 minutes or until browned.
7. Transfer to serving plates and garnish with the jalapeños before serving.

STORAGE: Store in an airtight container in the refrigerator for up to 4 days or in the freezer for up to 1 month.
REHEAT: Microwave, covered, until the desired temperature is reached or reheat in a frying pan or air fryer / instant pot, covered, on medium.
SERVE IT WITH: To make this a complete meal, serve with Baby Bok choy salad.
PER SERVING
calories: 428 | fat: 28.9g | total carbs: 8.4g | fiber: 3.0g | protein: 33.0g

BASIL-RUBBED PORK CHOPS

Macros: Fat 50% | Protein 49% | Carbs 1%
Prep time: 15 minutes | Cook time: 25 minutes | Serves 4

The refreshing basil and lime juice taste in these pork chops make them super tasty and special. Who knew that such a simple mix of ingredients could make a complete and warming meal for the table? But it is now all possible which quick oven-back recipe.

4 (8-ounce / 227-g) pork chops	Salt and freshly ground black
1 lime, juiced	pepper, to taste
¼ cup fresh basil, chopped	1 tablespoon olive oil
4 garlic cloves, minced	

1. Place the pork chops in a baking tray and drizzle lime juice over them to coat. Rub the basil, garlic, salt and black pepper over the chops.
2. Cover the chops and let stand for about 30 minutes.
3. Meanwhile, preheat an outdoor grill on medium heat, and lightly grease its grate with olive oil.
4. Transfer the marinated pork chops to the grill and cook for 10 minutes per side until the internal temperature reaches 145°F (63°C).
5. Let cool for about 5 minutes before serving.

STORAGE: Store in an airtight container in the fridge for up to 5 days or in your freezer for about 1 month.
REHEAT: Microwave, covered, until the desired temperature is reached or reheat in a frying pan or air fryer / instant pot, covered, on medium.
SERVE IT WITH: To add more flavors to this meal, serve the chops with creamy coleslaw on the side. They also taste great paired with sautéed green beans.
PER SERVING
calories: 512 | fat: 28.5g | total carbs: 2.1g | fiber: 0.2g | protein: 58.4g

CREAMY PORK LOIN AND MUSHROOMS

Macros: Fat 53% | Protein 45% | Carbs 3%
Prep time: 10 minutes | Cook time: 20 minutes | Serves 4

This is a healthy dish. It is easy to cook and has a delicious taste. The group of mushrooms and pork is classic and the best. The pork is infused in the mushroom's fragrance; it gives you an amazing eating experience.

2 pounds (907 g) pork loin	2 tablespoons butter
Salt and freshly ground black	1 cup white mushrooms
pepper, to taste	¾ cup sour cream

1. In a bowl, add the pork. Add black pepper and salt to season.
2. In a nonstick skillet, add butter and heat over medium heat. Add the pork and sauté for 3 minutes.
3. Pour mushroom and sour cream over the pork. Put the lid on and cook for 15 minutes until the pork is cooked through.
4. Transfer to serving plates and serve while hot.

STORAGE: Store in an airtight container in the refrigerator for up to 4 days or in the freezer for up to 1 month.
REHEAT: Microwave, covered, until the desired temperature is reached or reheat in a frying pan or air fryer / instant pot, covered, on medium.
SERVE IT WITH: To make this a complete meal, serve with egg mayo salad.
PER SERVING
calories: 573 | fat: 33.6g | total carbs: 3.8g | fiber: 0.2g | protein: 60.6g

CHEESY PORK CHOPS AND BACON

Macros: Fat 59% | Protein 40% | Carbs 1%
Prep time: 50 minutes | Cook time: 30 minutes | Serves 8

This recipe comes from the Swiss flavor. It is an easy recipe, but not a simple one. The combination of pork and bacon will give you a different palate enjoyment of the different texture of the meat in a single bite.

8 bone-in pork chops	2 tablespoons butter
Salt and freshly ground black	12 halved bacon strips
pepper, to taste	1 cup shredded Swiss cheese

1. In a clean bowl, add pork chops and season with black pepper and salt.
2. In a nonstick skillet, add butter and the seasoned pork chops.
3. Cook each side of the pork chops over medium heat for 3 minutes.
4. Add bacon and put the lid on. Cook over medium-low heat for 15 minutes until the bacon is crispy. Add the cheese and heat for 5 minutes until the cheese melts.
5. Transfer to serving plates to cool before serving.

STORAGE: Store in an airtight container in the refrigerator for up to 4 days or in the freezer for up to 1 month.
REHEAT: Microwave, covered, until the desired temperature is reached or reheat in a frying pan or air fryer / instant pot, covered, on medium.
SERVE IT WITH: To make this a complete meal, serve with ratatouille.
PER SERVING
calories: 496 | fat: 32.5g | total carbs: 1.1g | fiber: 0g | protein: 47.1g

LEMONY PORK BAKE

Macros: Fat 69% | Protein 31% | Carbs 0%
Prep time: 10 minutes | Cook time: 35 minutes | Serves 8

The easy to cook delicacy has a superb herb and citrus flavor. Citrus pork is crispy enough and tasty to enjoy and serve company. It also has an amazing outlook when served.

2 tablespoons melted butter, divided	Salt and freshly ground black pepper, to taste
1 tablespoon freshly grated lemon zest	2 pounds (907 g) boneless pork shoulder roast
1 tablespoon lemon juice	

1. Preheat the oven to 375°F (190°F) and grease the baking dish with 1 tablespoon butter lightly.
2. In a bowl, add lemon zest, lemon juice, remaining butter, black pepper and salt and mix to combine well.
3. Rub the pork with the mixture. Transfer the well-coated pork to the baking dish and bake in the oven for 30 minutes until an instant-read thermometer inserted in the center of the pork registers 165°F (74°C).
4. Transfer to serving plates and serve while hot.

STORAGE: Store in an airtight container in the refrigerator for up to 4 days or in the freezer for up to 1 month.
REHEAT: Microwave, covered, until the desired temperature is reached or reheat in a frying pan or air fryer / instant pot, covered, on medium.
SERVE IT WITH: To make this a complete meal, serve with an avocado shrimp salad.
PER SERVING
calories: 464 | fat: 34.1g | total carbs: 0.1g | fiber: 0g | protein: 34.1g

BEEF TENDERLOIN STEAKS WRAPPED

Macros: Fat 78% | Protein 22% | Carbs 0%
Prep time: 10 minutes | Cook time: 15 minutes | Serves 4

It is a zero carb dish that is best for lovers of beef. It is easy to cook and can share with your families and friends. The texture of the coated and seared beef steak will perfect fit your palate.

4 (4-ounce / 113-g) beef tenderloin steaks	8 bacon slices
Sea salt and ground black pepper to taste	1 tablespoon extra-virgin olive oil

1. Preheat the oven to 450°F (235°C) and line the baking sheet with parchment paper.
2. Arrange the steaks on a flat surface. Sprinkle with salt and pepper.
3. Wrap each steak tightly at the edges with 2 bacon slices and use toothpicks to secure.
4. Heat the olive oil in a skillet over medium-high heat.
5. Pan sear each side of the steaks for about 4 minutes and transfer to the baking sheet.
6. Roast the steaks in the preheated oven for 6 minutes until they are well browned on both sides.
7. Transfer the steaks to a flat surface to cool for about 10 minutes.
8. Remove the toothpicks before serving.

STORAGE: Store in an airtight container in the refrigerator for up to 4 days or in the freezer for up to 1 month.
REHEAT: Microwave, covered, until the desired temperature is reached or reheat in a frying pan or air fryer / instant pot, covered, on medium.
SERVE IT WITH: To make this a complete meal, serve with bacon cauliflower salad.
PER SERVING
calories: 564 | fat: 48.0g | total carbs: 0g | fiber: 0g | protein: 27.0g

SLOPPY JOES

Macros: Fat 71% | Protein 19% | Carbs 10%
Prep time: 15 minutes | Cook time: 40 minutes | Serves 8

The amount of ingredients creates a taste explosion in this dish. It is easy to cook and delicious. It is a low-carb dish that can suit you if you love fatty food. And you can also try to use the Sloppy Joes to make a keto burger with eggplant or tomato 'buns'.

¼ cup plus 1½ teaspoons refined avocado oil	1 teaspoon finely ground gray sea salt
1 teaspoon cumin seeds	⅓ cup raw macadamia nut halves
2 small minced cloves garlic	
1 minced piece fresh ginger root	1 tablespoon apple cider vinegar
¼ cup red onions, finely diced	½ cup unsweetened coconut milk
1 pound (454 g) ground beef	
1⅔ cups low-carb tomato sauce	¼ cup chopped fresh cilantro leaves, plus more for garnish
2 crushed whole dried chilis	
¾ cup water	4 endives, leaves separated, plus more for garnish
2 teaspoons curry powder	
½ teaspoon paprika	

1. Make Sloppy Joes: Add ¼ cup oil, cumin seeds, garlic, ginger, and onions in a saucepan. Cook over medium heat for about 3 minutes until the onions are fragrant.
2. Add the beef to cook for about 8 minutes until it loses the pink color. Stir occasionally to break the beef into small clumps.
3. Add the tomato sauce, crushed chilis, water, curry powder, paprika, and salt and stir thoroughly to mix. Cover the lid

partially to allow the steam to escape. Bring to a boil before adjusting the heat to medium-low to simmer for 25 minutes.
4. In a frying pan over medium-low heat, add the remaining oil and macadamia nuts. Roast for about 3 minutes until lightly golden. Toss constantly.
5. After 25 minutes of simmering, add the vinegar and coconut milk to the meat mixture. Adjust to medium-high heat and cook for about 5 minutes until thickened.
6. Add the cilantro and roasted nuts into the meat mixture. Stir well to mix.
7. Divide the endive leaves equally on 8 plates. Top with Sloppy Joes using a spoon.
8. Garnish the meal with extra cilantro and endives before serving.

STORAGE: Store in an airtight container in the refrigerator for up to 4 days or in the freezer for up to 1 month.
REHEAT: Microwave, covered, until the desired temperature is reached or reheat in a frying pan or air fryer / instant pot, covered, on medium.
SERVE IT WITH: To make this a complete meal, serve with a cabbage mushroom salad.
PER SERVING
calories: 340 | fat: 26.8g | total carbs: 8.1g | fiber: 2.7g | protein: 16.5g

SAUSAGE, BEEF AND CHILI RECIPE

Macros: Fat 57% | Protein 34% | Carbs 9%
Prep time: 20 minutes | Cook time: 8 hours | Serves 6

This is an easy, healthy, and hot delicacy. It can serve warm immediately or keep refrigerated for future use. It's very suitable for people who are busy and making this recipe will give you a wonderful memory.

1 pound (454 g) mild bulk sausage	1 (14½-ounce / 411-g) can diced tomatoes with juices
1 pound (454 g) ground beef	1½ teaspoons ground cumin
4 minced cloves garlic	1 tablespoon chili powder
½ chopped medium yellow onion	1 (6-ounce / 170-g) can low-carb tomato paste
1 diced green bell pepper	⅓ cup water

TOPPINGS:

1 cup sour cream	2 tablespoons sliced jalapeños
½ cup sliced green onions	½ cup shredded Cheddar cheese

1. In a pot, add sausage and beef. Cook until browned. Break the clumps with a wooden spoon. Pat dry with paper towels. Reserve half of the meat for drippings.
2. Transfer the meat to a slow cooker. Add the reserved drippings, garlic, onion, bell pepper, tomatoes with juices, cumin, chili powder, tomato paste, and water. Mix well to combine.
3. Put the slow cooker lid on, then cook for about 8 hours until the vegetables become soft.
4. Transfer them to serving plates. Top with sour cream, green onions, sliced jalapeños, and shredded cheese before serving.

STORAGE: Store in an airtight container in the refrigerator for up to 4 days or in the freezer for up to 1 month.
REHEAT: Microwave, covered, until the desired temperature is reached or reheat in a frying pan or air fryer / instant pot, covered, on medium.
SERVE IT WITH: To make this a complete meal, serve with a luscious green salad.
PER SERVING
calories: 388 | fat: 24.7g | total carbs: 10.6g | fiber: 2.9g | protein: 33.4g

BEEF MINI MEATLOAVES

Macros: Fat 65% | Protein 31% | Carbs 4%
Prep time: 10 minutes | Cook time: 30 minutes | Serves 8

This is an easy to cook delicacy. It is tasty and can serve as your lunch or dinner. You can try to use different keto-friendly wrappers to embrace the beef meatloaves, and you can also change the meat wrapped in the wrappers. The form of this recipe can make you warm about a recipe, a meal, or a family dinner.

1 pound (454 g) ground beef	mustard
⅓ cup nutritional yeast	¼ teaspoon ground black
¾ teaspoon ground gray sea salt	pepper
¼ cup low-carb tomato sauce	8 (1-ounce / 28-g) strips bacon
1 tablespoon prepared yellow	

1. Preheat the oven to 350°F (180°C).
2. In a bowl, add the beef, yeast, salt, tomato sauce, mustard, and pepper. Mix well with your hands.
3. Make the mini meatloaves: Scoop out 1 tablespoon portions and roll to form a cylinder. Repeat with the remaining mixture to make 8 cylinders. Wrap each of the cylinders with one strip of bacon. Transfer the wrapped cylinders to a cast-iron pan (loose ends of the bacon facing down) with a spacing of ½ inch (1.25 cm) between cylinders.
4. Bake in the preheated oven for about 30 minutes or until an instant-read thermometer inserted in the center registers 165°F (74°C).
5. Adjust the oven broiler to high. Allow the mini meatloaves to broil for 2 minutes until the bacon is crispy.
6. Transfer to a serving platter to cool before serving.

STORAGE: Store in an airtight container in the refrigerator for up to 4 days or in the freezer for up to 1 month.
REHEAT: Microwave, covered, until the desired temperature is reached or reheat in a frying pan or air fryer / instant pot, covered, on medium.
SERVE IT WITH: To make this a complete meal, serve with a keto caprese chicken salad.
PER SERVING
calories: 295 | fat: 21.2g | total carbs: 3.2g | fiber: 1.0g | protein: 21.9g

KETO BURGERS

Macros: Fat 76% | Protein 17% | Carbs 7%
Prep time: 15 minutes | Cook time: 15 minutes | Serves 6

It is a rich source of fat with low-carb content. You can try this recipe by changing the buns or the ingredients of making patties, maybe you can find the perfect burgers which suits your appetite.

BURGER PATTIES:

1 pound (454 g) ground beef	sea salt and ground black pepper
1½ teaspoons ground mustard	1 heaping tablespoon prepared
¼ teaspoon each ground gray	horseradish

BUNS:

1 (10½-ounce / 297-g edible portion) medium eggplant, chopped into ⅜-inch (1-cm)	thick rounds
	3 tablespoons refined avocado oil

FIXINGS:

1 (6-ounce / 170-g) peeled, mashed, and pitted large Hass avocado,	6 tablespoons keto-friendly mayonnaise
	6 lettuce leaves

1. Preheat the oven to 375°F (190°C) and line a baking sheet with parchment paper.

2. Make the burger patties: In a bowl, add the beef, mustard, salt, pepper, and horseradish. Mix well to combine using your hands.
3. Divide the burger mixture and pound with your hands to form 6 equal patties (½-inch / 1.25-cm thick).
4. Transfer the patties to the baking sheet, with a 1-inch (2.5-cm) spacing between the patties. Cook in the oven for about 15 minutes.
5. Make the buns: Preheat a frying pan over medium-high heat. In a bowl, add the eggplants, then drizzle with avocado oil. Turn them over to coat evenly.
6. Sear the coated eggplant slices in the pan for about 1 minute on each side until slightly golden and transfer to a cooling rack. Repeat the process until all the slices are done.
7. Make the burgers: Transfer one eggplant slice to a plate. Scoop a 1 ounce (28 g) of mashed avocado and top the slice. Top with a patty, a tablespoon of keto-friendly mayonnaise, a lettuce leaf, and a second eggplant slice. Do the same process with the remaining fixings before serving.

STORAGE: Store in an airtight container in the refrigerator for up to 3 days or in the freezer for up to 1 month.
REHEAT: Microwave, covered, until the desired temperature is reached or reheat in a frying pan or air fryer / instant pot, covered, on medium.
SERVE IT WITH: To make this a complete meal, serve with a cabbage and cucumber salad.
PER SERVING
calories: 492 | fat: 41.3g | total carbs: 8.3g | fiber: 4.5g | protein: 21.6g

PORK CHOPS WITH DIJON MUSTARD

Macros: Fat 51% | Protein 48% | Carbs 1%
Prep time: 20 minutes | Cook time: 50 minutes | Serves 4

The delicacy is perfect for an easy weeknight dinner. The tender and crispy nature of the pork chops with mustard will enlighten your palate. It is tasty with an amazing rosemary flavor.

1 tablespoon olive oil	coarsely chopped
4 pork chops	Salt and freshly ground black
2 tablespoons Dijon mustard	pepper, to taste
1 tablespoon fresh rosemary,	2 tablespoons butter

1. Preheat the oven to 350°F (180°C) and lightly grease a baking dish with olive oil.
2. In a bowl, add the pork chops. Add the mustard, rosemary, black pepper and salt. Toss to combine well. Wrap the bowl in plastic and refrigerate to marinate for at least 45 minutes.
3. Discard the marinade and transfer the pork chops to the baking dish and add the butter. Bake for 45 minutes until an instant-read thermometer inserted in the center of the pork registers at least 165°F (74°C).
4. Transfer to serving plates to serve while warm.

STORAGE: Store in an airtight container in the refrigerator for up to 4 days or in the freezer for up to 1 month.
REHEAT: Microwave, covered, until the desired temperature is reached or reheat in a frying pan or air fryer / instant pot, covered, on medium.
SERVE IT WITH: To make this a complete meal, serve with mushroom vegan kale salad.
PER SERVING
calories: 363 | fat: 21.0g | total carbs: 0.5g | fiber: 0.4g | protein: 40.5g

BEEF AND BUTTERED BRUSSELS SPROUTS

Macros: Fat 78% | Protein 18% | Carbs 4%
Prep time: 10 minutes | Cook time: 20 minutes | Serves 2

It is perfect for individuals who love simple meals as it has no complexities. The meal is easy to fix and with a tasty Brussels sprouts flavor.

1½ ounces (43 g) butter
5 ounces (142 g) ground beef
4½ ounces (128 g) Brussels sprouts

Salt and freshly ground black pepper, to taste
¼ cup keto-friendly mayonnaise

1. In a large pan, add 3 tablespoons of butter and melt over medium heat. Add the beef and cook until well browned for about 8 minutes.
2. Reduce the heat and add Brussels sprouts, black pepper, salt and the remaining butter. Cooks for 8 more minutes. Stir periodically.
3. Transfer the beef and Brussels sprouts to serving plates and top with keto-friendly mayonnaise before serving.

STORAGE: Store in an airtight container in the refrigerator for up to 4 days or in the freezer for up to 1 month.
REHEAT: Microwave, covered, until the desired temperature is reached or reheat in a frying pan or air fryer / instant pot, covered, on medium.
SERVE IT WITH: To make this a complete meal, serve with broccoli slaw.
PER SERVING
calories: 513 | fat: 44.8g | total carbs: 5.9g | fiber: 2.4g | protein: 22.3g

GARLICKY BEEF STEAK

Macros: Fat 70% | Protein 29% | Carbs 1%
Prep time: 15 minutes | Cook time: 30 minutes | Serves 6

It is easy to cook and with an amazing creamy taste. The crispy nature just brings joy into eating beef steak. The ingredients of this recipe also give you a large space to try your idea out, you can make this recipe luscious.

2 pounds (907 g) sirloin beef top steaks
4 minced garlic cloves
Salt and freshly ground black

pepper, to taste
½ cup butter
1½ cups cream

1. On a clean board, add the beefsteak and rub with garlic, black pepper and salt.
2. Mix butter and cream in a bowl. Add the beef to the mixture. Wrap the bowl in plastic and refrigerate to marinate for at least 45 minutes.
3. Preheat the grill to medium-high heat.
4. Transfer the steaks to the grill and allow each side to grill for 10 minutes.
5. Transfer to serving plates and serve while hot.

STORAGE: Store in an airtight container in the refrigerator for up to 4 days or in the freezer for up to 1 month.
REHEAT: Microwave, covered, until the desired temperature is reached or reheat in a frying pan or air fryer/instant pot, covered, on medium.
SERVE IT WITH: To make this a complete meal, serve with mushroom avocado tuna salad.
PER SERVING
calories: 485 | fat: 38.2g | total carbs: 1.5g | fiber: 0g | protein: 32.6g

SPICY LAMB MEAT

Macros: Fat 62% | Protein 33% | Carbs 5%
Prep time: 5 minutes | Cook time: 20 minutes | Serves 4

This is a versatile dish with low-carb content. It is keto-approved and easy to cook. It is the perfect dish to stay healthy.

1 tablespoon minced garlic
1 tablespoon minced ginger
2 tablespoons butter
1 cup chopped onions
½ teaspoon turmeric powder
½ teaspoon cayenne pepper

½ teaspoon ground coriander
1½ teaspoon cumin powder
1 teaspoon salt
1 pound (454 g) ground lamb meat

1. In a nonstick skillet, add garlic, ginger, butter, and onions and mix well. Sauté for approximately 3 minutes and add the turmeric powder, cayenne pepper, coriander, cumin powder, salt and lamb meat.
2. Put the lid on and cook on medium-high heat for 20 minutes until the lamb meat is cooked through.
3. Transfer into a serving platter to cool before serving.

STORAGE: Store in an airtight container in the refrigerator for up to 4 days.
REHEAT: Microwave, covered, until the desired temperature is reached or reheat in a frying pan or air fryer / instant pot, covered, on medium.
SERVE IT WITH: To make this a complete meal, serve with cabbage and egg salad.
PER SERVING
calories: 291 | fat: 20.1g | total carbs: 4.4g | fiber: 0.8g | protein: 23.8g

BAKED PORK GYROS

Macros: Fat 61% | Protein 36% | Carbs 3%
Prep time: 6 minutes | Cook time: 25 minutes | Serves 4

Such a delicious and nutritious dish! It has its origin in Greece and is perfect for a quick fix. The best cut of pork to make this dish is the neck or shoulder.

1 pound (454 g) ground pork meat
½ small chopped onion
1 teaspoon ground marjoram
1 teaspoon rosemary

4 garlic cloves
¼ teaspoon black pepper
¾ teaspoons salt
¾ cup water
1 teaspoon dried oregano

1. Preheat your oven to 400℉ (205℃).
2. In a food processor, add the ground pork meat, onions, marjoram, rosemary, garlic, black pepper, salt, water, and oregano and process to combine completely.
3. Tightly press to compact the meat mixture into a loaf pan. Cover with an aluminum foil and poking holes with a toothpick or a fork in the foil.
4. Bake the loaf in the oven for 25 minutes.
5. Transfer to a serving platter and serve while warm.

STORAGE: Store in an airtight container in the refrigerator for up to 4 days.
REHEAT: Microwave, covered, until the desired temperature is reached or reheat in a frying pan or air fryer / instant pot, covered, on medium.
SERVE IT WITH: To make this a complete meal, serve with tamari salmon and avocado salad.
PER SERVING
calories: 347 | fat: 23.6g | total carbs: 2.2g | fiber: 0.4g | protein: 29.5g

COCONUT PORK CHOPS

Macros: Fat: 71% | Protein: 26% | Carbs: 3%
Prep time: 10 minutes | Cook time: 27 minutes | Serves 4

A hit recipe of pork chops for the family and a friend's dinner gathering... These fabulous pork chops are so delicious that everyone would love to enjoy it.

¼ cup coconut oil, divided
1½ pounds (680 g) ¾-inch thick boneless pork chops
1 tablespoon fresh ginger, grated
2 teaspoons garlic, minced

1 cup unsweetened coconut milk
2 tablespoons fresh lime juice
1 teaspoon fresh basil, chopped
½ cup unsweetened coconut, shredded

1. In a large nonstick skillet, melt 2 tablespoons of coconut oil over medium heat and cook the pork chops for about 10 minutes, flipping occasionally, or until browned on both sides.
2. With a spatula, push the pork chops to the side of the skillet. In the center of the wok, add the remaining coconut oil and sauté the ginger and garlic for about 2 minutes. Add the coconut milk, lime juice and basil and stir to combine with the pork chops. Simmer covered for about 12 to 15 minutes.
3. Remove from the heat to serving plates. Serve with the garnishing of shredded coconut.

STORAGE: Store in an airtight container in the fridge for up to 4 days or in the freezer for up to 1 month.
REHEAT: Microwave, covered, until the desired temperature is reached or reheat in a frying pan or air fryer / instant pot, covered, on medium.
SERVE IT WITH: Enjoy these pork chops with fresh green salad.
PER SERVING
calories: 491 | fat: 39.0g | total carbs: 6.1g | fiber: 3.0g | protein: 32.0g

SPANISH BEEF EMPANADAS

Macros: Fat: 78% | Protein: 18% | Carbs: 4%
Prep time: 20 minutes | Cook time: 28 minutes | Serves 6

M ake your dinner table more tempting with this cheesy beef empanadas! These delicious empanadas are prepared with a cheesy dough made and spicy beef filling.

DOUGH:
1 cup Mozzarella cheese, shredded
5 tablespoons cream cheese, softened
¾ cup almond flour
1 tablespoon coconut flour

1 egg, beaten lightly
2 tablespoons unsweetened coconut milk
1 teaspoon garlic powder
½ teaspoon sea salt

FILLING:
¼ cup butter
1 pound (454 g) ground beef
1 onion, chopped
1 tablespoon garlic, minced
2 teaspoons dried oregano,

crushed
2 teaspoons ground cumin
1 teaspoon chili powder
Sea salt and freshly ground black pepper, to taste

1. Make the dough: In a small nonstick saucepan, add the Mozzarella and cream cheese over low heat and cook for about 2 to 3 minutes or until melted, stirring occasionally.
2. Remove from the heat to a heatproof mixing bowl. In the bowl of cheese mixture, add the flours, egg, coconut milk, garlic powder and salt. Mix well until a dough ball forms. Cover the bowl with plastic wrap, and then press it down slightly onto the surface of the dough. Refrigerate the bowl for about 30 minutes.

3. Make the filling: In a large nonstick skillet, melt the butter over medium-high heat and cook the beef for about 7 minutes until browned, breaking up the lumps of meat with a spatula. Add the onion and garlic and cook for about 4 to 5 minutes. Stir in the oregano, cumin, chili powder, salt and black pepper. Mix well and remove from the heat. Set the beef mixture aside to cool completely.
4. Preheat the oven to 425℉ (220ºC) and line a baking sheet with parchment paper.
5. Make the empanadas: Arrange a parchment paper on a flat surface. Place the dough over the parchment paper and with your hands, press into a thin layer. With a 3-inch round cutter, cut the dough into 12 circles. With a spoon, place the filling into the center of 1 dough circle. Fold the dough over and with a fork, then press the edges together to seal the filling. Repeat with remaining empanadas.
6. Arrange the empanadas on the prepared baking sheet in a single layer. Bake for about 10 to 12 minutes or until golden brown.
7. Remove the empanadas from the oven and serve on plates.

STORAGE: The assembled but unbaked empanadas can be covered in plastic and stored in the fridge for up to 2 days.
REHEAT: Microwave, covered, until the desired temperature is reached or reheat in a frying pan or air fryer / instant pot, covered, on medium.
SERVE IT WITH: Serve these empanadas with low-carb dressing.
PER SERVING
calories: 436 | fat: 38.1g | total carbs: 3.9g | fiber: 1.0g | protein: 19.0g

HEARTY CALF'S LIVER PLATTER

Macros: Fat: 75% | Protein: 21% | Carbs: 4%
Prep time: 15 minutes | Cook time: 25 minutes | Serves 4

A wonderful liver and onions recipe makes a dinner. Caramelized onions enhance the flavor of liver in a delish way.

½ cup butter
¼ cup extra-virgin olive oil
2 onions, sliced thinly
½ cup dry white wine
1 pound (454 g) calf's liver, trimmed and cut into strips

1 tablespoon balsamic vinegar
2 tablespoons fresh parsley, chopped
Sea salt and ground black pepper, to taste

1. In a large nonstick skillet, heat the butter and oil over medium heat until the butter melts. Sauté the onions for about 5 minutes. Stir in the white wine and immediately reduce the heat to medium-low. Cook covered for about 15 minutes, stirring occasionally. With a slotted spoon, transfer the onions to a plate.
2. Stir in the liver and vinegar and increase the heat to high. Cook for about 4 minutes more, stirring frequently. Add the cooked onions, parsley, salt and black pepper and stir to combine well.
3. Remove the liver mixture from heat and serve warm.

STORAGE: Store in an airtight container in the fridge for up to 4 days or in the freezer for up to 1 month.
REHEAT: Microwave, covered, until the desired temperature is reached or reheat in a frying pan or air fryer / instant pot, covered, on medium.
SERVE IT WITH: Broccoli mash is a great option to serve with this liver dish.
PER SERVING
calories: 497 | fat: 40.6g | total carbs: 7.9g | fiber: 3.0g | protein: 23.1g

BBQ PARTY PORK KABOBS

Macros: Fat: 58% | Protein: 38% | Carbs: 4%
Prep time: 15 minutes | Cook time: 12 minutes | Serves 4

One of the best recipes of pork kabobs that are so juicy and full of flavor. The versatile herbed marinade adds a terrific taste to pork cubes.

¼ cup olive oil
1 tablespoon garlic, minced
2 teaspoons dried oregano, crushed
1 teaspoon dried parsley, crushed
1 teaspoon dried basil, crushed

Sea salt and ground black pepper, to taste
1 (1-pound / 454-g) pork tenderloin, trimmed and cut into 1½-inch pieces
Olive oil cooking spray

SPECIAL EQUIPMENT:
4 metal skewers

1. In a mixing bowl, place the oil, garlic, dried herbs, salt, and black pepper and mix well. Add the pork pieces and coat with the marinade generously. Cover the bowl with plastic wrap and refrigerate for 2 to 4 hours.
2. Preheat your grill to medium-high heat and spray the grill grate with olive oil spray.
3. Remove the pork pieces from marinade and thread onto 4 metal skewers. Place the pork skewers onto the heated grill and cook for about 12 minutes, flipping occasionally, or until it reach the desired doneness.
4. Remove the skewers from the grill and place onto a platter for about 5 minutes before serving.

STORAGE: Store in an airtight container in the fridge for up to 4 days or in the freezer for up to 1 month.
REHEAT: Remove the skewers from the freezer and immediately grill, covered, over medium-high heat for about 15 minutes, flipping frequently.
SERVE IT WITH: Serve these pork kabobs over the bed of torn lettuce.
PER SERVING
calories: 261 | fat: 16.7g | total carbs: 2.2g | fiber: 1.0g | protein: 25.0g

ITALIAN METBALLS PARMIGIANA

Macros: Fat: 71% | Protein: 26% | Carbs: 3%
Prep time: 15 minutes | Cook time: 30 minutes | Serves 6

If you're looking for an elegant dish of ground pork, try this rich meatballs recipe! These tender meatballs are smothered in tomato sauce and then topped with Mozzarella cheese.

MEATBALLS:
1¼ pounds (567 g) ground pork
½ cup Parmesan cheese, shredded
½ cup almond flour
1 organic egg, beaten lightly
1 tablespoon fresh parsley, chopped

1 teaspoon fresh oregano, chopped
1 teaspoon garlic, minced
Sea salt and ground black pepper, to taste
2 tablespoons olive oil

TOPPING:
1 cup sugar-free tomato sauce
1 cup Mozzarella cheese, shredded

1. Preheat the oven 350℉ (180℃).
2. Make the meatballs: In a mixing bowl, add all ingredients except for oil and with your clean hands, mix until well combined. Make about 1½-inch meatballs from the pork mixture. In a large nonstick skillet, heat the oil over medium-high heat and cook the meatballs for about 15 minutes or until cooked through, flipping occasionally.
3. Remove the meatballs from the heat to a baking dish. Top with the tomato sauce evenly, followed by the Mozzarella cheese. Bake in the preheated oven for about 15 minutes or until the cheese is bubbly and golden.
4. Remove from the oven and serve hot.

STORAGE: Place the browned and then cooled meatballs in a resealable plastic bag. Seal the bag and freeze for about 3 to 4 days.
REHEAT: Microwave, covered, until the desired temperature is reached or reheat in a frying pan or air fryer / instant pot, covered, on medium.
SERVE IT WITH: Fresh veggie salad accompanies these meatballs nicely. **PER SERVING**
calories: 403 | fat: 32.2g | total carbs: 0.9g | fiber: 0g | protein: 26.0g

CHEESY LAMB SLIDERS

Macros: Fat 59% | Protein 34% | Carbs 7%
Prep time: 10 minutes | Cook time: 25 minutes | Serves 4

The dish of lamb sliders provides an interesting way to make your menu healthy and delicious. Cook the sliders with spices and serve with a feta cheese dressing. You can either serve them on top of lettuce leaves.

1 pound (454 g) ground lamb
½ teaspoon sea salt
½ teaspoon ground black pepper
2 garlic cloves, minced

2 teaspoons fresh oregano, leaves only
1 lemon, zested
¼ yellow onion, finely diced
1 tablespoon olive oil

FETA CHEESE DRESSING:
2 ounces (57 g) feta cheese
¼ cup plain Greek yogurt
1 garlic clove, pressed

Salt and ground black pepper, to taste

SERVING:
4 lettuce leaves
1 tomato, sliced

½ red onion, sliced into rings

1. Preheat the grill to medium-high heat.
2. In a medium mixing bowl, and add ground lamb, salt, black pepper, minced garlic, oregano, lemon zest, and diced onion.
3. Thoroughly mix these ingredients together and keep it aside.
4. Make about 6 small sized lamb meat patties out of this mixture and keep them on a plate.
5. Lightly grease the grill grates with olive oil and grill the patties for 4 minutes per side until cooked through.
6. Meanwhile, mix all the feta cheese dressing ingredients in a separate bowl.
7. Spread the lettuce leaves on four serving plates and top with grilled patties.
8. Drizzle the feta cheese dressing over them. Garnish with tomato and onion, then serve.

STORAGE: Store in a sealed airtight container in the fridge for up to 2 days or in your freezer for about 1 month.
REHEAT: Microwave, covered, until the desired temperature is reached or reheat in a frying pan or air fryer / instant pot, covered, on medium.
SERVE IT WITH: To add more flavors to this meal, serve this dish with cream cheese dip.
PER SERVING
calories: 320 | fat: 21.0g | total carbs: 6.6g | fiber: 1.3g | protein: 27.6g

WINE BRAISED LAMB SHANKS

Macros: Fat 65% | Protein 29% | Carbs 5%
Prep time: 10 minutes | Cook time: 2 hours 20 minutes | Serves 4

These wine braised lamb shanks are a simple way to make your ketogenic menu more interesting. The lamb shanks are first seared and then cooked well in a garlicky wine sauce, which gives them a unique flavor and hearty aroma. Use fresh herbs to garnish the shanks, and it will taste even better.

3 tablespoons olive oil
4 lamb shanks
5 garlic cloves, sliced
1 small onion, chopped
Salt and freshly ground black

pepper, to taste
1 cup dry white wine
2 teaspoons fresh rosemary, chopped
Rosemary sprigs, for garnish

1. Heat the olive oil in a large frying pan over medium-high heat.
2. Add lamb shanks to the hot pan, then sear them for 6 minutes per side. Transfer the seared shanks to a plate.
3. Add garlic to the same pan and sauté for 30 seconds over medium-low heat.
4. Toss in onion and cook for about 5 minutes until soft and translucent. Return the seared shanks to the pan.
5. Add salt, black pepper, rosemary, and wine. Mix well and cook covered on low heat for 2 hours, stirring occasionally. Add water if needed.
6. Garnish with rosemary sprigs and serve warm.

STORAGE: Store in a sealed airtight container in the fridge for up to 3 days or in your freezer for about 1 month.
REHEAT: Microwave, covered, until the desired temperature is reached or reheat in a frying pan or air fryer / instant pot, covered, on medium.
SERVE IT WITH: To add more flavors to this meal, serve the lamb shanks with tomato-cucumber salad. It also tastes great paired with cauliflower mash on the side.
PER SERVING
calories: 361 | fat: 23.3g | total carbs: 4.3g | fiber: 0.5g | protein: 23.6g

KETO BEEF BURGER

Macros: Fat 74% | Protein 20% | Carbs 6%
Prep time: 15 minutes | Cook time: 35 minutes | Serves 4

With this keto burger recipe, you can make your own low-carb burger buns. You can keep these buns ready and serve them with a simple beef burger, mayonnaise, sliced tomatoes, and onions to make a complete burger and enjoy fresh.

KETO BUNS:
1¼ cups super fine almond flour
5 tablespoons ground psyllium husk powder
2 teaspoons baking powder
1 teaspoon of sea salt

1¼ cups water, hot
3 egg whites
2 teaspoons white wine vinegar or apple cider vinegar
1 tablespoon sesame seeds

HAMBURGER:
5 ounces (142 g) bacon
1¾ pounds (794 g) ground beef
Salt and black pepper, to taste
1 ounce (28 g) butter or olive oil, for frying

2 ounces (57 g) lettuce, shredded
1 tomato, thinly sliced
1 red onion, thinly sliced
½ cup mayonnaise, keto-friendly

1. Preheat the oven to 350°F (180°C).
2. Make the buns: Mix almond flour, husk powder, baking powder, and salt in a large mixing bowl.
3. Slowly pour in hot water and mix this well with a hand mixer. Add egg whites and vinegar. Mix again until all the ingredients are combined, and it forms a smooth dough.
4. Divide the dough into 4 equal-sized pieces and wet your hands to roll these pieces into a smooth bun.
5. Arrange the buns on the baking sheet lined with parchment paper and sprinkle sesame seeds on top.
6. Cover the buns with plastic wrap and leave them at room temperature until the buns have doubled in size.
7. Bake them for 20 to 25 minutes in the preheated oven until golden brown.
8. Meanwhile, place a suitable skillet over medium heat and add the bacon. Cook for 3 to 4 minutes per side until evenly crispy and browned.
9. Remove from the skillet to a paper towel-lined plate. Crumble the bacon into pieces in a bowl, then mix in the ground beef, salt, and pepper. Make four burger patties out of this beef mixture with your hands.
10. Melt the butter in the skillet over medium heat. Add the burger patties and cook for 8 minutes until slightly charred and golden brown, flipping occasionally.
11. Remove the buns from the oven to a large platter. Slice the baked buns in half and spoon mayonnaise inside the buns.
12. Divide the patties among the buns. Top each patty evenly with the lettuce, tomato, and onion. Serve warm.

STORAGE: Store in a sealed airtight container in the fridge for up to 2 days or freeze the uncooked patties in your freezer for about 1 month.
REHEAT: Microwave, covered, until the desired temperature is reached or reheat in a frying pan or air fryer / instant pot, covered, on medium.
SERVE IT WITH: To add more flavors to this meal, serve the keto burgers with coleslaw on the side. They also taste great paired with spinach cheese dip.
PER SERVING
calories: 1063 | fat: 87.0g | total carbs: 16.0g | fiber: 10.0g | protein: 54.0g

ONE-PAN SAUSAGE & BROCCOLI

Macros: Fat: 79% | Protein: 17% | Carbs: 4%
Prep time: 10 minutes | Cook time: 20 minutes | Serves 4

A recipe that pairs up the sausage and broccoli for an indulgent meal. This delicious dish is easy to make and everyone will eat it up with happiness.

2 tablespoons olive oil
1 pound (454 g) mild Italian sausage, casing removed
4 cups small broccoli florets

1 tablespoon garlic, minced
Freshly ground black pepper, as required

1. In a large nonstick skillet, heat the oil over medium heat. Cook the sausage for about 8 to 10 minutes or until browned completely, stirring frequently. With a slotted spoon, transfer the sausage meat onto a plate and set aside.
2. In the same skillet, add the broccoli and cook for about 6 minutes, stirring frequently. Stir in the garlic and cook for about 3 minutes, stirring frequently. Add the cooked sausage meat and black pepper and cook for about 1 minute.
3. Remove from the heat and serve hot.

STORAGE: Store in an airtight container in the fridge for up to 4 days or in the freezer for up to 1 month.
REHEAT: Microwave, covered, until the desired temperature is reached or reheat in a frying pan or air fryer / instant pot, covered, on medium.
SERVE IT WITH: Serve this dish with cooked cauliflower rice.
PER SERVING
calories: 487 | fat: 43.2g | total carbs: 7.0g | fiber: 2.0g | protein: 18.9g

LEMONY PORK LOIN ROAST

Macros: Fat 38% | Protein 59% | Carbs 3%
Prep time: 5 minutes | Cook time: 30 minutes | Serves 10

This pork loin roast is known for its special marinade, which is made of onion with lemon juice, coconut aminos, garlic, and dried herbs. The roast is then dipped in this marinade for an hour, which enhances its taste and texture. Once cooked, the roast can be served with a range of low-carb veggies.

⅓ cup coconut aminos
½ cup lemon juice
1 red onion, sliced
1½ teaspoons garlic, chopped

1 tablespoon dried rosemary
¼ cup olive oil
1 (5-pound / 2.3-kg) boneless
pork loin roast

1. Preheat the oven to 350°F (180°C).
2. In a medium bowl, add coconut aminos, lemon juice, red onion slices, garlic, rosemary, and olive oil. Mix these ingredients well.
3. Pour this marinade into a Ziploc bag.
4. Place the pork loin roast in this bag and seal. Shake the bag well to coat the pork loin roast.
5. Transfer the roast and its marinade to a roasting pan and bake it for about 2 hours until the internal temperature of the pork reaches 165°F (74°C).
6. Once roasted, remove the pork from the oven and allow to rest for 10 minutes. Slice and serve hot.

STORAGE: Store in a sealed airtight container in the fridge for up to 5 days or in your freezer for about 1 month.
REHEAT: Microwave, covered, until the desired temperature is reached or reheat in a frying pan or air fryer / instant pot, covered, on medium.
SERVE IT WITH: To add more flavors to this meal, serve the pork roast with crispy cauliflower pops. It also tastes great paired with sautéed spinach.
PER SERVING
calories: 346 | fat: 14.7g | total carbs: 2.7g | fiber: 0.1g | protein: 50.9g

PORK CHOPS WITH CARAMELIZED ONION

Macros: Fat 60% | Protein 39% | Carbs 1%
Prep time: 10 minutes | Cook time: 30 minutes | Serves 4

With the crispy and crunchy caramelized onion on the side, these pork chops offer a rich mix of flavors. Crispy bacon with creamy sauce makes a balanced combination of flavor, which nicely complements these pork chops.

4 ounces (113 g) bacon, chopped
1 yellow onion, thinly sliced
¼ teaspoon salt
¼ teaspoon pepper

4 pork chops
½ cup chicken broth
¼ cup heavy whipping cream

1. Heat a large skillet over medium heat until hot.
2. Add bacon to the hot skillet and cook for 3 to 4 minutes on each side until crispy, then transfer to a bowl. Leave the bacon grease in the skillet.
3. Toss in onion, along with salt and black pepper, then sauté for 2 minutes until golden brown.
4. Transfer the sautéed onion to the bacon bowl and keep it aside.
5. Increase the heat to medium-high and add pork chops.
6. Sprinkle the salt and black pepper to season the chops. Cook for 5 minutes then flips them. Cook for 6 minutes more until the internal temperature reaches 145°F (63°C).

7. Remove the chops from the pan and place them on a plate. Cover them with aluminum sheet and keep them aside.
8. Pour broth into the same skillet and scrape off the brown bits. Stir in cream and cook for 3 minutes until mixture is thickened.
9. Return the bacon and onions to the skillet and mix well.
10. Pour this mixture over the cooked pork chops and serve warm.

STORAGE: Store in a sealed airtight container in the fridge for up to 2 days or in your freezer for about 1 month.
REHEAT: Microwave, covered, until the desired temperature is reached or reheat in a frying pan or instant pot, covered, on medium.
SERVE IT WITH: To add more flavors to this meal, serve the pork chops with cucumber dill cream salad. They also taste great paired with roasted cauliflower florets.
PER SERVING
calories: 485 | fat: 32.4g | total carbs: 1.5g | fiber: 0.2g | protein: 44.2g

PORK CHOPS STUFFED WITH CHEESE-BACON MIX

Macros: Fat 56% | Protein 43% | Carbs 1%
Prep time: 15 minutes | Cook time: 20 minutes | Serves 2

Now you can enjoy the pork loin chops with a rich and cheesy filling inside. The blue cheese is mixed with crispy bacon, chives, and basic seasonings, then filled in the pork chops pockets. You can add other varieties of cheese.

1 teaspoon olive oil
2 bacon slices, cooked and crumbled
2 tablespoons chopped fresh chives
4 ounces (113 g) crumbled blue cheese

2 boneless pork loin chops, butterflied
Salt and freshly ground black pepper, to taste
Freshly chopped parsley, for garnish

SPECIAL EQUIPMENT:
Toothpicks, soaked for at least 30 minutes

1. Preheat the oven to 325°F (160°C). Lightly grease a shallow baking dish with olive oil and set aside.
2. In each pork loin chop, cut a slit about 2 inches deep and 3 inches long to form a pocket.
3. In a small bowl, add bacon, chives, and blue cheese. Stir well. Make two equal sized balls out of this mixture with your hands. Stuff each ball into the pork chop pockets.
4. Secure the edges of the chops with a toothpick and rub them with garlic salt and black pepper on the outside.
5. Arrange the stuffed chops in the greased baking dish and bake for 20 minutes in the preheated oven, or until a meat thermometer inserted into the thickest part of pork loin chops reaches 145°F (63°C).
6. Garnish with chopped parsley and serve warm.

STORAGE: Store in a sealed airtight container in the fridge for up to 2 days or in your freezer for about 1 month.
REHEAT: Microwave, covered, until the desired temperature is reached or reheat in a frying pan or air fryer / instant pot, covered, on medium.
SERVE IT WITH: To add more flavors to this meal, serve the pork chops with roasted cauliflower. It also tastes great paired with a tomato-cucumber salad.
PER SERVING
calories: 562 | fat: 35.1g | total carbs: 1.7g | fiber: 0.1g | protein: 57.0g

MINT OIL BRAISED LAMB CHOPS

Macros: Fat 63% | Protein 25% | Carbs 12%
Prep time: 20 minutes | Cook time: 10 minutes | Serves 4

The classic minty flavor is here to make your day. These lamb chops offer you a rich combination of healthy ingredients. The chops are cooked with basic seasoning and herbs, then it is served with special mint oil, which gives it a refreshing mint aroma and unique taste.

8 lamb chops
2 tablespoons olive oil, divided
Salt and freshly ground black

pepper, to taste
2 teaspoons fresh rosemary, chopped

MINT OIL:
¼ cup mint leaves
2 tablespoons extra-virgin olive oil

1 teaspoon lemon zest
1 tablespoon lemon juice

1. Place the lamb chops in a shallow tray and rub them evenly with 1 tablespoon olive oil, black pepper, salt, and rosemary.
2. Cover the seasoned lamb chops with a plastic sheet and refrigerate them for 20 minutes to 2 hours to marinate.
3. Heat 1 tablespoon of olive oil over medium heat.
4. Place the rosemary lamb chops in the skillet and sear them for 3 minutes per side until the internal temperature reaches 145°F (63°C).
5. Pulse mint leaves with olive oil, lemon zest, and lemon juice in a food processor until smooth.
6. Drizzle the mint mixture over the seared chops on a plate and serve warm.

STORAGE: Store in a sealed airtight container in the fridge for up to 3 days or in your freezer for about 1 month.
REHEAT: Microwave, covered, until the desired temperature is reached or reheat in a frying pan or air fryer / instant pot, covered, on medium.
SERVE IT WITH: To add more flavors to this meal, serve the lamb chops with cauliflower mash. It also tastes great paired with guacamole on the side.
PER SERVING
calories:278 | fat: 19.3g | total carbs: 14.0g | fiber: 5.1g | protein: 17.1g

THAI PORK MEAL

Macros: Fat 55% | Protein 43% | Carbs 2%
Prep time: 15 minutes | Cook time: 30 minutes | Serves 4

It's time to serve delicious Thai meal at the table. The thinly sliced pork is first seared in butter for a crispy texture and then cooked in a mixture of wine and stock. It is seasoned with basic seasonings and makes a good serving for people looking for some protein-rich meal.

1 pound (454 g) thinly sliced pork loin
Salt and freshly ground black pepper, to taste
1 tablespoon extra-virgin olive oil

1 tablespoon unsalted butter
1 cup chicken stock
1 cup dry white wine
3 tablespoons fresh cilantro, chopped

1. Place the sliced pork in a bowl and mix it with salt and black pepper. Set aside.
2. In a large skillet over medium heat, add olive oil and butter to melt.
3. Add the pork slices to the skillet and cook until browned on both sides.

4. Pour in chicken stock and cook until it thickens, stirring frequently.
5. Add dry white wine and cook on low heat until the liquid is reduced to half.
6. Once cooked, remove the hot skillet from the heat.
7. Garnish with cilantro and serve warm.

STORAGE: Store in a sealed airtight container in the fridge for up to 3 days or in your freezer for about 1 month.
REHEAT: Microwave, covered, until the desired temperature is reached or reheat in a frying pan or air fryer / instant pot, covered, on medium.
SERVE IT WITH: To add more flavors to this meal, serve the pork loin with zucchini fries. It also tastes great paired with Brussels sprout salad.
PER SERVING
calories: 336 | fat: 18.0g | total carbs: 1.5g | fiber: 0g | protein: 29.6g

CLASSIC SAUSAGE & BEEF MEATLOAF

Macros: Fat: 66% | Protein: 32% | Carbs: 2%
Prep time: 15 minutes | Cook time: 1 hour 15 minutes | Serves 6

A great-tasting baked feast of meatloaf for family and friend's dinner party! This meatloaf is flavored with the combo of ground beef, sausage meat, whipping cream, egg, veggies and herbs.

1½ pounds (680 g) Italian sausage, casing removed
1 pound (454 g) ground beef
½ cup almond flour
1 egg, beaten lightly
¼ cup heavy whipping cream
½ red bell pepper, seeded and chopped

½ of onion, chopped finely
2 teaspoons garlic, minced
1 teaspoon dried oregano, crushed
¼ teaspoon sea salt
⅛ teaspoon freshly ground black pepper

1. Preheat the oven to 400℉ (205ºC).
2. Make the meatloaf: In a large bowl, place all ingredients and mix thoroughly until well combined.
3. Place the beef mixture into a loaf pan evenly and press lightly to smooth the top with your hands. Bake for about 1 hour to 1 hour 15 minutes, or until the internal temperature reaches 165℉ (74ºC) on a meat thermometer.
4. Remove from the oven and drain off any grease. Let it cool for about 10 minutes before slicing to serve.

STORAGE: Store in an airtight container in the fridge for up to 4 days or in the freezer for about 1 month.
REHEAT: Microwave, covered, until the desired temperature is reached or reheat in a frying pan or air fryer / instant pot, covered, on medium.
SERVE IT WITH: This meatloaf goes well with mashed broccoli.
PER SERVING
calories: 479 | fat: 35.0g | total carbs: 4.0g | fiber: 1.5g | protein: 38.7g

ROASTED VIETNAMESE LAMB CHOPS

Macros: Fat 57% | Protein 39% | Carbs 4%
Prep time: 10 minutes | Cook time: 25 minutes | Serves 3

If you haven't yet tried the Vietnamese lamb chops, then here is your chance to try them at home. All you need to make this delicious meal is a mixture of some spices and citrus juices to season the lamb loin chops. Then enjoy them with a hearty salad on the side.

5 (3-ounce / 85-g) lamb loin chops (1-inch thick)
1 teaspoon garlic powder, or to taste
2 garlic cloves, sliced
½ teaspoon liquid stevia
1 pinch chili powder
Freshly ground black pepper, to taste
1 tablespoon coconut aminos
2 tablespoons olive oil
1 tablespoon fresh lime juice
¼ cup fresh cilantro, chopped
2 lime wedges
2 lemon wedges

1. Set the lamb chops in a roasting pan and combine with garlic powder, garlic, stevia, chili powder, black pepper, salt, and pepper.
2. Evenly sprinkle coconut aminos, olive oil, and 1 tablespoon of lime juice over the chops. Cover them with a plastic sheet and refrigerate overnight to marinate.
3. Preheat the oven to 400°F (205°C) and leave the lamb chops at room temperature for 10 minutes.
4. Uncover these chops and roast them for 25 minutes in the preheated oven.
5. Serve with cilantro, lemon and lime juice on top.

STORAGE: Store in a sealed airtight container in the fridge for up to 3 days or in your freezer for about 1 month.
REHEAT: Microwave, covered, until the desired temperature is reached or reheat in a frying pan or air fryer / instant pot, covered, on medium.
SERVE IT WITH: To add more flavors to this meal, serve the lamb chops with salad greens. It also tastes great paired with sautéed asparagus sticks.
PER SERVING
calories: 299 | fat: 18.9g | total carbs: 3.7g | fiber: 0.4g | protein: 28.8g

HERBED LAMB LEG

Macros: Fat 67% | Protein 33% | Carbs 0%
Prep time: 5 minutes | Cook time: 2 hours | Serves 10

Have you tried a lamb leg roasted busting with a peculiar garlicky aroma and soothing herb's flavors? Well, this recipe will offer you all of this. By using these basic ingredients, you can add a perfect balance of flavors to your lamb leg while roasting.

1 (5-pound / 2.3-kg) leg of lamb
3 garlic cloves, cut into slivers
1 teaspoon dried rosemary, crushed
1½ teaspoons salt
3 teaspoons dried dill weed
½ teaspoon ground black pepper

1. Preheat the oven to 325°F (160°C).
2. Using a sharp knife to make a few holes in the lamb leg and stuff them with garlic slivers.
3. Thoroughly mix rosemary, salt, black pepper and dill in a small bowl and rub the mixture over the lamb.
4. Place the prepared and seasoned lamb in a roasting pan.
5. Roast the lamb uncovered for about 2 hours in the preheated oven. Then cover it with aluminum foil. Leave the loosely wrapped lamb for 20 minutes at room temperature.
6. Let cool for 8 minutes before slicing to serve.

STORAGE: Store in a sealed airtight container in the fridge for up to 5 days or in your freezer for about 1 month.
REHEAT: Microwave, covered, until the desired temperature is reached or reheat in a frying pan or air fryer / instant pot, covered, on medium.
SERVE IT WITH: To add more flavors to this meal, serve the lamb leg with cauliflower rice. It also tastes great paired with roasted broccoli florets.
PER SERVING
calories: 524 | fat: 38.8g | total carbs: 0.6g | fiber: 0.1g | protein: 40.8g

TANGY LAMB PATTIES

Macros: Fat 60% | Protein 36% | Carbs 4%
Prep time: 10 minutes | Cook time: 15 minutes | Serves 4

This effortless lamb patties recipe can give you a hearty meal. You can cook these patties for dinner, or stuff them in low-carb buns or bread to make burgers or sandwiches, respectively.

3 green onions, minced
1 pound (454 g) ground lamb
1 teaspoon ground cumin
4 garlic cloves, minced
1 tablespoon curry powder
Salt and freshly ground black pepper, to taste
¼ teaspoon dried red pepper flakes
1 tablespoon olive oil

1. Preheat the grill to high heat.
2. Add green onion, lamb, cumin, garlic, curry powder, black pepper, red pepper flakes, and salt into a bowl, and mix them well.
3. Make 4 equal sized patties out of this mixture with your hands.
4. Lightly grease the grill grates with olive oil and grill the patties for 5 minutes per side until golden brown and slightly charred.
5. Let cool for 5 minutes before serving.

STORAGE: Store in a sealed airtight container in the fridge for up to 2 days or freeze the uncooked patties in your freezer for about 3 months.
REHEAT: Microwave, covered, until the desired temperature is reached or reheat in a frying pan or air fryer / instant pot, covered, on medium.
SERVE IT WITH: To add more flavors to this meal, serve the patties with tomato and avocado salad.
PER SERVING
calories: 264 | fat: 17.8g | total carbs: 3.0g | fiber: 1.3g | protein: 23.8g

OVEN-BAKED LAMB LEG

Macros: Fat 67% | Protein 33% | Carbs 0%
Prep time: 15 minutes | Cook time: 2 hours | Serves 10

The time to serve the lamb leg is here! The roasted lamb leg is perfect servings for a large family, or you can serve it at a fancy festive dinner to treat your guests with its tempting aromas and flavors. By using just these 5 ingredients, you can cook yourself a complete low-carb meal.

5 pounds (2.3 kg) leg of lamb
4 garlic cloves, sliced
Salt and freshly ground black
pepper, to taste
2 tablespoons fresh rosemary

1. Preheat the oven to 350°F (180°C).
2. Using a sharp knife, cut several 3- to 4-inch slits in the top of the lamb leg, then stuff the garlic into the slits.
3. Sprinkle salt, black pepper over the leg and place it in a roasting pan. Place the rosemary sprigs on top.
4. Roast the rosemary lamb for 2 hours in the preheated oven or until desired doneness.
5. Once roasted, leave the lamb at room temperature for 10 minutes before carving.

STORAGE: Store in a sealed airtight container in the fridge for up to 5 days or in your freezer for about 1 month.
REHEAT: Microwave, covered, until the desired temperature is reached or reheat in a frying pan or air fryer / instant pot, covered, on medium.
SERVE IT WITH: To add more flavors to this meal, serve the lamb leg on top salad green. It also tastes great paired with a bowl of cucumber cream salad.
PER SERVING
calories: 524 | fat: 38.7g | total carbs: 0.5g | fiber: 0.1g | protein: 40.7g

ZESTY LAMB LEG

Macros: Fat 35% | Protein 64% | Carbs 1%
Prep time: 20 minutes | Cook time: 3 hours | Serves 10

Aroasted lamb leg tastes even better when it is cooked with an herb and zesty filling. In this recipe, the lamb leg is infused with all the spices like mustard, cardamom, and marjoram, and its slits are stuffed with lemon peel to give it better taste and aroma.

1 teaspoon salt	½ teaspoon dried marjoram
1 teaspoon seasoned salt	5 pounds (2.3 kg) leg of lamb
½ teaspoon black pepper	1 lemon peel, cut into slivers
¼ teaspoon dry mustard	½ teaspoon dried thyme
⅛ teaspoon ground cardamom	Fresh mint, optional

1. Preheat the oven to 325°F (160°C).
2. Add salt, seasoned salt, black pepper, mustard, cardamom, and marjoram in a bowl.
3. Mix well and rub the mixture over the lamb liberally. Cut 16 deep slits in this seasoned lamb roast with a sharp knife.
4. Mix lemon peel and thyme in a separate bowl and insert this dry mixture into the slits.
5. Place the prepared lamb roast in a roasting pan, fat-side up. Roast the lamb roast for 3 hours in the prepared oven until its internal temperature reaches 180°F (82°C) on a meat thermometer.
6. Remove from the oven to a plate and garnish with fresh mint, if desired.

STORAGE: Store in a sealed airtight container in the fridge for up to 5 days or in your freezer for about 1 month.
REHEAT: Microwave, covered, until the desired temperature is reached or reheat in a frying pan or air fryer / instant pot, covered, on medium.
SERVE IT WITH: To add more flavors to this meal, serve the lamb leg on top of cauliflower rice. It also tastes great paired with sautéed Brussels sprouts.
PER SERVING
calories: 306 | fat: 12.0g | net carbs: 0.4g | fiber: 0.2g | protein: 45.9g

KALE PORK PLATTER WITH FRIED EGGS

Macros: Fat 85% | Protein 10% | Carbs 5%
Prep time: 5 minutes | Cook time: 15 minutes | Serves 4

Now you can enjoy a delicious pork meal in the morning as a breakfast or serve it on the side and make your menu more nutritious and healthier. It has every nutrient that you need on your ketogenic diet. Smoked pork belly with kale and pecans is a combination that you will never forget.

3 ounces (85 g) butter	1 ounce (28 g) pecans or walnuts
½ pound (227 g) kale	1 ounce (28 g) frozen cranberries
6 ounces (170 g) smoked pork belly or bacon	4 eggs
	Salt and black pepper, to taste

1. Add ⅔ of the butter to a frying pan and melt it over medium-high heat.
2. Toss in kale leaves and sauté until their edges are slightly browned.
3. Remove the kale from the pan and keep it in a bowl. Set aside for a while.
4. Add pork belly to the pan and cook until it is crispy.
5. Reduce the heat and return the kale to the pan. Add nuts and cranberries and cook for 2 minutes.
6. Transfer the pork mixture to two serving plates.

7. Increase the heat and melt the remaining butter in the frying pan.
8. Crack the eggs one at a time into the pan and fry for about 3 minutes until set.
9. Top each plate of the pork and kale mixture with two fried eggs. Season as desired with salt and pepper. Serve while still warm.

STORAGE: Store in a sealed airtight container in the fridge for 1 day.
SERVE IT WITH: To add more flavors to this meal, serve this dish with the sliced avocados on top.
PER SERVING
calories: 533 | fat: 49.1g | total carbs: 7.8g | fiber: 2.8g | protein: 17.2g

SWEET AND SPICY PORK

Macros: Fat: 36% | Protein: 62% | Carbs: 2%
Prep time: 15 minutes | Cook time: 20 minutes | Servings: 6

Have you ever seen a pork dish that has the perfect combination of being a low-carb and a low-fat dish? This scrumptious sweet and spicy pork is the best dish for anyone craves that meaty goodness. This melt-in-your-mouth pork is perfect for any dinner party, brunch, or family gathering.

2 pounds (907 g) pork tenderloin	½ cup Dijon mustard
½ teaspoon liquid stevia	¼ teaspoon chili powder
¼ teaspoon salt	2 tablespoons olive oil, divided

1. Put the pork in a Ziploc bag.
2. Mix the stevia, salt, mustard, and chili powder in a bowl, then pour it inside the Ziploc bag with the pork tenderloin.
3. Seal the bag and give it a shake, then put it in the refrigerator to marinate for 4 hours.
4. Preheat the grill to high heat and lightly grease the grill grates with 1 tablespoon olive oil.
5. Remove the meat from the marinade and discard the marinade. Put the meat on a preheated grill and brush the meat with remaining olive oil.
6. Grill for 10 to 20 minutes, flipping the meat halfway through, or until the meat is cooked to your desired doneness.
7. Remove the pork from the grill, cut into slices, and serve on a plate.

STORAGE: Store in an airtight container in the fridge for up to 4 days or in the freezer for up to 1 month.
REHEAT: Microwave, covered, until the desired temperature is reached or reheat in a frying pan or air fryer / instant pot, covered, on medium.
SERVE IT WITH: To make this a complete meal, serve it with a glass of sparkling water and a veggie salad.
PER SERVING
calories: 200 | fat: 8.0g | total carbs: 1.0g | fiber: 0g | protein: 31.0g

COLORFUL SAUSAGE & BELL PEPPERS COMBO

Macros: Fat: 80% | Protein: 17% | Carbs: 3%
Prep time: 15 minutes | Cook time: 32 minutes | Serves 6

Such a satisfying and colorful combo! With the combo of sweet Italian sausage, bell peppers and onion, this recipe is bursting with delish flavors.

1½ pounds (680 g) sweet Italian sausages
2 tablespoons olive oil
1 red onion, sliced thinly
1 orange bell pepper, seeded and cut into 3-inch long strips
1 red bell pepper, seeded and cut into 3-inch long strips

1 yellow bell pepper, seeded and cut into 3-inch long strips
1 tablespoon garlic, minced
½ cup white wine
Sea salt and ground black pepper, to taste
Olive oil cooking spray

1. Preheat a grill to medium-high and spray the grill grate with olive oil spray.
2. Place the sausage links onto the heated grill and cook for about 12 minutes, flipping occasionally. Transfer the sausages onto a plate and set aside for about 15 minutes. Then cut each sausage into 2-inch pieces.
3. In a large nonstick skillet, heat the oil over medium-high heat and stir in the onion, bell peppers and garlic. Cook for about 10 minutes, stirring occasionally. Add the cooked sausage slices and wine. Cook for about 10 minutes, stirring occasionally. Sprinkle with salt and black pepper to taste.
4. Remove from the heat and serve hot.

STORAGE: Store in an airtight container in the fridge for up to 4 days or in the freezer for up to 1 month.
REHEAT: Microwave, covered, until the desired temperature is reached or reheat in a frying pan or air fryer / instant pot, covered, on medium.
SERVE IT WITH: Fresh baby spinach goes great with this sausage meal.
TIP: For a nice presentation, cut the bell peppers into uniform slices.
PER SERVING
calories: 450 | fat: 39.9g | total carbs: 5.1g | fiber: 1.0g | protein: 18.0g

BAKED BRUSSELS SPROUTS AND PINE NUT WITH BACON

Macros: Fat: 76% | Protein: 12% | Carb: 12%
Prep time: 5 minutes | Cook time: 10 minutes | Serves 6

Do you want to make a salad which only needs 5 minutes to prepare it? The keto Brussels sprouts are best suited for people with a hectic lifestyle. It will go with any of the roasted or fried meals as a side dish. The keto food can use for an extended period if it can refrigerate in a tight container. It will look fresh for 4 or 5 days, and you can consume like a freshly made side dish.

8 ounces (227 g) bacon, sliced into pieces
¼ cup butter
⅔ cup pine nuts
3 medium green onions, finely grated

2 pounds (907 g) Brussels sprouts, cored and coarsely chopped
½ teaspoon salt
½ teaspoon ground black pepper

1. Put the sliced bacon into a nonstick skillet and sauté over medium-high heat for 3 to 4 minutes on each side or until it becomes crisp. Crumble the bacon with a spatula and set aside. Reserve 2 tablespoons of bacon grease for later use.
2. Melt the butter in the same skillet over medium heat and add the reserved bacon grease. Add pine nuts and sauté for 2 minutes or until it becomes brown. Put sliced green onions and coarsely chopped Brussels sprouts into the skillet. Add salt and pepper. Continue cooking for 10 to 15 minutes or until the sprouts become fork-tender.
3. Serve on a plate by garnishing with crumbled bacon.

STORAGE: You can refrigerate it in a tight container and keep for 4 to 5 days.
REHEAT: The keto salad can microwave as per the instructions or also reheat by an air fryer or frying pan or in an instant pot on low-medium heat.
SERVE IT WITH: Side dishes are always a great combination when served with fried / roasted non-veg meals.
PER SERVING
calories: 410 | fat: 34.7g | total carbs: 19.6g | fiber: 7.8g | protein: 12.5g

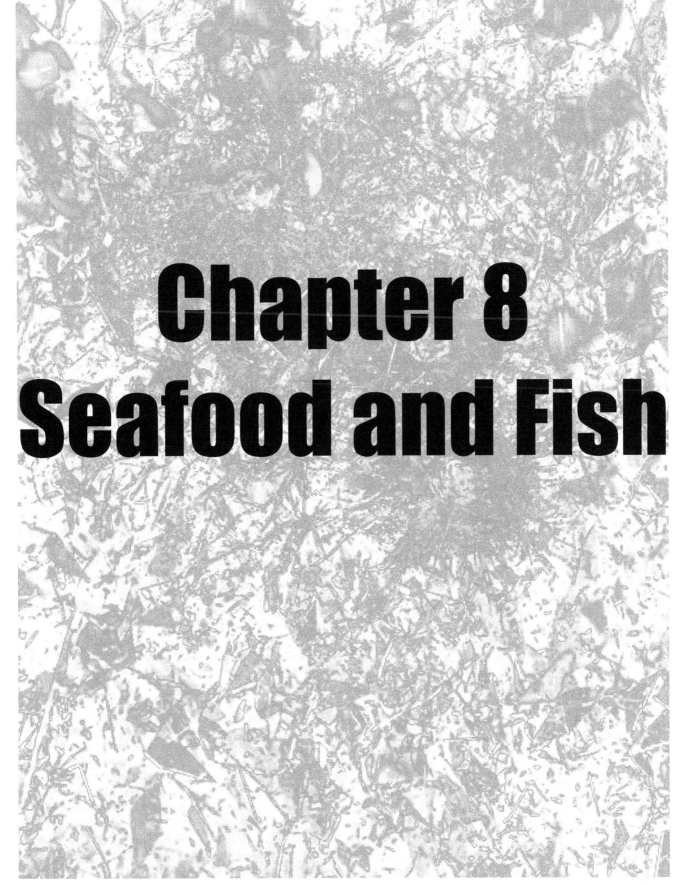

Chapter 8
Seafood and Fish

LEMONY GRILLED CALAMARI

Macros: Fat: 46% | Protein: 43% | Carbs: 11%
Prep time: 15 minutes | Cook time: 3 minutes | Serves 4

This recipe is one of the best ways to prepare calamari tubes for your dining table. The marinade of lemon, fresh oregano, garlic, and seasoning gives a lusciously tangy flavor.

2 pounds (907 g) calamari tubes and tentacles, cleaned
2 tablespoons olive oil
4 tablespoons fresh lemon juice
2 to 3 teaspoons lemon zest, grated

2 tablespoons fresh oregano, chopped
1 tablespoon garlic, minced
Sea salt and ground black pepper, to taste
Olive oil cooking spray

1. Preheat the grill to high heat.
2. Using a knife, score the top layer of the calamari tubes about 2 inches (5 cm) apart. Set aside.
3. In a large bowl, add the oil, lemon juice, lemon zest, oregano, garlic, salt, and black pepper and mix well.
4. Add the calamari tubes to the bowl and coat with the mixture generously. Refrigerate to marinate for at least 30 minutes or up to 1 hour.
5. Grease the grill grates with olive oil cooking spray.
6. Place the calamari tubes on the grill and cook for about 1½ minutes per side or until lightly charred.
7. Let cool for about 5 minutes before serving.

STORAGE: Wrap the cooked and cooled calamari in food-safe plastic wrap, pressing out any excess air. Place the wrapped calamari in a sealable plastic freezer bag and freeze for up to 1 month.
REHEAT: Reheat by spreading on a foil-lined baking sheet and baking at 400°F (205°C) for 8 to 10 minutes.
SERVE IT WITH: To make this a complete meal, serve it with grilled vegetables or sliced avocado.
PER SERVING
calories: 427 | fat: 22.2g | total carbs: 12.5g | fiber: 1.4g | protein: 42.7g

BROWNED SALMON CAKES

Macros: Fat 61% | Protein 35% | Carbs 4%
Prep time: 10 minutes | Cook time: 15 minutes | Serves 4

1 (15-ounce / 425-g) can salmon, deboned, flaked and drained
2 beaten eggs

1 medium onion, diced finely
1 teaspoon ground black pepper
3 tablespoons olive oil

1. In a mixing bowl, add the beaten eggs, salmon, diced onion, and pepper. Stir thoroughly to combine.
2. Make the salmon cakes: Scoop out equal-sized portions of the salmon mixture and shape into patties with your palm, about 2 inches in diameter.
3. Heat the olive oil in a large skillet over medium heat. Add the salmon patties and fry for 4 to 5 minutes per side until lightly golden brown around the edges.
4. Remove from the heat and serve on a plate.

STORAGE: You can refrigerate the cakes with either in an airtight container or wrap with plastic wrap. But be careful, it can't be stored in the freezer as it doesn't taste good afterward.
REHEAT: Microwave, covered, until the desired temperature is reached or reheat in a frying pan or air fryer/instant pot, covered, on medium.
SERVE IT WITH: To make it a complete meal, you can serve it with green beans or grilled vegetables.
PER SERVING
calories: 330 | fat: 22.6g | total carbs: 3.5g | fiber: 0.7g | protein: 26.8g

SNOW CRAB CLUSTERS WITH GARLIC BUTTER

Macros: Fat 16% | Protein 82% | Carbs 2%
Prep time: 5 minutes | Cook time: 15 minutes | Serves 2

These perfect Crab Clusters with Garlic Butter will melt in your mouth with every bite! The combination of seasonings and succulent taste of the crab will be the only way you'll ever cook crab clusters again!

1 pound (454 g) snow crab clusters, thawed if necessary
¼ cup butter
1 clove garlic, minced

1½ teaspoons dried parsley
⅛ teaspoon salt
¼ teaspoon ground black pepper

1. On the cutting board, cut a slit lengthwise into the shell of each crab. Set aside.
2. In a skillet, melt the butter over medium heat. Add the garlic and cook for 2 minutes until tender. Add the parsley, salt, and pepper, then cook for 1 minute more. Stir in the crab and simmer for 5 to 6 minutes.
3. Remove from the heat and serve on a plate.

STORAGE: Store in an airtight container in the fridge for up to 2 days. Not recommend freezing.
REHEAT: Microwave, covered, until it reaches the desired temperature.
SERVE IT WITH: To make this a complete meal, you can serve it with cabbage and asparagus salad.
PER SERVING
calories: 222 | fat: 4.0g | total carbs: 0.8g | fiber: 0.1g | protein: 45.7g

SPICED FISH CURRY

Macros: Fat: 68% | Proteins: 22% | Carbs: 10%
Prep time: 30 minutes | Cook time: 10 minutes | Serves 4

Prepare fish curry in your instant pot to enjoy all the flavors. With a wide range of spices, enjoy this unique recipe for lunch or dinner with friends and relatives. You can add more onions to improve the taste.

2 tablespoons olive oil
6 curry leaves, or bay leaves
1 tablespoon ginger, grated
2 garlic cloves, granulated
2 medium onions, chopped
½ teaspoon ground turmeric
1 teaspoon ground coriander
2 teaspoons ground cumin
1 teaspoon chili powder
½ teaspoon ground fenugreek

2 cups unsweetened coconut milk
1 pound (454 g) cod fillets, rinsed and cut into bite-sized pieces
2 green chilies, deseeded and chopped
1 tomato, chopped
Salt, to taste

1. Heat the olive oil in a large saucepan over medium heat.
2. Add the curry leaves and fry for 1 minute. Mix in the ginger, garlic cloves, and onions, then cook for 3 minutes until tender.
3. Stir in the turmeric, coriander, cumin, chili powder, and fenugreek. Cook for 2 minutes, then pour in the coconut milk. Add the fish, green chilies, and tomatoes.
4. Reduce the heat to medium-low and simmer uncovered for about 10 to 12 minutes, or until you can flake the fish easily with a fork.
5. Add the salt to taste, then serve on a platter.

STORAGE: Store in an airtight container in the fridge for up to 3 days.
REHEAT: Microwave, covered, until the desired temperature is reached or reheat in a frying pan/instant pot, covered, on medium.
SERVE IT WITH: To make this a complete meal, serve the fish curry with Marinated Bok Choy Salad.
PER SERVING
calories: 456 | fat: 36.1g | total carbs: 12.1g | fiber: 2.1g | protein: 25.0g

DEVILED EGG WITH SHRIMP

Macros: Fat 73% | Protein 24% | Carbs 3%
Prep time: 5 minutes | Cook time: 10 minutes | Serves 4

This keto deviled egg meal is so delicious and is perfect for a group or your family gathering. This signature appetizer dish is also keto-friendly and ready in no time. A classic family favorite! The best deviled eggs with creamy filling! These super simple, easy keto deviled eggs use common ingredients and take just 20 minutes.

54 eggs	1 teaspoon tabasco
¼ cup keto-friendly mayonnaise	8 peeled and cooked shrimp
1 pinch herbal salt	Fresh dill, for garnish

1. Put the eggs in a pot of water and bring to a boil for 10 minutes.
2. Take the eggs from the pot and put them in a bowl of cold water. Peel and slice the eggs in half, then spoon the yolks to a bowl. Reserve the egg whites on a clean plate.
3. Mash the yolks with a fork and add the mayonnaise, herbal salt, and tabasco. Stir to combine well.
4. Fill each egg white evenly with the egg yolk mixture, then top with the cooked shrimp.
5. Garnish with dill and serve warm.

STORAGE: Hard-boiled and peeled eggs can be made 1 day in advance and stored in the refrigerator. You can also make the fillings up to 1 day ahead and store in the fridge.
REHEAT: Microwave, covered, until the desired temperature is reached or reheat in a frying pan/instant pot, covered, on medium.
SERVE IT WITH: To make this a complete meal, serve with buttery cauliflower rice and keto egg salad.
PER SERVING
calories: 178 | fat: 14.4g | total carbs: 1.5g | fiber: 0.2g | protein: 9.9g

SALMON PIE

Macros: Fat 77% | Protein 12% | Carbs 11%
Prep time: 15 minutes | Cook time: 40 minutes | Serves 8

This Salmon pie is made with leftover baked salmon, eggs, cheese, and a super flaky low-carb crust. The filling is a breeze to make, so this quiche one of those easy and tasty keto recipes. Salmon and dill adore each other so much. And you'll swoon over them together, too, in this hearty and cheesy keto pie.

PIE CRUST:

¾ cup almond flour	husk powder
1 beaten egg	3 tablespoons olive oil
1 pinch salt	4 tablespoons water
1 teaspoon baking powder	4 tablespoons sesame seeds
1 tablespoon ground psyllium	4 tablespoons coconut flour

FILLING:

¼ teaspoon ground black pepper	3 eggs
½ teaspoon onion powder	5 ounces (142 g) cream cheese
1 cup keto-friendly mayonnaise	5 ounces (142 g) Cheddar cheese, shredded
2 tablespoons fresh dill, chopped finely	
	8 ounces (227 g) smoked salmon

SPECIAL EQUIPMENT:
A 10-inch (25-cm) springform pan

1. Preheat the oven to 350°F (180°C).
2. Put all the ingredients for the pie crust in a food processor, and process until the pie crust mixture is sticky and forms a ball.
3. Line a 10-inch (25-cm) springform pan with parchment paper. Using an oiled spatula, press the pie crust mixture evenly into the bottom of the springform pan.
4. Bake in the preheated oven for about 10 minutes until lightly browned.
5. Meanwhile, in a bowl, stir together all the ingredients for the filling until well combined.
6. Remove the pan from the oven. Add the filling and salmon to the pie crust mixture, smoothing the top with a spatula.
7. Return the pan to the oven and bake for about 30 minutes, or until the filling is set, and the top is golden brown.
8. Remove from the oven and allow to cool for 8 minutes before serving.

STORAGE: Store in an airtight container in the fridge for up to 3 days or in the freezer for up to 3 months.
REHEAT: Place it in the microwave until the desired temperature, or reheat in a frying pan.
SERVE IT WITH: To make this a complete meal, serve drizzled with lemon dill sauce. It also tastes great paired with roasted asparagus.
PER SERVING
calories: 635 | fat: 54.1g | total carbs: 18.5g | fiber: 0.9g | protein: 19.4g

PAN SEARED TILAPIA WITH ALMOND CRUST

Macros: Fat 51% | Protein 43% | Carbs 6%
Prep time: 20 minutes | Cook time:10 minutes | Serves 8

If you're looking to cook tilapia with a unique twist, look no further. Almonds give this recipe a crunchy, buttery taste that goes well with the mild flavor of the tilapia. This easy recipe will yield restaurant-quality results!

2 eggs	cheese, divided
½ tablespoon lemon pepper seasoning	8 (6-ounce / 170-g) tilapia fillets
½ tablespoon garlic pepper seasoning	⅛ cup coconut flour
	6 tablespoons butter
1 cup ground almonds	Salt, to taste
2 cups freshly grated Parmesan	8 sprigs parsley
	8 lemon wedges

1. In a bowl, beat the eggs with the lemon pepper and garlic pepper seasoning until blended. Set aside.
2. On a plate, stir together ground almonds with 1 cup of Parmesan cheese.
3. Dust the tilapia fillets with flour and shake off excess. Dip the tilapia in the egg mixture, then press into the almond mixture until coated well.
4. Melt the butter in a large skillet over medium-high heat. Cook tilapia in melted butter until golden brown on both sides, 2 to 3 minutes per side.
5. Reduce heat to medium, and season fillets with salt if desired. Sprinkle the tilapia with the remaining Parmesan cheese, cover, and continue cooking until the Parmesan cheese has melted, about 5 minutes.
6. Transfer the tilapia fillets to eight serving plates. Garnish with parsley springs and lemon wedges to serve.

STORAGE: Place fish fillets in an airtight container and store in the fridge for up to 3 days.
REHEAT: Microwave, covered, until the desired temperature is reached or reheat in a frying pan or air fryer/instant pot, covered, on medium.
SERVE IT WITH: This dish goes well with warm kale salad, cauliflower rice, or zucchini noodles.
PER SERVING
calories: 428 | fat: 24.1g | total carbs: 7.8g | fiber: 1.5g | protein: 46.5g

TASTY MAHI MAHI CAKES

Macros: Fat: 58% | Proteins: 40% | Carbs: 2%
Prep time: 30 minutes | Cook time: 15 minutes | Serves 4

A perfect combination of uniquely chosen ingredients, a considerable amount of canned Mahi Mahi along with garnishing ingredients proves the sweetness that can be acquired from mahi mahi to make fulfilling seafood for dinner.

1 (12-ounce / 340-g) can Mahi Mahi	¼ cup onions minced
2 teaspoons primal palate seafood seasoning	3 tablespoons olive oil
3 egg yolks	1 teaspoon chives, for garnish
	2 teaspoons parsley, for garnish
	4 lemon wedges, for garnish

1. Start by preheating the oven to 350°F (180°C).
2. In a mixing bowl, mix the fish, seafood seasoning, egg yolks, and onions.
3. Make the mahi mahi cakes: Scoop out 2 tablespoons of the fish mixture and using your hands to shape it into a patty, about ½ inch thick. Repeat with the remaining fish mixture. Place them on a greased baking dish.
4. Put the baking dish in the preheated oven and bake until the cakes are cooked through, about 15 minutes.
5. Remove the patties from the oven to a plate.
6. Heat the olive oil in a skillet over medium-high heat. Add the patties and cook for about 5 minutes, flipping occasionally.
7. Sprinkle the chives, parsley, and lemon wedges on top for garnish and serve.

STORAGE: Store in an airtight container in the fridge for up to 3 days.
REHEAT: Microwave, covered, until the desired temperature is reached or reheat in a frying pan or air fryer/instant pot, covered, on medium.
SERVE IT WITH: To make this a complete meal, serve the mahi mahi cakes with a crispy asparagus salad.
PER SERVING
calories: 223 | fat: 14.3g | total carbs: 1.6g | fiber: 0.2g | protein: 22.2g

KETO TACO FISHBOWL

Macros: Fat 77% | Protein 13% | Carbs 10%
Prep time: 5 minutes | Cook time: 10 minutes | Serves 4

A re you tired of eating daily repeated dishes? Just try to make keto taco fishbowl yourself. It doesn't take much time to be prepared. This recipe is very simple to be prepared and it's also rich in the ingredients.

DRESSING:

½ cup keto-friendly mayonnaise	½ teaspoon garlic powder
2 tablespoons lime juice	Salt and freshly ground black pepper, to taste
1 teaspoon hot sauce	

MAIN MEAL:

½ pound (227 g) green cabbage or red cabbage	3 tablespoons olive oil, divided
½ yellow onion	10 ounces (284 g) white fish, patted dry
1 tomato	1 tablespoon Tex-Mex seasoning
1 avocado	Fresh cilantro, for garnish
Salt and ground black pepper, to taste	Lime, for garnish

1. In a bowl, mix the ingredients for the dressing before frying the fish, so the flavors have time to develop. Allow to sit at room temperature or keep in the refrigerator.
2. With a sharp knife or mandolin, shred or slice all vegetables finely except the avocado. Split the avocado in half and remove the pit. Slice the avocado thinly and using a spoon to scoop avocado slices out of the skin. Season the vegetables and avocado slices with salt and pepper on a plate, then drizzle with 2 tablespoons olive oil. Toss well and set aside.
3. Rub both sides of white fish with salt, pepper, and Tex-Mex seasoning.
4. In a skillet, add the remaining olive oil. Fry the fish in olive oil over medium heat for 3 to 4 minutes on both sides, or until the fish flakes easily with a fork.
5. Transfer the vegetable mixture to a serving bowl. Top with the fish and pour over the dressing. Garnish with fresh cilantro and lime before serving.

STORAGE: Store the leftovers in an airtight container in the fridge for up to 3 days.
REHEAT: Wrap the fish in a foil with a little olive oil to keep it moist and then put it into the oven at about 200°F (93°C) for 5 to 7 minutes.
SERVE IT WITH: To make this a complete meal, serve it with mushroom soup or vegetable roasted salad.
PER SERVING
calories: 489 | fat: 42.9g | total carbs: 14.2g | fiber: 5.6g | protein: 15.1g

GRILLED WHITE FISH WITH ZUCCHINI

Macros: Fat 52% | Protein 39% | Carbs 9%
Prep time: 10 minutes | Cook time: 15 minutes | Serves 4

W ould you like to brighten your dinner up, this is the best choice for you and your friends after a busy day. If you're a seafood person, you will love it.

KALE PESTO:

3 ounces (85 g) kale, chopped	½ teaspoon salt
1 garlic clove	¼ teaspoon ground black pepper
3 tablespoons lemon juice	2 teaspoons olive oil
2 ounces (57 g) walnuts, shelled	

FISH AND ZUCCHINI:

2 zucchinis, rinsed and drained, cut into slices	1 teaspoon lemon juice
2 tablespoons olive oil, divided	1½ pounds (680 g) white fish (such as cod), thawed at room temperature, if frozen
Salt and freshly ground black pepper, to taste	

1. Make the kale pesto: Add the kale to the food processor with the garlic, lemon juice, and walnuts and blend, then sprinkle with salt and pepper for seasoning, and then add the olive oil and blend until the mixture becomes creamy and set aside until ready to serve.
2. Rub the zucchini slices with 1 tablespoon of olive oil, salt, pepper, and lemon juice and set aside.
3. Grease a nonstick skillet with remaining olive oil, and heat over medium-high heat.
4. Grill the fish in the skillet for 3 minutes on each side. Sprinkle with salt and black pepper, and serve with zucchini and kale pesto immediately.

STORAGE: We can store the leftovers in an airtight container in the freezer for up to 4 days. Pesto can be stored in the refrigerator for 3 to 4 days or in the freezer for up to 1 month.
REHEAT: Reheat the leftovers in the oven until warmed thoroughly.
SERVE IT WITH: To enjoy the meal, serve this dish with cauliflower rice and tangy cucumber salad.
PER SERVING
calories: 321 | fat: 19.5g | total carbs: 8.1g | fiber: 2.8g | protein: 30.3g

SALMON WITH TOMATO AND BASIL

Macros: Fat 48% | Protein 49% | Carbs 3%
Prep time: 10 minutes | Cook time: 20 minutes | Serves 2

Salmon with tomatoes and basil is your choice; it's really fun to cook it. Besides, it's so yummy! When salmon with tomato and basil, there's no room for leftovers!

2 (6-ounce / 170-g) salmon fillets, skinless, boneless
1 tablespoon dried basil
1 tomato, sliced thinly

1 tablespoon olive oil
2 tablespoons Parmesan cheese, finely grated
Nonstick cooking spray

1. Preheat the oven to 375°F (190°C). Using an aluminum foil, line a baking sheet, and spray it with nonstick cooking spray.
2. Arrange the salmon fillets on the baking sheet. Sprinkle the fillets with basil, then top them with tomato slices. Drizzle with olive oil and scatter the Parmesan cheese over them.
3. Bake in the preheated oven for about 15 to 20 minutes until the salmon becomes opaque in the middle and the cheese is melted.
4. Remove from the oven and cool for 5 minutes before serving.

STORAGE: Store in an airtight container in the fridge for up to 4 days or in the freezer for up to 1 month.
REHEAT: Microwave, covered, until the desired temperature is reached or reheat in a frying pan or air fryer/instant pot, covered, on medium.
SERVE IT WITH: To make this a complete meal, serve with roasted broccoli or leafy greens.
PER SERVING
calories: 332 | fat: 17.9g | total carbs: 2.5g | fiber: 0.6g | protein: 38.1g

GRILLED SPICY SHRIMP

Macros: Fat 23% | Protein 74% | Carbs 3%
Prep time: 15 minutes | Cook time: 6 minutes | Serves 6

When it comes to having a remarkable, flavorful meal, shrimp on the grill is almost always unquestionable. A meal of a huge store of protein and nearly no fat. It would be just perfect for your keto balance.

1 large garlic clove, crushed
1 teaspoon coarse salt
1 teaspoon paprika
½ teaspoon cayenne pepper
¼ cup lemon juice

2 tablespoons olive oil, plus more for greasing the grill grates
2 pounds (907 g) large shrimp, deveined and peeled
8 lemon wedges, for garnish

1. Preheat the grill to medium heat.
2. In a bowl, add the garlic, salt, paprika, cayenne pepper, lemon juice, and olive oil. Stir well with a fork until a paste forms.
3. In a separate bowl, toss the shrimp, garlic paste until evenly coated.
4. Lightly grease the grill grates with olive oil. Cook shrimp on the grill for 2 to 3 minutes on each side until opaque.
5. Squeeze the lemon wedges on top of the shrimp and serve hot.

STORAGE: Store in an airtight container in the fridge for up to 4 days or in the freezer for up to 1 month.
REHEAT: Microwave, covered, until the desired temperature is reached or reheat in a frying pan or air fryer/instant pot, covered, on medium.
SERVE IT WITH: To make this a complete meal, serve it with zucchini noodle salad or roasted asparagus with Parmesan.
PER SERVING
calories: 198 | fat: 5.0g | total carbs: 2.0g | fiber: 0.2g | protein: 36.4g

SALMON FILLETS WITH DILL AND LEMON

Macros: Fat 64% | Protein 32% | Carbs 4%
Prep time: 10 minutes | Cook time: 25 minutes | Serves 4

Thinking about what to cook on lunch and, in the meantime, want something fast, flavorful and suitable to your keto style? Here's Salmon fillets with Dill and Lemon, the dish that will be, tens of times, repeatable. Your family, friends and everyone to taste it, would ask for more!

1 pound (454 g) salmon fillets
¼ cup melted butter
¼ cup lemon juice
1 tablespoon dried dill weed

¼ teaspoon garlic powder
Sea salt and fresh ground black pepper, to taste

1. Preheat the oven to 350°F (180°C).
2. Place the salmon fillets on a lightly greased baking dish.
3. Combine the melted butter and lemon juice in a bowl. Drizzle the mixture over the fillets. Sprinkle with dill, garlic powder, sea salt, and pepper.
4. In the preheated oven, bake the fillets for 25 minutes until the fish flakes easily with a fork.
5. Remove the fish from the oven and serve warm.

STORAGE: Store in an airtight container in the fridge for up to 4 days or in the freezer for up to 1 month.
REHEAT: Microwave, covered, until the desired temperature is reached or reheat in a frying pan or air fryer/instant pot, covered, on medium.
SERVE IT WITH: To make this a complete meal, serve it with sautéed green beans or roasted broccoli.
PER SERVING
calories: 321 | fat: 20.8g | total carbs: 1.6g | fiber: 0.2g | protein: 69.5g

EASY SALMON STEAKS WITH DILL

Macros: Fat 35% | Protein 64% | Carbs 1%
Prep time: 5 minutes | Cook time: 25 minutes | Serves 4

When it comes to maintaining your keto routine, salmon steaks with dill is your best friend. It contains almost no carbs! Besides, the out of this world taste that would make you repeat it so many times.

1 pound (454 g) salmon fillets
1 teaspoon dried dill weed
½ teaspoon ground black pepper

Salt, to taste
1 teaspoon onion powder
2 tablespoons melted butter

1. Preheat the oven to 400°F (205°C).
2. Arrange the salmon fillets on a lightly greased baking dish.
3. Sprinkle dill, pepper, salt, and onion powder over the fillets. Rub the butter over the steaks evenly.
4. Bake the fillets in the preheated oven for 20 minutes or until flaky.
5. Remove from the oven and serve warm on a platter.

STORAGE: Store in an airtight container in the fridge for up to 4 days or in the freezer for up to 1 month.
REHEAT: Microwave, covered, until the desired temperature is reached or reheat in a frying pan or air fryer/instant pot, covered, on medium.
SERVE IT WITH: The salmon steaks perfectly go well with crunchy cabbage slaw or grilled zucchini.
PER SERVING
calories: 431 | fat: 16.9g | total carbs: 0.9g | fiber: 0.2g | protein: 69.1g

SALMON BLACKENED FILLETS

Macros: Fat 49% | Protein 49% | Carbs 2%
Prep time: 15 minutes | Cook time: 10 minutes | Serves 4

Wondering what to cook for lunch.? Want something tasty, filled with protein, and keto keeper? Salmon blackened fillets will be there for you; it would be so desired on your feast. Your family will beg to cook it again and again. Enjoy it while making it, to enjoy it when having it!

1 tablespoon ground cayenne pepper	1 tablespoon onion powder
2 tablespoons ground paprika	2 teaspoons salt
½ teaspoon ground white pepper,	¼ teaspoon dried basil
½ teaspoon ground black pepper,	¼ teaspoon dried thyme
	¼ teaspoon dried oregano
	½ cup melted butter
	4 salmon fillets

1. In a bowl, combine the cayenne pepper, paprika, white pepper, black pepper, onion powder, salt, basil, thyme, and oregano.
2. Brush both sides of each salmon fillets with ¼ cup of butter, and sprinkle with the cayenne pepper mixture. Then drizzle the remaining butter over the fillets.
3. Cook the salmon fillets in a skillet over high heat, buttered side down, for 3 or 4 minutes or until blackened. Flip the fillets halfway through the cooking time or until opaque.
4. Remove the fillets from the skillet and serve warm.

STORAGE: Store in an airtight container in the fridge for up to 4 days or in the freezer for up to 1 month.
REHEAT: Microwave, covered, until the desired temperature is reached or reheat in a frying pan or air fryer/instant pot, covered, on medium.
SERVE IT WITH: To maintain your keto routine, highly recommend serving it with broccoli rice, green salad, or a dollop of plain Greek yogurt.
PER SERVING
calories: 629 | fat: 37.7g | total carbs: 4.5g | fiber: 2.0g | protein: 66.3g

CRISPY KETO CREAMY FISH CASSEROLE

Macros: Fat 70% | Protein 23% | Carbs 8%
Prep time: 25 minutes | Cook time: 30 minutes | Serves 4

Once you finish your hard work, you need a crunchy meal to indulge yourself with. Crispy keto creamy fish casserole will hit the spot as it's so easy to make by yourself. With a few ingredients, you will get this fabulous dish!

1 head broccoli, cut into florets	1 tablespoon parsley, finely chopped
2 tablespoons olive oil	
1 teaspoon salt	1¼ cups heavy whipping cream
¼ teaspoon freshly ground black pepper	1 tablespoon Dijon mustard
6 scallions, chopped	1½ pounds (680 g) white fish, in serving- pieces
1 ounce (28 g) melted butter, for greasing the casserole dish	3 ounces (85 g) butter slices, under room temperature

1. Preheat the oven to 400℉ (205℃).
2. Heat the olive oil in a nonstick skillet over medium heat.
3. Add the broccoli to the skillet and sauté for 5 to 7 minutes or until tender, then season the broccoli with salt and ground black pepper, add the finely chopped scallions, and sauté for 1 to 2 minutes more.
4. Prepare a casserole dish and grease it with butter to add a tasty level of flavors to the meal. Then pour the sautéed broccoli and scallions in the casserole dish, stir them well until they have a delicious butter smell.
5. In a bowl, mix finely chopped parsley with cream and Dijon mustard and pour the mixture over the casserole dish. Stir until fully incorporated. Then nestle the white fish in the casserole dish. Top them with the butter slices.
6. Cook in the preheated oven for 20 to 30 minutes, or until the fish exudes tender and takes in the flavor from the delicious butter.
7. Remove the casserole dish from the oven and serve the fish and vegetables warm.

STORAGE: We can store the leftovers in an airtight container in the freezer for up to 4 days. Use it as a side dish in the coming days.
REHEAT: Reheat the recipe by wrapping the leftovers in aluminum foil and reheating in the oven for 5 to 7 minutes.
SERVE IT WITH: Serve it warm with creamy spinach and dill or with fresh salad to enjoy your meal to utmost.
PER SERVING
calories: 611 | fat: 48.3g | total carbs: 13.2g | fiber: 4.8g | protein: 34.4g

COCONUT KETO SALMON AND NAPA CABBAGE

Macros: Fat 74% | Protein 22% | Carbs 4%
Prep time: 10 minutes | Cook time: 20 minutes | Serves 4

The soft palate of shredded coconut combines with tender salmon. This dish will bring you a delightful experience of eating. Simple but crisp taste of Napa cabbage, and this recipe embraces all the nutrients you need.

1¼ pounds (567 g) salmon	4 tablespoons olive oil, for frying
1 tablespoon coconut oil	1¼ pounds (567 g) Napa cabbage
1 teaspoon sea salt	
½ teaspoon onion powder	Salt and freshly ground black pepper, to taste
1 teaspoon turmeric	
2 ounces (57 g) unsweetened shredded coconut	4 ounces (113 g) butter
	Lemon, for serving

1. On a wooden board, cut the salmon into 1×1-inch pieces. Then rub coconut oil on salmon pieces. Place the pieces in a medium bowl and set aside.
2. Prepare a mixture of salt, onion powder, turmeric, and unsweetened shredded coconut, finely mix the mixture. Meanwhile, put the salmon pieces into this creamy mixture to get a good coating.
3. In a nonstick frying pan with 4 tablespoons of olive oil on medium heat. Fry the seasoned salmon pieces with coconut mixture for about 4 to 7 minutes in a pan, stirring every 2 minutes. Leave it in the pan until golden brown, or until soft.
4. Meanwhile, prepare and cut the cabbage into wedges. Fry the cabbage in a saucepan with butter until it turns into a light creamy liquid. On a platter, pour the cabbage liquid and generously season with salt and pepper.
5. In a dish decorated with lemon slices, place the fried salmon and pour the creamy cabbage liquid and top with wedges of lemon. Serve warm!

STORAGE: Store in an airtight container in the fridge for up to 4 days or in the freezer for up to 1 month.
REHEAT: You can reheat the extras smoothly in a light skillet on medium-low heat until warmed through.
SERVE IT WITH: Serve it immediately with vegetable soup or crispy salad to be a perfect meal. Enjoy to the full!
PER SERVING
calories: 628 | fat: 52.9g | total carbs: 7.1g | fiber: 1.6g | protein: 32.7g

PARCHMENT BAKED SALMON

Macros: Fat 49% | Protein 49% | Carbs 2%
Prep time: 15 minutes | Cook time: 25 minutes | Serves 3

Wondering what to cook on dinner and afraid to spoil your keto routine? The rich meal is, usually, lopsided- full of protein and full of fat at the same time.
Now, Parchment Baked Salmon has solved it for you. A cow protein meal with approximately no fat! If you look to keep your keto routine up, it'll be your cup of tea.

1 (8-ounce / 227-g) boneless
salmon fillet
Salt and freshly ground black
pepper, to taste

¼ cup basil leaves, chopped
Olive oil cooking spray
1 lemon, sliced thinly

1. Preheat the oven to 400°F (205°C). Line a baking sheet with parchment paper and coat the bottom with cooking spray.
2. Arrange the salmon fillet, skin-side down, in the middle of the parchment paper.
3. Using a sharp knife, cut 2 to 3-inch slits into the salmon fillet. Stuff the basil leaves into the slits. Spray the salmon fillet with cooking spray and top with sliced lemon.
4. Fold the edges of parchment paper over the salmon fillet several times to seal it into an airtight packet.
5. Bake in the preheated oven for about 25 minutes, or until the fish reaches at least 145°F (63°C) on a meat thermometer.
6. Remove from the oven, and cool for 8 minutes before clipping the parchment paper. Remove the lemon slices and serve.

STORAGE: Store in an airtight container in the fridge for up to 4 days or in the freezer for up to 1 month.
REHEAT: Microwave, covered, until the desired temperature is reached or reheat in a frying pan or air fryer/instant pot, covered, on medium.
SERVE IT WITH: To make this a complete meal, serve it with roasted Brussels sprouts or cucumber salad.
PER SERVING
calories: 165 | fat: 9.0g | total carbs: 1.6g | fiber: 0.2g | protein: 20.0g

CLASSIC SHRIMP SCAMPI

Macros: Fat 9% | Protein 88% | Carbs 3%
Prep time:30 minutes | Cook time: 15 minutes | Serves 4

A restaurant-quality seafood dish that will impress even the pickiest of eaters! These shrimps are sautéed in garlic, butter, and dry white wine, and best enjoyed immediately.

2 cloves garlic, minced
½ cup butter, melted
½ cup dry white wine

2 pounds (907 g) medium
shrimp, peeled and deveined
3 green onions, chopped

1. Preheat the oven to 400°F (205°C).
2. In a bowl, combine the garlic, butter, wine, and shrimp. Stir thoroughly.
3. Arrange the shrimp in a greased baking dish. Place the baking dish in the oven and bake for about 8 minutes until the shrimp is opaque.
4. Remove from the oven and serve the shrimp with green onions on top.

STORAGE: Store in an airtight container in the fridge for up to 3 to 4 days or in the freezer for up to 1 month.
REHEAT: Microwave, covered, until the desired temperature is reached or reheat in a frying pan or air fryer / instant pot, covered, on medium.
SERVE IT WITH: To make this a complete meal, serve with cauliflower rice.
PER SERVING
calories: 209 | fat: 2.2g | total carbs: 1.6g | fiber: 0.2g | protein: 45.9g

STUFFED MEDITERRANEAN SWORDFISH

Macros: Fat 58% | Protein 36% | Carbs 6%
Prep time: 15 minutes | Cook time: 20 minutes | Serves 2

Flavorful, protein full, and super toothsome. The Stuffed Mediterranean Swordfish is a true masterpiece on your table. The best in summer!

1 (8-ounce / 227-g) swordfish (2-
to 3-inch thick)
1 tablespoon fresh lemon juice
1 tablespoon plus 1 teaspoon
olive oil, plus more for greasing

the grill grates
1 garlic clove, minced
1 cup fresh spinach, rinsed,
drained, and finely minced
¼ cup crumbled feta cheese

1. Preheat the grill to high heat and grease the grill grates lightly with olive oil.
2. Cut a slit in swordfish to create a pocket open from one side. Then, in a small bowl, mix together the lemon juice and 1 tablespoon of olive oil; brush finely on both sides of the swordfish. Set aside.
3. In a small skillet over medium-low heat, heat 1 teaspoon of olive oil.
4. Add the garlic clove to the skillet and sauté for 30 seconds or until fragrant.
5. Add the spinach and cook for 3 to 5 minutes or until wilted.
6. Remove from the heat, and stuff the spinach into the swordfish pocket. Scatter the feta cheese over spinach.
7. Arrange the swordfish on the grill grates, and cook for about 9 minutes. Turn them over and keep cooking until opaque.
8. Remove the swordfish from the grill and serve warm.

STORAGE: Store in an airtight container in the fridge for no more than 2 days, or in the freezer, uncooked, for up to 1 month.
REHEAT: Reheat by placing the swordfish in microwave, cover, until it reaches the desired temperature.
SERVE IT WITH: For a complete meal, we recommend you to serve it with sautéed vegetables, spicy kale Caesar with roasted garlic, avocado salad or low-carb blueberries juice.
PER SERVING
calories: 317 | fat: 20.8g | total carbs: 5.2g | fiber: 2.2g | protein: 27.8g

LOW CARB POACHED EGGS WITH TUNA SALAD

Macros: Fat 68% | Protein 27% | Carbs 5%
Prep time: 10 minutes | Cook time: 10 minutes | Serves 2

When you make this colorful recipe, don't forget to take a shot and post it to your Instagram to let your friends know how gorgeous you are! Low-carb poached eggs with tuna salad is an elegant dish to go with any main meal.

TUNA SALAD:
4 ounces (113 g) tuna in olive oil,
rinsed and drained
⅓ cup chopped celery stalks
½ red onion
½ cup mayonnaise, keto-

friendly
1 teaspoon Dijon mustard
Juice and zest of ½ lemon
Salt and freshly ground black
pepper, to taste

POACHED EGGS:
4 eggs
1 teaspoon salt
2 teaspoons white wine vinegar
or white vinegar
2 tablespoons olive oil

2 ounces (57 g) leafy greens or
lettuce
2 ounces (57 g) cherry tomatoes,
chopped

1. Chop the tuna and mix it in a bowl with the other ingredients for the salad. You can make it ahead of time and keep it in the refrigerator. The flavor will enhance with time.
2. Bring a pot of water to a boil over medium heat. Add the vinegar and salt, then stir the water in circles to create a swirl using a spoon. Crack the eggs into the pot, one at a time.
3. Let simmer for 3 minutes and use a slotted spoon to remove it from the water.
4. Transfer the eggs to the bowl of tuna salad and drizzle with olive oil. Gently toss until everything is combined.
5. Serve them with leafy greens and cherry tomatoes on the side.

STORAGE: Store in an airtight container in the fridge for up to 3 days.
REHEAT: Microwave, covered, until the desired temperature is reached or reheat in a frying pan or air fryer / instant pot, covered, on medium.
PER SERVING
calories: 534 | fat: 40.5g | total carbs: 7.2g | fiber: 1.4g | protein: 34.0g

CABBAGE PLATE WITH KETO SALMON

Macros: Fat 73% | Protein 12% | Carbs 16%
Prep time: 5 minutes | Cook time: 0 minutes | Serves 4

You do not have enough time to prepare dinner after work, confused about the recipe you want to prepare. Don't worry! With the avocado plate with cream salmon, you can amaze you with its great taste. With only four ingredients, you can prepare a cool, speedy, and splendid dinner!

7 ounces (198 g) fresh salmon
2 avocados
2 teaspoons coconut oil
6 teaspoons olive oil, divided
½ teaspoon onion powder,
1 teaspoon turmeric
2 cups shredded coconut,

unsweetened
12 ounces (340 g) cabbage, chopped
2 teaspoons butter
1 pinch of lemon zest
Salt and freshly ground black pepper, to taste

1. Cut the salmon into 1×1-inch pieces. Then drizzle the coconut oil and 2 teaspoons of olive oil on salmon pieces. Place the pieces in a medium bowl and set aside.
2. Mix the salt, onion powder, turmeric, and unsweetened shredded coconut in a separate bowl. Meanwhile, dunk the pre-prepared salmon pieces into this mixture.
3. In a nonstick frying pan with 4 teaspoons of olive oil on medium heat. Fry the seasoned salmon pieces with coconut mixture for about 4 to 7 minutes in a pan, stirring every 2 minutes. Leave it in the pan until golden brown and soft.
4. Meanwhile, fry the cabbage in a saucepan with butter until it is lightly caramelized. In a third bowl, pour the cabbage liquid and generously season with salt and pepper.
5. On a dish with lemon slices, place the fried salmon and pour the creamy cabbage over it. Serve warm.

STORAGE: Store in an airtight container in the fridge for up to 4 days or in the freezer for up to 1 month.
REHEAT: You can reheat the extras in a light skillet on medium-low heat until warmed through.
SERVE IT WITH: Serve it immediately with roasted vegetable soup or avocado crunchy fries to be a splendid meal.
PER SERVING
calories: 502 | fat: 42.8g | total carbs: 21.2g | fiber: 12.7g | protein: 14.8g

KETO MAUI WOWIE SHRIMP

Macros: Fat 68% | Protein 31% | Carbs 1%
Prep time: 15 minutes | Cook time: 10 minutes | Serves 6

A quick, easy, and delicious grilled shrimp recipe. These Maui wowie shrimp will be on your table in under 20 minutes, which makes them excellent for a busy night!

1 tablespoon olive oil
2 pounds (907 g) medium-sized raw shrimp, peeled and deveined

¼ teaspoon garlic salt
Freshly ground pepper, to taste
1 cup keto-friendly mayonnaise
1 large lemon, sliced

SPECIAL EQUIPMENT:
Bamboo skewers, soaked for at least 30 minutes

1. Preheat the grill to medium heat and grease the grill grates lightly with olive oil.
2. Thread 3 to 4 shrimp onto the bamboo skewers. Make sure the shrimp are all in the same direction.
3. Season the shrimp with salt and pepper on both sides.
4. Using a silicone brush, generously coat the shrimp with mayonnaise on both sides.
5. Place the shrimp on the preheated grill and cook for about 5 minutes per side, or until the shrimp are pink and opaque.
6. Transfer the shrimp to a plate and serve with lemon slices.

STORAGE: Store in an airtight container in the fridge for up to 4 days or in the freezer for up to 1 month.
REHEAT: Microwave, covered, until the desired temperature is reached or reheat in a frying pan or air fryer/instant pot, covered, on medium.
SERVE IT WITH: This dish goes well with warm kale salad, cauliflower rice, or zucchini noodles.
PER SERVING
calories: 401 | fat: 30.5g | total carbs: 0.8g | fiber: 0g | protein: 30.8g

SMOKED SALMON AND LETTUCE BITES

Macros: Fat 73% | Protein 20% | Carbs 7%
Prep time: 20 minutes | Cook time: 0 minutes | Serves 6

After finishing your work with relaxation and let your little brother prepare this dish for the whole family. How is that! Yes, this is the smoked salmon bites that need no oven to be prepared. Simple, speedy, and suitable for any main dish.

7 ounces (198 g) smoked salmon, cut into small pieces
8 ounces (227 g) cream cheese
⅓ tablespoon mayonnaise, keto-friendly
4 tablespoons chopped fresh dill

or fresh chives
½ lemon, zested
¼ teaspoon ground black pepper
2 ounces (57 g) lettuce, for serving

1. Add the cream cheese, mayonnaise, fresh dill, lemon zest, and pepper in a bowl. Stir to combine well.
2. Lay the lettuce on a clean work surface. Top with the salmon pieces and pour the cream cheese mixture over. Serve immediately.

STORAGE: Store in an airtight container in the fridge for up to 3 days.
REHEAT: Microwave the salmon, covered, until the desired temperature is reached or reheat in a frying pan or air fryer / instant pot, covered, on medium.
SERVE IT WITH: You can serve with thinly sliced and toasted low-carb keto bread or crunchy vegetables.
PER SERVING
calories: 179 | fat: 15.0g | total carbs: 3.3g | fiber: 1.1g | protein: 8.6g

AHI TUNA STEAKS

Macros: Fat 61% | Protein 39% | Carbs 0%
Prep time: 5 minutes | Cook time: 10 minutes | Serves 2

If you're up to air and want something fast, tasty, and keto saver, this ahi tuna steak is made for you. It's filled with protein and almost no carbs in it!

2 (5-ounce / 142-g) ahi tuna steaks	1 teaspoon ground paprika
¼ teaspoon cayenne pepper	½ tablespoon butter
A pinch kosher salt	2 tablespoons olive oil
	1 teaspoon whole peppercorns

1. Sprinkle the ahi tuna steaks with cayenne pepper, salt and paprika in a bowl.
2. In a medium skillet over medium heat, melt the butter, then add the olive oil. Cook the peppercorns in the mixture for 5 minutes or until softened.
3. Gently place the spiced tuna in the skillet. Cook for 1 to 2 minutes per side or until cooked your desired doneness.
4. Remove them from the skillet and serve hot.

STORAGE: Store in an airtight container in the fridge for up to 4 days or in the freezer for up to 1 month.
REHEAT: Microwave, covered, until the desired temperature is reached or reheat in a frying pan or air fryer/instant pot, covered, on medium.
SERVE IT WITH: The tuna steaks taste great paired with tomato and cucumber salad.
PER SERVING
calories: 669 | fat: 45.1g | total carbs: 0.8g | fiber: 0.5g | protein: 65.5g

SALMON WITH GARLIC DIJON MUSTARD

Macros: Fat 39% | Protein 57% | Carbs 4%
Prep time:15 minutes | Cook time: 20 minutes | Serves 4

Try this elegant salmon dish that is full of flavor. The mustard keeps the salmon moist and tender, and gives it an incredibly delicious taste!

1 tablespoon olive oil	4 large cloves garlic, thinly sliced
⅓ cup Dijon mustard	Salt and freshly ground black pepper, to taste
4 (6-ounce / 170-g) salmon fillets	1 teaspoon dried tarragon
1 red onion, thinly sliced	

1. Preheat the oven to 400°F (205°C) and grease a baking pan with olive oil.
2. Generously rub the Dijon mustard all over the salmon, then place the salmon in the pan, skin-side down.
3. Put the onion slices and garlic cloves on the salmon fillets. Sprinkle with salt, pepper, and tarragon.
4. Arrange the pan in the preheated oven and bake for 20 minutes, or until the salmon easily flakes when tested with a fork.
5. Remove from the heat and serve on a plate.

STORAGE: Store in an airtight container in the fridge for up to 2 days. Not recommend freezing.
REHEAT: Microwave the salmon and cucumber sauce, covered, until it reaches the desired temperature.
SERVE IT WITH: To make this a complete meal, you can serve it with rich chicken and mushroom broth and roasted asparagus.
PER SERVING
calories: 265 | fat: 11.6g | total carbs: 2.8g | fiber: 1.1g | protein: 36.0g

GRILLED TUNA SALAD WITH GARLIC SAUCE

Macros: Fat 61% | Protein 31% | Carbs 8%
Prep time: 10 minutes | Cook time: 15 minutes | Serves 4

A crisp, pretty salad topped with grilled tuna. Our creamy garlic dressing pulls it all together. It's simple to make so you can enjoy a tasty keto meal and the warm sunshine!

GARLIC DRESSING:

⅔ cup keto-friendly mayonnaise	Salt and freshly ground black pepper, to taste
2 tablespoons water	
2 teaspoons garlic powder	

TUNA SALAD:

2 eggs	4 ounces (113 g) leafy greens
8 ounces (227 g) green asparagus	2 ounces (57 g) cherry tomatoes
1 tablespoon olive oil	½ red onion
¾ pound (340 g) fresh tuna, in slices	2 tablespoons pumpkin seeds
	Salt and freshly ground black pepper, to taste

1. Mix the ingredients together for the garlic dressing. And set them aside.
2. Put the eggs in boiling water for 8 to 10 minutes. Cooling in cold water would facilitate the peeling.
3. Slice the asparagus into lengths and rapidly fry them inside a hot pan with no oil or butter. Then set them aside.
4. Rub the tuna with oil and fry or grill for 2 to 3 minutes on each side. Season with salt and pepper.
5. Put the leafy greens, asparagus, peeled eggs cut in halves, tomatoes and thinly sliced red onion into a plate.
6. Finally, cut the tuna into slices and spread the slices evenly over the salad. Pour the dressing on top and add some pumpkin seeds.

STORAGE: Store in an airtight container in the fridge for up 2 to 4 days.
SERVE IT WITH: To make this a complete meal, serve with a roasted chicken thigh.
PER SERVING
calories: 397 | fat: 27.1g | total carbs: 8.3g | fiber: 2.8g | protein: 30.0g

ASPARAGUS SEARED SALMON

Macros: Fat 74% | Protein 23% | Carbs 3%
Prep time: 10 minutes | Cook time: 20 minutes | Serves 4

Do you watch movies with your friends, but feel very boring! Try eating asparagus Seared salmon with easy Hollandaise while watching your favorite movies and you will feel the difference. It can be prepared fast and easily with your friends at your sweet home.

1 tablespoon butter	pepper, to taste
20 ounces (567 g) salmon fillets	14 ounces (397 g) green asparagus, rinsed and trimmed
Salt and freshly ground black	

HOLLANDAISE:

1 egg	1 tablespoon lemon juice
7 ounces (198 g) butter, melted	1 lemon, sliced

1. Melt the butter in a large skillet over medium heat.
2. Add the salmon fillets and cook for 14 minutes or until opaque. Flip the fillets halfway through the cooking time.
3. Add the asparagus gradually to the skillet while cooking the fillets and season with salt and pepper. Sauté the asparagus for 10 minutes or until soft and wilted.
4. Reduce the heat to low to keep the salmon and asparagus warm while making the Hollandaise..

HOLLANDAISE:

1. Break the egg in a bowl, then melt the butter in the microwave
2. Pour slowly melted butter into the egg in the mixing bowl. Keep stirring to mix until creamy.
3. Add lemon juice and salt.
4. Serve the salmon with creamy Hollandaise and soft asparagus. Decorate with slices of lemon for extra flavor and color.

STORAGE: Store the leftovers of salmon in an airtight container in the fridge for up to 5 days or in the freezer for up to 1 month.
REHEAT: You can reheat the extras in a lightly oiled skillet on medium-low heat until the salmon moistened through.
SERVE IT WITH: To make this a complete meal, you can serve it with roasted cauliflower.
PER SERVING
calories: 639 | fat: 53.7g | total carbs: 5.3g | fiber: 2.2g | protein: 35.2g

GRILLED RED LOBSTER TAILS

Macros: Fat 43% | Protein 56% | Carbs 1%
Prep time:15 minutes | Cook time: 12 minutes | Serves 2

Treat your family and friends to this delicious and easy version of grilled red lobster tails! This recipe uses a special blend of lemon, garlic, and paprika, which perfectly complements the sweetness of the lobsters.

1 tablespoon freshly squeezed lemon juice	Pinch of white pepper
½ cup extra virgin olive oil	2 (10-ounce / 284-g) red lobster tails
½ tablespoon salt	
Pinch of garlic powder	1 teaspoon olive oil, for greasing the grill grates
½ tablespoon paprika	

1. Preheat the grill to high heat.
2. In a bowl, whisk together the lemon juice, olive oil, salt, garlic powder, paprika, and white pepper.
3. Using a large knife, cut open lobster tails and slice lengthwise. Brush the flesh side of lobster tail with the marinade.
4. Lightly grease the grill grates with olive oil. Place the tails on the preheated grill, flesh-side down. Grill for about 10 minutes, flipping once, or until the lobster is opaque. Frequently baste tails with the marinade.
5. Let cool for 5 minutes before serving.

STORAGE: Place lobster tails in an airtight container and store in the fridge for up to three days.
REHEAT: Microwave, covered, until the desired temperature is reached or reheat in an air fryer or instant pot, covered, on medium.
SERVE IT WITH: This dish goes well with warm kale salad, cauliflower rice, or zucchini noodles.
PER SERVING
calories: 416 | fat: 20.1g | total carbs: 1.7g | fiber: 0.7g | protein: 57.8g

LOW CARB SEAFOOD CHOWDER

Macros: Fat 66% | Protein 26% | Carbs 8%
Prep time: 20 minutes | Cook time: 20 minutes | Serves 4

You have no time to prepare a great meal for your friends and guests. Here's the low-carb seafood chowder, a perfect rich recipe that you can prepare it in minimal time. Let your guests relish during the day.

4 tablespoons butter	2 garlic cloves, minced
5 ounces (142 g) celery stalks, sliced	4 ounces (113 g) cream cheese
	1 cup clam juice

1½ cups heavy whipping cream	8 ounces (227 g) shrimp, peeled and deveined
2 teaspoons dried sage or dried thyme	2 ounces (57 g) baby spinach
½ lemon, juiced and zested	Salt and freshly ground black pepper, to taste
1 pound (454 g) salmon fillets, cut into 1-inch pieces	Fresh sage, for garnish

1. Melt the butter in a large pot over medium heat. Add celery and garlic. Cook for about 5 minutes, stirring occasionally. Add clam juice, cream, cream cheese, sage, lemon juice and lemon zest. Let it simmer for about 10 minutes without a lid.
2. Add the salmon and shrimp. Simmer for 3 minutes or until salmon is opaque. Add the baby spinach and stir until wilted. Season with salt and pepper.
3. Garnish with fresh sage before serving for extra flavor.

STORAGE: The rest of the mixture can be kept in an airtight container in the fridge for 4 days, and it can also be kept in the freezer for 10 days.
REHEAT: Microwave, covered, until the desired temperature is reached or reheat in a frying pan or instant pot, covered, on medium.
SERVE IT WITH: You can serve this recipe with keto sesame salmon and cucumber and fennel salad.
PER SERVING
calories: 622 | fat: 46.7g | total carbs: 12.5g | fiber: 1.6g | protein: 38.8g

CHEESY BROCCOLI WITH KETO FRIED SALMON

Macros: Fat 61% | Protein 34% | Carbs 5%
Prep time:10 minutes | Cook time: 25 minutes | Serves 4

Cheesy broccoli with keto fried salmon is a magical recipe to cook with your family members and take turns in each step. This delicious recipe is one of the easiest recipes to make at home, far away from unhealthy fast food!

1 pound (454 g) broccoli, cut into florets	5 ounces (142 g) grated Cheddar cheese
3 ounces (85 g) butter	1½ pound (680 g) salmon
Salt and freshly ground black pepper, to taste	1 lime

1. Preheat the oven to 400°F (205°C).
2. Put the broccoli florets into a pot of lightly salted water. Bring to a simmer. Make sure the broccoli maintains its chewy texture and delicate color.
3. Drain the broccoli and discard the boiling water. Set aside, uncovered, for a minute or two to allow the steam to evaporate.
4. Place the drained broccoli in a well-greased baking dish. Add pepper and butter to taste.
5. Sprinkle cheese on top of the broccoli and bake in the oven for 15 to 20 minutes or until the cheese turns a golden color.
6. In the meantime, season the salmon with salt and pepper and fry in plenty of butter, a few minutes on each side. The lime can be fried in the same pan or be served raw.

STORAGE: Store the left dressing in an airtight container in the fridge for 5 days, and it can also be kept in the freezer for 30 days.
REHEAT: Reheat it with greased skillet over medium-low heat for 6 to 8 minutes until warm through.
SERVE IT WITH: Serve it with Cauliflower Soup, or serve it with a dish of warm Broccoli Cheddar Soup. Splendid!
PER SERVING
calories: 580 | fat: 39.2g | total carbs: 9.0g | fiber: 3.0g | protein: 48.2g

KETO CHILI-COVERED SALMON WITH SPINACH

Macros: Fat 55% | Protein 38% | Carbs 7%
Prep time: 5 minutes | Cook time: 20 minutes | Serves 4

This chili-covered salmon with spinach is elegant, spicy, easy, delicious, and keto. What more can you want out of dinner?

¼ cup olive oil
1½ pounds (680 g) salmon, in pieces
Salt and freshly ground black pepper, to taste
1 ounce (28 g) Parmesan cheese, grated finely
1 tablespoon chili paste
½ cup sour cream
1 pound (454 g) fresh spinach

1. Preheat oven to 400°F (205°C).
2. Grease the baking dish with half of the olive oil, season the salmon with pepper and salt, and put in the baking dish, skin-side down.
3. Combine Parmesan cheese, chili paste and sour cream. Then spread them on the salmon fillets.
4. Bake for 20 minutes, or until the salmon flakes easily with a fork or it becomes opaque.
5. Heat the remaining olive oil in a nonstick skillet, sauté the spinach until it's wilted, about a couple of minutes, and season with pepper and salt.
6. Serve with the oven-baked salmon immediately.

STORAGE: This recipe is freezer friendly, so it can be stored in the freezer for up to 3 months. To freeze, cover each quiche slice tightly in aluminum foil and freeze for up to 3 months.
REHEAT: Place it in the microwave until the desired temperature, or reheat in a frying pan.
SERVE IT WITH: To make this a complete meal, serve with riced cauliflower and a green salad.
PER SERVING
calories: 461 | fat: 28.5g | total carbs: 8.0g | fiber: 2.8g | protein: 42.6g

KETO EGG BUTTER AND SMOKED SALMON

Macros: Fat 84% | Protein 11% | Carbs 5%
Prep time: 5 minutes | Cook time: 15 minutes | Serves 4

This is what we call a breakfast for champions! If you want a keto meal that will keep you on top of your game for hours and hours, this is it!

4 eggs
½ teaspoon sea salt
¼ teaspoon ground black pepper
5 ounces (142 g) butter, at room temperature
4 ounces (113 g) smoked salmon
1 tablespoon fresh parsley, chopped finely
2 avocados
2 tablespoons olive oil

1. Put the eggs in a pot and cover them with cold water. Then put the pot on the stove without a lid and bring it to a boil.
2. Lower the heat and let it simmer for 6 to 9 minutes. Then remove eggs from the water and put them in a bowl with cold water.
3. Peel the eggs and cut them finely. Use a fork to mix the eggs and butter. Then season to taste with pepper, salt.
4. Serve the egg butter with slices of smoked salmon, finely chopped parsley, and a side of diced avocado tossed in olive oil.

STORAGE: Store in an airtight container in the fridge for up to 2 days.
REHEAT: Place it in the microwave until it reaches the desired temperature.
SERVE IT WITH: To make this a complete meal, serve with cauliflower rice and a green salad.
PER SERVING
calories: 638 | fat: 61.1g | total carbs: 9.8g | fiber: 6.8g | protein: 16.5g

KETO BAKED SALMON WITH BUTTER

Macros: Fat 71% | Protein 29% | Carbs 0%
Prep time: 10 minutes | Cook time: 25 minutes | Serves 6

This lemon salmon is out-of-this-world delicious. With only a few ingredients, it's easy and quick to make. This lemon butter sauce and salmon recipe is good enough for company but easy enough for a weeknight dinner!

1 tablespoon olive oil
2 pounds (907 g) salmon
1 teaspoon sea salt
Freshly ground black pepper, to
taste
7 ounces (198 g) butter
1 lemon

1. Start by preheating the oven to 425°F (220°C).
2. In a large baking dish, spray it with olive oil. Then add the salmon, skin-side down. Season with salt and pepper.
3. Cut the lemon into thin slices and place them on the upper side of the salmon. Cut the butter in thin slices and spread them on top of the lemon slices.
4. Put the dish in the heated oven and bake on the middle rack for about 25 to 30 minutes, or until the salmon flakes easily with a fork.
5. Melt the rest of the butter in a small saucepan until it bubbles. Then remove from heat and let cool a little. Consider adding some lemon juice on the melted cool butter.
6. Serve the fish with the lemon butter.

STORAGE: Store in an airtight container in the fridge for up to 2 days.
REHEAT: Microwave, covered, until the desired temperature is reached or reheat in a frying pan or air fryer / instant pot, covered, on medium.
SERVE IT WITH: To make this a complete meal, serve with riced broccoli and a green salad.
PER SERVING
calories: 474 | fat: 37.6g | total carbs: 0.7g | fiber: 0.1g | protein: 32.6g

CHEESY VERDE SHRIMP

Macros: Fat 45% | Protein 50% | Carbs 5%
Prep time: 10 minutes | Cook time: 10 minutes | Serves 4

Ten minutes is all you need to create this delicious, healthy, and super tasty shrimp dish. These shrimps are thoroughly mixed with olive oil and garlic and topped with lots of Parmesan cheese.

2 tablespoons olive oil
2 garlic cloves, minced
¼ cup scallions, chopped
1 pound (454 g) fresh shrimps,
deveined, and peeled
½ cup parsley, chopped
½ cup Parmesan cheese, grated

1. In a large skillet, heat the olive oil over medium heat.
2. Add the garlic and chopped scallions and sauté briefly, making sure the garlic does not turn brown.
3. Add the shrimps and cook until they become opaque. Sprinkle chopped parsley over the shrimp.
4. Remove cooked shrimps from heat. Serve on a dish and sprinkle with grated cheese.

STORAGE: Place the cooked shrimp in an airtight container and store in the fridge for up to 3 days.
REHEAT: Preheat the oven to 300°F (150°C). Arrange shrimps in a single layer on a cooking tray, and cover with aluminum foil. Place the covered tray in the oven and cook for around 15 minutes.
SERVE IT WITH: This dish goes well with warm kale salad, cauliflower rice, or zucchini noodles.
PER SERVING
calories: 215 | fat: 10.9g | total carbs: 3.2g | fiber: 0.4g | protein: 26.8g

BEST MARINATED GRILLED SHRIMP

Macros: Fat 47% | Protein 52% | Carbs 1%
Prep time:15 minutes | Cook time:6 minutes | Serves 6

A very simple and easy marinade that makes your shrimps so yummy and it doesn't even need any cocktail dressings. It's super easy, delicious and quick to make.

⅓ cup olive oil
3 cloves garlic, minced
2 tablespoons chopped fresh basil
2 tablespoons red wine vinegar
½ teaspoon salt

¼ teaspoon cayenne pepper
2 pounds (907 g) fresh shrimp, peeled and deveined
1 tablespoon olive oil, for greasing

SPECIAL EQUIPMENT:
6 wooden skewers, soaked for at least 30 minutes

1. Mix the olive oil, garlic, basil, red wine vinegar, salt, and cayenne in a large bowl. Stir in the shrimp and toss to coat well.
2. Cover the bowl with plastic wrap, then place in the refrigerator to marinate for 1 hour.
3. Preheat the grill to medium heat and lightly spray the grill grates with olive oil spray.
4. Thread the shrimp onto skewers, piercing once near the tail and once near the head, discarding the marinade.
5. Grill for 6 minutes, flipping occasionally, or until the shrimp is opaque.
6. Allow to cool for about 3 minutes and serve hot.

STORAGE: Store in an airtight container in the fridge for up to 3 days.
REHEAT: Microwave, covered, until the desired temperature is reached or reheat in a frying pan or air fryer / instant pot, covered, on medium.
SERVE IT WITH: To make this a complete meal, serve the shrimp with a glass of green smoothie.
PER SERVING
calories: 278 | fat: 14.6g | total carbs: 0.9g | fiber: 0.1g | protein: 36.4g

CHEESY KETO TUNA CASSEROLE

Macros: Fat 78% | Protein 18% | Carbs 4%
Prep time: 10 minutes | Cook time: 20 minutes | Serves 6 to 8

If you're a seafood person, you will enjoy this recipe to the utmost. You can freely make the cheesy keto tuna casserole yourself. With not much time, you will amaze your family members that you are the top chef in your family. Don't underestimate your abilities in making new dishes.

2 ounces (57 g) butter, divided
1 yellow onion
1 green bell pepper
5½ ounces (156 g) celery stalks
Salt and freshly ground black pepper, to taste

1 pound (454 g) tuna in olive oil, drained
1 teaspoon chili flakes
1 cup mayonnaise, keto-friendly
4 ounces (113 g) freshly shredded Parmesan cheese

SERVING:
6 ounces (170 g) baby spinach, sliced
2 tablespoons olive oil

1. Preheat the oven to 400℉ (205°C).
2. On a board, finely chop the yellow onion, green pepper, and celery, then sauté in a large skillet with 1 ounce (28 g) butter

until softened. Sprinkle with salt and pepper.
3. Mix the drained tuna, chili flakes, mayonnaise, Parmesan cheese, and pepper in a butter greased baking dish, add the seasoned fried vegetables to it, stir well.
4. Cook in the preheated oven for 15 to 20 minutes or until the tuna is opaque and the cheese melts.
5. Serve tuna and fried vegetables with sliced spinach and olive oil.

STORAGE: With ease, you can store the leftovers of keto tuna in an airtight bag in the fridge for up to 3 days or in the freezer for up to 5 days.
REHEAT: You can reheat the extras with a piece of cake by using a heavy skillet with a little butter or oil as desired on medium-low heat until tuna moistened through.
SERVE IT WITH: Serve it with the crunchy vegetable salad to enjoy eating the meal with your friends, or serve it with Savory Pork Salad.
PER SERVING
calories: 493 | fat: 40.1g | total carbs: 5.5g | fiber: 1.4g | protein: 20.4g

CREAMY SALMON SAUCE ZOODLES

Macros: Fat 66% | Protein 26% | Carbs 8%
Prep time: 15 minutes | Cook time: 15 minutes | Serves 4

It's an enjoyable time to challenge your friends to try this rich recipes. Creamy salmon sauce zoodles will be your challenging game to make, it's easy to make it at all. The winner will take a priceless prize from his friends.

2 pounds (907 g) zucchini
Salt and freshly ground black pepper, to taste
4 ounces (113 g) cream cheese
1 cup heavy whipping cream

¼ cup chopped fresh basil
1 pound (454 g) smoked salmon
1 lime, juiced
2 tablespoons olive oil

1. Cut the zucchini after washing it thoroughly into thin slices with a sharp knife.
2. Prepare a colander to filter the zucchini, add a little salt and toss to coat well. Leave them sit for 7 to 12 minutes. Gently press the mixture to get rid of excess salted water.
3. Meanwhile, mix the cream cheese with lemon juice, chopped fresh basil in a bowl. Set aside until ready to serve.
4. Cut the salmon into thin slices and sprinkle with salt and pepper. Add the salmon to an oiled skillet and fry over medium-high heat for 8 minutes or until the salmon is opaque and tender on both sides. Then add zucchini spirals and cook for 2 minutes until soft.
5. Serve the recipe on a large plate with the cream sauce.

STORAGE: We can store extras or the leftovers of this recipe in an airtight container in the refrigerator for up to 5 days, because the recipe contains fish and it will go off if it exceeds this period.
REHEAT: To keep the salmon moist, reheat it inside a foil with a little of olive oil for 5 to 8 minutes in the oven.
SERVE IT WITH: Serve it warm with Italian Sausage and Zucchini Soup or with Creamy Paprika Pork.
PER SERVING
calories: 444 | fat: 33.4g | total carbs: 10.1g | fiber: 2.6g | protein: 29.3g

SALMON FILLETS BAKED WITH DIJON

Macros: Fat 40% | Protein 58% | Carbs 2%
Prep time: 10 minutes | Cook time: 15 minutes | Serves 4

Are you into seafood and want something fast, full of protein and keeping your keto routine? Salmon Fillets with Dijon is the one. A super rich dish that would be a true masterpiece on your table. Only in max 20 minutes.

4 (4-ounce / 113-g) salmon fillets
¼ cup butter, melted
3 tablespoons Dijon mustard
Salt and freshly ground black pepper, to taste
⅛ cup coconut flour

1. Preheat the oven to 400°F (205°C) and line a baking pan with aluminum foil.
2. In a bowl, mix the salmon fillets, butter, mustard, salt and pepper. Stir well until the salmon is fully coated.
3. Place the salmon in the baking pan, then evenly sprinkle the coconut flour on top.
4. Transfer the pan into the preheated oven and bake until the salmon easily flakes when tested with a fork, about 15 minutes.
5. Remove from the oven and cool for 5 minutes before serving.

STORAGE: Store in an airtight container in the fridge for up to 3 to 4 days or in the freezer for up to 1 month.
REHEAT: Microwave, covered, until the desired temperature is reached or reheat in a frying pan or air fryer / instant pot, covered, on medium.
SERVE IT WITH: You can serve it alongside cauliflower rice.
PER SERVING
calories: 484 | fat: 21.6g | total carbs: 2.7g | fiber: 0.5g | protein: 70.1g

BLACKENED TROUT

Macros: Fat 68% | Protein 31% | Carbs 1%
Prep time: 20 minutes | Cook time: 10 minutes | Serves 6

Looking for an easy seafood dish that tastes great? Give this blackened trout recipe a try! The recipe calls for trout, but you can substitute for red snapper or catfish.

2 teaspoons dry mustard
1 tablespoon paprika
1 teaspoon ground cumin
1 teaspoon cayenne pepper
1 teaspoon white pepper
1 teaspoon black pepper
1 teaspoon dried thyme
1 teaspoon salt
¾ cup unsalted butter, melted
6 (4-ounce / 113-g) trout fillets
1 tablespoon olive oil

1. Combine the dry mustard, paprika, cumin, cayenne pepper, white pepper, black pepper, thyme, and salt in a medium bowl. Stir to combine and set aside.
2. Put ¾ cup butter on a platter, then dredge the trout fillets into the butter to coat evenly. Sprinkle with the spicy mixture, gently pressing the mixture into the fillets.
3. Heat the olive oil in a skillet over medium-high heat, then add the fillets. Cook the fish for about 2 to 3 minutes per side, turning occasionally, or until the fish is lightly browned on the edges.
4. Remove from the heat and serve warm.

STORAGE: Store in an airtight container and store in the fridge for 3 to 4 days or up to a month in the freezer.
REHEAT: Microwave, covered, until the desired temperature is reached or reheat in a frying pan or air fryer / instant pot, covered, on medium.
SERVE IT WITH: To make this a complete meal, you can serve it with beef stew, and kale and spinach salad.
PER SERVING
calories: 328| fat: 25.0g | total carbs: 1.7g | fiber: 0.8g | protein: 24.0g

TROUT FILLETS WITH LEMONY YOGURT SAUCE

Macros: Fat 36% | Protein 57% | Carbs 7%
Prep time: 12 minutes | Cook time: 8 to 10 minutes | Serves 4

Enjoy this tender trout that is served with a tangy, lemony yogurt sauce! This is definitely a recipe you will make several times for your family.

1 cup plain Greek yogurt
1 cucumber, shredded
1 teaspoon lemon zest
1 tablespoon extra-virgin olive oil
Salt and freshly ground black
pepper, to taste
2 tablespoons fresh dill weed, chopped
1 pinch lemon pepper
4 (6-ounce / 170-g) rainbow trout fillets

1. Mix the yogurt, cucumber, lemon zest, olive oil, salt, and pepper in a bowl. Stir thoroughly and set aside.
2. Preheat the oven to 400°F (205°C).
3. Sprinkle the lemon pepper on top and arrange the fillets in a greased baking dish.
4. Bake in the preheated oven for about 8 to 10 minutes or until fork-tender.
5. Remove from the oven and serve the fish alongside the yogurt sauce.

STORAGE: Store in an airtight container in the fridge for up to 2 days. Not recommend freezing.
REHEAT: Microwave the fillets, covered, until the desired temperature is reached.
SERVE IT WITH: To make this a complete meal, you can serve it with fresh cucumber soup.
PER SERVING
calories: 281 | fat: 11.4g | total carbs: 5.3g | fiber: 0.7g | protein: 37.6g

DELICIOUS KETO CEVICHE

Macros: Fat 39% | Protein 50% | Carbs 11%
Prep time: 15 minutes | Cook time: 0 minutes | Serves 4

What a colorful fish! You always have plenty of time to make this easy but incredible recipe. ceviche with its simple ingredient will make your table full of splendid colors.

1 pound (454 g) skinless white fish, cut into ½-inch cubes
½ red onion, thinly sliced
1 fresh jalapeño, deseeded and thinly sliced
¼ red bell pepper, thinly sliced
1 tablespoon salt
¾ cup lime juice, plus more as needed

FOR SERVING:
2 tablespoons lime juice
1 lime, cut into wedges
2 tablespoons olive oil
4 tablespoons fresh cilantro, minced

1. Prepare a dish with a lid to put the skinless white fish, then add the onions, jalapeño, thinly sliced bell pepper, and salt. Toss to coat the fish well. Pour the lime juice over.
2. Leave the fish in the fridge for about 3 hours for infusing.
3. Take the fish and vegetables out of the fridge and discard the marinade. Rinse the fish and vegetables thoroughly with cold water.
4. Place the fish on a serving dish, then drizzle with olive oil and lemon juice. Spread the fresh cilantro for topping. Serve cold with lime.

STORAGE: You can easily store extras or the leftovers of keto ceviche in an airtight bag in the freezer for up to 3 days.
SERVE IT WITH: Serve it chilled with creamy paprika pork to let your dinner perfect.
PER SERVING
calories: 174 | fat:7.6g | total carbs: 6.3g | fiber: 0.6g | protein: 20.7g

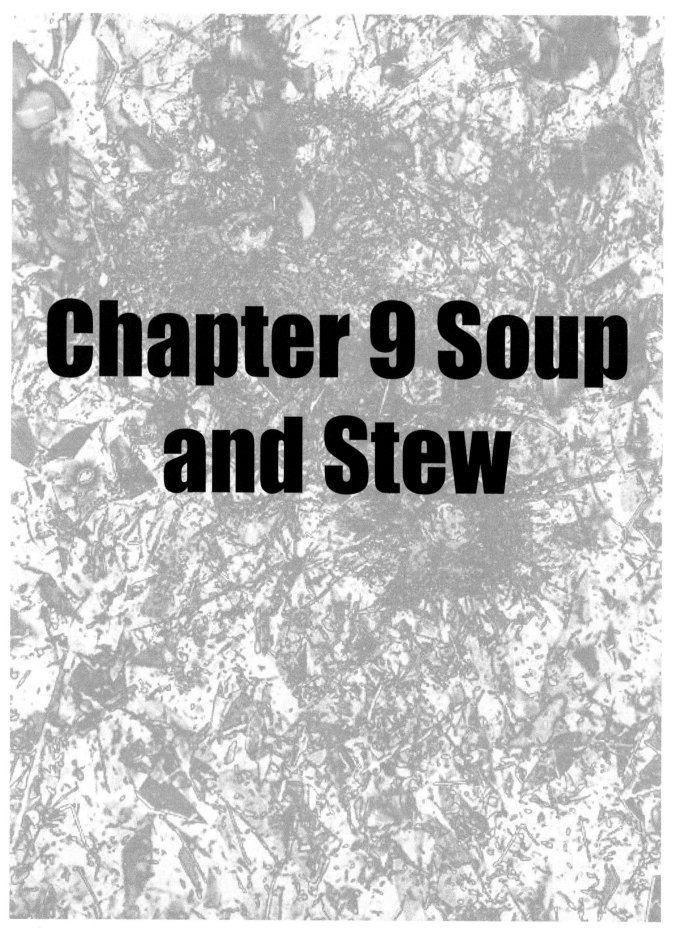

Chapter 9 Soup and Stew

CHEESY CAULIFLOWER SOUP

Macros: Fat 68% | Protein 17% | Carbs 15%
Prep time: 10 minutes | Cook time: 30 minutes | Serves 8

Awarming bowl of cauliflower soup is a perfect serving for every dinner table. The cheese rich recipe offers you a mix of healthy fat and protein. All the ingredients, including cauliflower, are cooked into a smooth and creamy soup, which is mixed with cream and cheese.

¼ cup butter
1 head cauliflower, chopped
½ onion, chopped
½ teaspoon ground nutmeg
4 cups chicken stock

1 cup heavy whipping cream
Salt and freshly ground black pepper, to taste
1 cup Cheddar cheese, shredded

SPECIAL EQUIPMENT:
An immersion blender

1. Take a large stockpot and place it over medium heat.
2. Add butter to this pot and let it melt.
3. Add cauliflower and onion to the melted butter and sauté for 10 minutes until these veggies are soft.
4. Add nutmeg and chicken stock to the pot and bring to a boil.
5. Reduce the heat to low and allow it to simmer for 15 minutes.
6. Remove the stockpot from the heat and then add heavy cream.
7. Purée the cooked soup with an immersion blender until smooth.
8. Sprinkle this soup with salt and black pepper.
9. Garnish with Cheddar cheese and serve warm.

STORAGE: Store in an airtight container in the fridge for up to 3 days or in the freezer for up to 1 month.
REHEAT: Microwave, covered, until the desired temperature is reached or reheat in a saucepan or slow cooker / instant pot, covered, on medium.
SERVE IT WITH: To make this a complete meal, serve the cauliflower soup with roasted cheesy asparagus on the side.**PER SERVING**
calories: 224 | fat: 16.8g | total carbs: 10.8g | fiber: 2.2g | protein: 9.6g

CAULIFLOWER CREAM SOUP

Macros: Fat 78% | Protein 16% | Carbs 6%
Prep time: 15 minutes | Cook time: 4 hours 10 minutes | Serves 5

Cauliflower makes a good serving for every healthy diet plan, and this creamy cauliflower bacon soup will make a delicious meal to serve at the table. The smooth and creamy soup is mixed with crispy bacon bits, which give it a unique taste and texture.

10 slices bacon
3 small heads cauliflower, cored and cut into florets
4 cups chicken broth
¼ cup (½ stick) salted butter
3 cloves garlic, pressed

½ large yellow onion, chopped
1 cup heavy whipping cream
2 cups Cheddar cheese, shredded
Salt and black pepper, to taste
Freshly chopped chives or green onions, for garnish

SPECIAL EQUIPMENT:
An immersion blender

1. Take a large skillet and place it over medium heat.
2. Add bacon to the skillet and cook for about 8 minutes until brown and crispy.
3. Transfer the cooked bacon to a paper towel-lined plate to absorb the excess grease.
4. Allow the bacon to cool, then chop it. Wrap the plate of chopped bacon in plastic and refrigerate it.

5. Add the cauliflower florets to the food processor and pulse until chopped thoroughly.
6. Add chicken broth, butter, garlic, onion, and chopped cauliflower to the slow cooker.
7. Give all these ingredients a gentle stir, then put on the lid.
8. Cook the cauliflower soup for 4 hours on high heat.
9. Once the cauliflower is tender, purée the soup with an immersion blender until smooth.
10. Add chopped bacon, heavy cream, cheese, salt, and black pepper. Mix well and let the cheese melt in the hot soup.
11. Garnish with green onions or chives, then serve warm.

STORAGE: Store in an airtight container in the fridge for up to 2 days or in the freezer for up to 1 month.
REHEAT: Microwave, covered, until the desired temperature is reached or reheat in a saucepan or instant pot, covered, on medium.
SERVE IT WITH: To make this a complete meal, serve the cauliflower cream soup with crispy bacon strips on the side.
PER SERVING
calories: 627 | fat: 54.3g | total carbs: 13.7g | fiber: 3.7g | protein: 24.6g

SHRIMP MUSHROOM CHOWDER

Macros: Fat 76% | Protein 18% | Carbs 6%
Prep time: 10 minutes | Cook time: 40 minutes | Serves 6

It's about time to add some seafood to the menu and enjoy a delicious bowl of soup mixed with tasty shrimp. The combination of shrimp with mushrooms and onions becomes irresistible when these ingredients are cooked in a mixture of coconut milk and bone broth.

¼ cup refined avocado oil
⅓ cup diced yellow onions
1⅔ cups diced mushrooms
10½ ounces (298 g) small raw shrimp, shelled and deveined
1 can (13½-ounce / 383-g) unsweetened coconut milk
⅓ cup chicken bone broth
2 tablespoons apple cider vinegar
1 teaspoon onion powder
1 teaspoon paprika

1 bay leaf
¾ teaspoon finely ground gray sea salt
½ teaspoon dried oregano leaves
¼ teaspoon ground black pepper
1 medium zucchini (7-ounce / 198-g), cubed
12 radishes (6-ounce / 170-g), cubed

1. Add avocado oil to a large saucepan and place it over medium heat.
2. Add onions and mushrooms to the pan and sauté for 10 minutes or until onions are soft and mushrooms are lightly browned.
3. Stir in shrimp, coconut milk, chicken broth, apple cider vinegar, onion powder, paprika, bay leaf, sea salt, oregano leaves, and black pepper.
4. Cover the soup mixture with a lid and cook for 20 minutes on low heat.
5. Add zucchini and radishes to the soup and cook for 10 minutes.
6. Remove the bay leaf from the soup and divide the soup into 6 small serving bowls. Serve hot.

STORAGE: Store in an airtight container in the fridge for up to 3 days or in the freezer for up to 1 month.
REHEAT: Microwave, covered, until the desired temperature is reached or reheat in a slow cooker or instant pot, covered, on medium.
SERVE IT WITH: To make this a complete meal, serve the shrimp mushroom soup with roasted green beans on the side.
PER SERVING
calories: 311 | fat: 26.3g | total carbs: 7.7g | fiber: 2.9g | protein: 13.7g

EGG BROTH

Macros: Fat 76% | Protein 17% | Carbs 7%
Prep time: 5 minutes | Cook time: 5 minutes | Serves 4

It is the simplest egg soup recipe that you can find. If you have chicken broth left in your refrigerator, then you can make food use of it by making a comforting and warming soup. Simply cook the broth with beaten eggs and add some seasonings as per your taste and Voila!

2 tablespoons unsalted butter	Salt and black pepper, to taste
4 cups chicken broth	1 sliced green onion, for garnish
3 large eggs	

1. Take a medium stockpot and place it over high heat.
2. Add butter and chicken broth to the pot and bring to a boil.
3. Break eggs into a bowl and beat them for 1 minute with a fork until frothy.
4. Once the broth boils, slowly pour in beaten eggs while stirring the broth with a spoon.
5. Cook for 1 minute with continuously stirring, then sprinkle salt and black pepper to season.
6. Garnish with sliced green onion, then serve warm.

STORAGE: Store in an airtight container in the fridge for up to 2 days or in the freezer for up to 1 month.
REHEAT: Microwave, covered, until the desired temperature is reached or reheat in a saucepan or slow cooker / instant pot, covered, on medium.
SERVE IT WITH: To make this a complete meal, serve the egg broth soup with tomato cheese salad on the side.
PER SERVING
calories: 93 | fat: 7.8g | total carbs: 1.8g | fiber: 0.1g | protein: 3.9g

PORK TARRAGON SOUP

Macros: Fat 66% | Protein 28% | Carbs 6%
Prep time:10 minutes | Cook time: 1 hour 20 minutes | Serves 6

Have you tried a pork soup which has a distinct taste of turnips and dried herbs? The recipe is perfect for all those who are looking for a complete package of nutrients in a single meal. It is prepared out of pork, bacon, lard, broth, herbs, and spices.

⅓ cup lard	¼ cup dry white wine
1 pound (454 g) pork loin, cut into ½-inch (1.25-cm) pieces	1¾ cups chicken bone broth
10 strips bacon (about 10-ounce / 284-g), cut into ½-inch (1.25-cm) pieces	4 sprigs fresh thyme
	2 tablespoons unflavored gelatin
¾ cup sliced shallots	2 tablespoons apple cider vinegar
3 medium turnips (about 12½-ounce / 354-g), cubed	½ cup unsweetened coconut milk
1 tablespoon yellow mustard	1 tablespoon dried tarragon leaves

1. Take a large saucepan and place it over medium heat.
2. Add lard to the saucepan and allow it to melt.
3. Add pork pieces to the melted lard and sauté for 8 minutes until golden brown.
4. Add bacon pieces and sliced shallots and sauté for 5 minutes or until fragrant.
5. Add turnips, mustard, wine, bone broth, and thyme sprigs to the soup.
6. Mix these ingredients gently and cover this soup with a lid.
7. Bring the soup to a boil, then reduce the heat to medium-low. Cook this soup for 1 hour.

8. Remove and discard the thyme sprigs from the soup then add gelatin, vinegar, coconut milk, and tarragon.
9. Increase the heat to medium and bring the soup to a boil. Cover to cook for 10 minutes.
10. Divide the cooked soup into 6 serving bowls and serve warm.

STORAGE: Store in an airtight container in the fridge for up to 4 days or in the freezer for up to 1 month.
REHEAT: Microwave, covered, until the desired temperature is reached or reheat in a slow cooker or instant pot, covered, on medium.
SERVE IT WITH: To make this a complete meal, serve the pork tarragon soup with fresh avocado guacamole on the side.
PER SERVING
calories: 566 | fat: 41.5g | total carbs: 9.7g | fiber: 1.2g | protein: 39.6g

CREAMY BROCCOLI AND CAULIFLOWER SOUP

Macros: Fat 80% | Protein 10% | Carbs 10%
Prep time:20 minutes | Cook time:15 minutes | Serves 6

If you have been wondering about novel ways to add broccoli to your diet, then this soup is the perfect way to have more broccoli every other day. This cream soup is made of a puréed mixture of cooked cauliflower and broccoli, which is then mixed with a pleasant combination of seasonings.

1 (13½-ounce / 383-g) can unsweetened coconut milk	roughly chopped
	1 large head broccoli, cored and cut into large florets
2 cups vegetable stock	
1 (14-ounce / 397-g) small head cauliflower, cored and cut into large florets	¼ teaspoon ground black pepper
	¼ teaspoon ground white pepper
2 medium celery sticks, chopped	⅓ cup butter-infused olive oil
1 teaspoon finely ground gray sea salt	1 chopped green onion, for garnish
6 green onions, green parts only,	

1. Take a large saucepan and place it over medium heat.
2. Add coconut milk, vegetable stock, cauliflower florets, chopped celery, salt, and green onions.
3. Mix them gently, then cover and bring the soup to a boil.
4. Continue cooking the soup for 15 minutes until the cauliflower florets are soft.
5. Meanwhile, blanch the broccoli in a pot of boiling water for 1 minute until soft but still crisp, then drain on a paper towel. Set aside on a plate.
6. When the cauliflower soup is cooked, transfer it to a blender.
7. Add black pepper, white pepper, and olive oil. Blend the soup for 1 minute until smooth.
8. Add the soft broccoli and blend again for 30 seconds.
9. Divide the cooked broccoli and cauliflower soup into 6 serving bowls.
10. Garnish with chopped green onions and serve warm.

STORAGE: Store in an airtight container in the fridge for up to 2 days or in the freezer for up to 1 month.
REHEAT: Microwave, covered, until the desired temperature is reached or reheat in a slow cooker or instant pot, covered, on medium.
SERVE IT WITH: To make this a complete meal, serve the broccoli soup with roasted artichoke hearts on the side.
PER SERVING
calories: 264 | fat: 23.3g | total carbs: 10.3g | fiber: 3.6g | protein: 6.9g

CHICKEN TURNIP SOUP

Macros: Fat 66% | Protein 33% | Carbs 1%
Prep time: 10 minutes | Cook time: 6 to 8 hours | Serves 5

The low-carb chicken turnip soup is just the right recipe for a light and healthy diet. You can use cooked leftover chicken to make this soup in no time. As long as you have water, onions, turnips, and some basic seasonings, you can get it ready in a slow cooker within 8 hours.

12 ounces (340g) bone-in chicken
¼ cup turnip, chopped
¼ cup onions, chopped
4 garlic cloves, smashed
4 cups water

3 sprigs thyme
2 bay leaves
Salt, to taste
¼ teaspoon freshly ground black pepper

1. Put the chicken, turnip, onions, garlic, water, thyme springs, and bay leaves in a slow cooker.
2. Season with salt and pepper, then give the mixture a good stir.
3. Cover and cook on low for 6 to 8 hours until the chicken is cooked through.
4. When ready, remove the bay leaves and shred the chicken with a fork.
5. Divide the soup among five bowls and serve.

STORAGE: Store in an airtight container in the fridge for up to 4 days or in the freezer for up to 1 month.
REHEAT: Microwave, covered, until the desired temperature is reached or reheat in a saucepan or instant pot, covered, on medium.
SERVE IT WITH: To make this a complete meal, serve the chicken turnip soup with sautéed spinach on the side.
PER SERVING
calories: 186 | fat: 13.6g | total carbs: 3.3g | fiber: 2.6g | protein: 15.2g

SPINACH MUSHROOM SOUP

Macros: Fat 83% | Protein 6% | Carbs 11%
Prep time: 10 minutes | Cook time: 5 minutes | Serves 3

With this classic spinach-mushroom recipe, you can enjoy a clear vegetable soup mixed with the goodness of sesame seeds and garlic. Flavored with tamari sauce, this spinach soup stands out from the rest for its unique taste and aroma.

1 tablespoon olive oil
1 teaspoon garlic, finely chopped
1 cup spinach, torn into small pieces
½ cup mushrooms, chopped

Salt and freshly ground black pepper, to taste
½ teaspoon tamari
3 cups vegetable stock
1 teaspoon sesame seeds, roasted

1. Place a saucepan over medium heat and add olive oil to heat.
2. Add garlic to the hot oil and sauté for 30 seconds or until fragrant.
3. Add spinach and mushrooms, then sauté for 1 minute or until lightly tender.
4. Add salt, black pepper, tamari, and vegetable stock. Cook for another 3 minutes. Stir constantly.
5. Garnish with sesame seeds and serve warm.

STORAGE: Store in an airtight container in the fridge for up to 4 days or in the freezer for up to 1 month.
REHEAT: Microwave, covered, until the desired temperature is reached or reheat in a slow cooker or instant pot, covered, on medium.
SERVE IT WITH: To make this a complete meal, serve the spinach mushrooms soup with roasted asparagus sticks on the side.
PER SERVING
calories: 80 | fat: 7.4g | total carbs: 3.2g | fiber: 1.1g | protein: 1.2g

GARLICKY CHICKEN SOUP

Macros: Fat 83% | Protein16% | Carbs 1%
Prep time:10 minutes | Cook time: 10 minutes | Serves 4

This creamy chicken soup is a valuable addition to your nutritious menu. And it can be served as a fancy meal on the table. It has a unique combination of flavors for the use of Garlic Gusto Seasoning with heavy cream and cream cheese.

2 tablespoons butter
1 large chicken breast cut into strips
4 ounces (113 g) cream cheese, cubed
2 tablespoons Garlic Gusto

Seasoning
½ cup heavy cream
14½ ounces (411 g) chicken broth
Salt, to taste

1. Place a saucepan over medium heat and add butter to melt.
2. Add chicken strips and sauté for 2 minutes.
3. Add cream cheese and seasoning, and cook for 3 minutes, stirring occasionally.
4. Pour in the heavy cream and chicken broth. Bring the soup to a boil, then lower the heat.
5. Allow the soup to simmer for 4 minutes, then sprinkle with salt.
6. Let cool for 5 minutes and serve while warm.

STORAGE: Store in an airtight container in the fridge for up to 2 days or in the freezer for up to 1 month.
REHEAT: Microwave, covered, until the desired temperature is reached or reheat in a slow cooker or instant pot, covered, on medium.
SERVE IT WITH: To make this a complete meal, serve the garlicky chicken soup with roasted green beans on the side.
PER SERVING
calories: 243 | fat: 22.5g | total carbs: 7.0g | fiber: 6.6g | protein: 9.6g

STEWED MAHI MAHI

Macros: Fat 63% | Protein 29% | Carbs 8%
Prep time: 15 minutes | Cook time: 33 minutes | Serves 2

Mahi mahi is a special fish that will satisfy your craving as you follow the keto diet. You can add your favorite keto-friendly spices to improve the taste. The recipe is perfect for lunch or dinner.

¾ pound (340 g) cubed Mahi Mahi fillets
Salt and freshly ground black pepper, to taste

1½ tablespoons butter
½ chopped onion
¾ cup homemade fish broth
Fresh cilantro, for garnish

1. In a bowl, season the mahi mahi fillets with black pepper and salt.
2. Melt the butter in a pressure cooker, then stir in the onions.
3. Cook the onions until soft for about 3 minutes.
4. Pour in the fish broth and then add the mahi mahi fillets.
5. Cook covered for 30 minutes at high pressure.
6. Release the pressure naturally and serve hot with fresh cilantro sprinkled on top.

STORAGE: Store in an airtight container in the fridge for up to 1 week
REHEAT: Microwave, covered, until the desired temperature is reached.
SERVE IT WITH: To make this a complete meal, serve the stewed mahi mahi with roasted cabbage with bacon.
PER SERVING
calories: 571 | fat 39.9g | total carbs: 22.6g | fiber: 11.4g | protein 34.5g

CAULIFLOWER CURRY SOUP

Macros: Fat 77% | Protein 9% | Carbs 14%
Prep time:15 minutes | Cook time: 26 minutes | Serves 4

This cauliflower curry soup is loved for its tangy flavors. The cauliflower florets are cooked with a spicy mixture of broth, Serrano pepper, curry powder, and other spices. You can adjust the proportion of spices according to your taste preference. The coconut milk in the recipe brings the much-needed balance in the flavors.

2 tablespoons avocado oil	½ teaspoon black pepper
1 white onion, chopped	1 teaspoon salt
4 garlic cloves, chopped	1 cup of water
½ Serrano pepper, seeds removed and chopped	1 large cauliflower, cut into florets
1-inch ginger, chopped	1 cup chicken broth
¼ teaspoon turmeric powder	1 can unsweetened coconut milk
2 teaspoons curry powder	Cilantro, for garnish

1. Place a saucepan over medium heat and add oil to heat.
2. Add onions to the hot oil and sauté them for 3 minutes.
3. Add garlic, Serrano pepper, and ginger, then sauté for 2 minutes.
4. Add turmeric, curry powder, black pepper, and salt. Cook for 1 minute after a gentle stir.
5. Pour water into the pan, then add cauliflower.
6. Cover this soup with a lid and cook for 10 minutes. Stir constantly.
7. Remove the soup from the heat and allow it to cool at room temperature.
8. Transfer this soup to a blender and purée the soup until smooth.
9. Return the soup to the saucepan and add broth and coconut milk. Cook for 10 minutes more and stir frequently.
10. Divide the soup into four bowls and sprinkle the cilantro on top for garnish before serving.

STORAGE: Store in an airtight container in the fridge for up to 4 days or in the freezer for up to 1 month.
REHEAT: Microwave, covered, until the desired temperature is reached or reheat in a slow cooker or instant pot, covered, on medium.
SERVE IT WITH: To make this a complete meal, serve the cauliflower curry soup with avocado fries on the side.
PER SERVING
calories: 342 | fat: 29.1g | total carbs: 18.3g | fiber: 5.5g | protein: 7.17g

RED GAZPACHO CREAM SOUP

Macros: Fat 78% | Protein 15% | Carbs 7%
Prep time: 15 minutes | Cook time:20 minutes | Serves 10

The Gazpacho soup is known for its roasted bell pepper taste, which is then enhanced by the combination of pepper with basil, spring onion, tomatoes, and other vegetables and seasonings. With this recipe, you can get to enjoy so many nutrients in a single meal.

1 large red bell pepper, halved	2 tablespoons apple cider vinegar
1 large green bell pepper, halved	2 garlic cloves
2 tablespoons basil, freshly chopped	2 tablespoons fresh lemon juice
4 medium tomatoes	1 cup extra virgin olive oil
1 small red onion	Salt and black pepper, to taste
1 large cucumber, diced	1¼ pounds (567 g) feta cheese, shredded
2 medium spring onions, diced	

1. Preheat the oven to 400°F (205°C) and line a baking tray with parchment paper.
2. Place all the bell peppers in the baking tray and roast in the preheated oven for 20 minutes.
3. Remove the bell peppers from the oven. Allow to cool, then peel off their skin.
4. Transfer the peeled bell peppers to a blender along with basil, tomatoes, red onions, cucumber, spring onions, vinegar, garlic, lemon juice, olive oil, black pepper, and salt. Blend until the mixture smooth.
5. Add black pepper and salt to taste.
6. Garnish with feta cheese and serve warm.

STORAGE: Store in an airtight container in the fridge for up to 4 days or in the freezer for up to 1 month.
REHEAT: Microwave, covered, until the desired temperature is reached or reheat in a saucepan or slow cooker / instant pot, covered, on medium.
SERVE IT WITH: To make this a complete meal, serve the bell pepper soup with deviled eggs on the side.
PER SERVING
calories: 248 | fat: 21.6g | total carbs: 8.3g | fiber: 4.1g | protein: 9.3g

SOUR AND SPICY SHRIMP SOUP WITH MUSHROOMS

Macros: Fat: 45% | Protein: 41% | Carbs: 14%
Prep time: 10 minutes | Cook time: 39 minutes | Serves 6

This sour and spicy shrimp soup with mushrooms is a delicious dish laden with body-cleansing spices. This spicy soup can be a variety of things for anyone. From comfort food to a warm bowl, this shrimp soup brings seafood to your taste buds in unexplored ways.

3 tablespoons butter	1 tablespoon coconut oil
1 pound (454 g) shrimp, peeled and deveined	1 small green zucchini
1 piece ginger root, peeled	½ pound (227 g) cremini mushrooms, sliced into wedges
½ teaspoon fresh lime zest	2 tablespoons fish sauce
1 medium onion, diced	2 tablespoons fresh lime juice
4 garlic cloves	¼ cup fresh Thai basil, coarsely chopped
1 stalk lemongrass	¼ bunch fresh cilantro, coarsely chopped
1 red Thai chili, roughly chopped	
Salt and black pepper, to taste	
5 cups chicken broth	

1. Heat the butter in a pot over medium heat and add the shrimps. Cook for 1 minute.
2. Mix it well with a wooden spoon and add the ginger root, lime zest, onion, garlic, lemongrass stalk, red Thai chili, salt, and pepper. Cook, covered, for 3 minutes.
3. Pour the broth into the pot and let it cook for 30 minutes. Drain the liquid from the ingredients in the pot.
4. Put a pan over high heat and add the coconut oil, zucchini, and mushrooms to the pan, then season it with salt and pepper. Let fry for 3 minutes, then add the shrimp mixture.
5. Mix the contents of the pan and let it cook for 2 minutes, then add the fish sauce, lime juice, salt, and black pepper.
6. Let it cook for 1 minute and mix in the basil and cilantro.
7. Serve immediately.

STORAGE: Store in an airtight container in the fridge for up to 4 days or in the freezer for up to 1 month.
REHEAT: Microwave, covered, until the desired temperature is reached or reheat in a frying pan or instant pot, covered, on medium.
PER SERVING
calories: 180| fat: 9.1g | total carbs: 7.6g | fiber: 1.4g | protein: 18.4g

RICH BEEF STEW WITH DUMPLING

Macros: Fat 42% | Protein 46% | Carbs 12%
Prep time: 10 minutes | Cook time: 4 hours | Serves 8

Comforting, cozy, and warming, this highly indulgent fare is a delightfully tender stew with melt in your mouth tender beef pieces. And the daikon radish is a delicious and perfect vegetable in making a keto-friendly soup. The flavor explosion when you take the first bite is so good and indisputable. Though I eat this by itself, if you want to make, you can replace the dumplings to mashed cauliflower.

2 tablespoons olive oil, divided
2 pounds (907 g) stew beef
1 red onion, chopped
1 daikon radish, chopped
3½ ounces (99-g) pumpkin, chopped
3 sprigs of fresh rosemary

3 bay leaves
2 cloves garlic, minced
½ cup dry red wine
2 cups beef stock
¾ teaspoon sea salt
¼ teaspoon black pepper

DUMPLINGS:
¾ cup almond flour
⅓ cup sesame seed flour
1 tablespoon fresh thyme
1 tablespoon psyllium husk powder
1 cup water, boiling
¼ cup coconut flour
1½ teaspoons gluten-free baking powder

1 tablespoon chopped rosemary
¼ teaspoon of sea salt
1 pinch black pepper
3 large egg whites
1 large beaten egg
1 teaspoon fresh lemon zest, for garnish
Fresh parsley, for garnish

1. Preheat the oven to 325°F (160°C).
2. Heat a large saucepan over medium heat and place 1 tablespoon of olive oil and beef in it.
3. Sear the meat for 4 minutes on each side or until browned. Transfer to a paper-lined plate.
4. Pour the remaining oil to it along with onion, radish, and pumpkin.
5. Sauté the vegetables for 8 minutes and add rosemary, bay leaves, garlic, and browned meat.
6. Cook for a further 2 minutes and pour the wine. Lower the heat and continue cooking for an additional 4 minutes.
7. Stir in the stock, salt, and pepper. Mix well and allow it to boil. Pour the mixture to the baking dish.
8. Roast the mixture for 3 hours. Remove from the oven and increase the temperature of the oven to 350°F (180°C).
9. In the meantime, combine almond flour, sesame seed flour, thyme, husk powder, water, coconut flour, baking powder, rosemary, salt, pepper, egg whites and egg. Make dumplings out of this dough.
10. Keep the dumplings in greased cupcake tins and bake in the oven for 23 minutes.
11. Flip with a spoon and bake for another 4 minutes.
12. Gently place the dumplings into the stew and gently stir.
13. Serve in bowls and enjoy it hot. Garnish with lemon zest and parsley.

STORAGE: Store in an airtight container in the refrigerator for up to 3 days. If you are planning to freeze, make, and add the dumplings on day before.
REHEAT: Microwave, covered, until the desired temperature is reached or reheat in a pan / instant pot, covered, on low.
SERVE IT WITH: To make this a complete meal, you can serve it with a cherry tomato and mushroom salad and fried pork chop.
PER SERVING
calories: 282 | fat: 10.8g | total carbs: 9.8g | fiber: 1.2g | protein: 32.2g

ZUCCHINI CREAM SOUP

Macros: Fat 43% | Protein 51% | Carbs 6%
Prep time: 15 minutes | Cook time: 20 minutes | Serves 4

Zucchini is known for its fiber-rich juicy content, and when it is added to the meal, it is super healthy. In this soup, the zucchini chunks are cooked with a mixture of sour cream, broth, cheese, and butter. The cooked soup is blended well to get a smooth and creamy mixture to serve.

2 tablespoons butter
2 pounds (907 g) chicken broth
2 garlic cloves
2 medium zucchinis, cut into large chunks

½ small onion, quartered
4 tablespoons sour cream
Salt and black pepper, to taste
1 cup Parmesan cheese, freshly grated

1. Place a medium pot over medium heat and add butter, chicken broth, garlic, zucchini, and onion.
2. Bring the mixture to a boil, then reduces the heat to medium-low. Simmer the soup for 20 minutes.
3. Remove the pot from the heat and allow it to cool for 10 minutes.
4. Use an immersion blender to purée the soup until smooth.
5. Add sour cream, salt, cheese and black pepper, and stir well. Serve warm.

STORAGE: Store in an airtight container in the fridge for up to 2 days or in the freezer for up to 1 month.
REHEAT: Microwave, covered, until the desired temperature is reached or reheat in a saucepan or slow cooker / instant pot, covered, on medium.
SERVE IT WITH: To make this a complete meal, serve the zucchini soup with sautéed zucchini noodles on the side.
PER SERVING
calories: 425 | fat: 20.2g | total carbs: 7.0g | fiber: 0.5g | protein: 54.3g

SWISS CHARD EGG SOUP

Macros: Fat 80% | Protein 12% | Carbs 8%
Prep time: 5 minutes | Cook time: 15 minutes | Serves 4

There is no better way to make use of Swiss chard than this delicious and healthy low-carb soup. In this recipe, the Swiss chard is cooked with broth, butter, eggs, and other seasonings. Serve it warm with your favorite green herbs.

3 cups beef bone broth
2 eggs, whisked
2 tablespoons coconut amino
3 tablespoons butter

2 cups Swiss chard, chopped
1 teaspoon ground oregano
1 teaspoon ginger, grated
Salt and black pepper, to taste

1. Take a large-sized saucepan and place it over medium heat.
2. Add bone broth to the pan and allow it to heat for 5 minutes.
3. Add whisked eggs to the broth. Stir constantly.
4. Add coconut amino, butter, Swiss chard, oregano, ginger, black pepper, and salt.
5. Mix well and cook the soup for 10 minutes.
6. Serve warm and fresh.

STORAGE: Store in an airtight container in the fridge for up to 2 days or in the freezer for up to 1 month.
REHEAT: Microwave, covered, until the desired temperature is reached or reheat in a saucepan or slow cooker / instant pot, covered, on medium.
SERVE IT WITH: To make this a complete meal, serve the egg chard soup with roasted cauliflower florets on the side.
PER SERVING
calories: 237 | fat: 21.0g | total carbs: 6.6g | fiber: 1.8g | protein: 7.3g

ASPARAGUS CREAM SOUP

Macros: Fat 63% | Protein 16% | Carbs 21%
Prep time: 15 minutes | Cook time:22 minutes | Serves 6

If you are living on a low-carb healthy diet, then nothing is more perfect than this asparagus soup. We enjoy asparagus in a variety of its recipes; in this one, the green sticks are cooked with onion, broth, butter, and sour cream to make a rich and creamy soup.

4 tablespoons butter	Salt and black pepper, to taste
1 small onion, chopped	2 pounds (907g) asparagus, cut
6 cups low-sodium chicken	in half
broth	½ cup sour cream

1. Place a large pot over low heat and add butter to melt.
2. Add onion to the melted butter and sauté for 2 minutes or until soft.
3. Add chicken broth, salt, black pepper, and asparagus.
4. Bring the soup to a boil, then cover the lid and cook for 20 minutes.
5. Remove the pot from the heat and allow it to cool for 5 minutes.
6. Transfer the soup to a blender and blend until smooth.
7. Add sour cream and pulse again to mix well.
8. Serve fresh and warm.

STORAGE: Store in an airtight container in the fridge for up to 2 days or in the freezer for up to 1 month.
REHEAT: Microwave, covered, until the desired temperature is reached or reheat in a saucepan or slow cooker / instant pot, covered, on medium.
SERVE IT WITH: To make this a complete meal, serve the asparagus cream soup with crispy zucchini chips on the side.
PER SERVING
calories: 138 | fat: 10.5g | total carbs: 10.2g | fiber: 3.5g | protein: 5.9g

KETO BEEF SOUP

Macros: Fat 67% | Protein 26% | Carbs 7%
Prep time: 10 minutes | Cook time: 19 minutes | Serves 6

Within a few minutes in the kitchen, you can easily prepare the keto beef soup. The ingredients used are readily available. Follow the directions given and enjoy the tasty soup while on a keto diet.

3 tablespoons butter	shredded
2 diced celery stalks	Salt and freshly ground black
1 diced onion	pepper, to taste
2 minced garlic cloves	1 pound (454 g) corned beef,
6 cups beef stock	chopped
1 teaspoon caraway seeds	1½ cups shredded Swiss cheese
1 cup low-carb sauerkraut,	2 cups heavy whipping cream

1. In a large saucepan, melt the butter over medium heat.
2. Stir in the celery and onion. Sauté for about 3 minutes until tender.
3. Add the garlic and cook for 1 minute more until soft.
4. Add the beef stock, caraway seeds, sauerkraut, black pepper, and salt. Stir well and allow to boil.
5. Mix in the corned beef and cook for 15 minutes over low heat.
6. Add the cheese and heavy cream, then cook for 1 minute more.
7. Remove from the heat and serve warm.

STORAGE: Store in an airtight container in the fridge for up to 1 week
REHEAT: Microwave, covered, until the desired temperature is reached or reheat in a frying pan or instant pot, covered, on medium.
PER SERVING
calorie: 451 | fat: 34.4g | total carbs: 9.2g | fiber: 1.1g | protein: 30.6g

BEEF TACO SOUP

Macros: Fat 58% | Protein 35% | Carbs 7%
Prep time: 15 minutes | Cook time:24 minutes | Serves 8

This beef taco soup will melt your heart with its creamy, delicious flavors. It is cooked out of beef mixed with tomatoes and chilies. Cream cheese, cream, and broth are all mixed to make a rich combination of taste and nutrients.

2 garlic cloves, minced	2 (10-ounce / 284-g) cans diced
½ cup onions, chopped	tomatoes and green chilies
1 pound (454 g) ground beef	½ cup heavy cream
1 teaspoon chili powder	2 teaspoons salt
1 tablespoon ground cumin	2 (14½-ounce / 411-g) cans beef
1 (8-ounce / 227-g) package	broth
cream cheese, softened	

1. Take a large saucepan and place it over medium-high heat.
2. Add garlic, onions, and ground beef to the soup and sauté for 7 minutes until beef is browned.
3. Add chili powder and cumin, then cook for 2 minutes.
4. Add cream cheese and cook for 5 minutes while mashing the cream cheese into the beef with a spoon.
5. Add diced tomatoes and green chilies, heavy cream, salt and broth then cook for 10 minutes.
6. Mix gently and serve warm.

STORAGE: Store in an airtight container in the fridge for up to 3 days or in the freezer for up to 1 month.
REHEAT: Microwave, covered, until the desired temperature is reached or reheat in a slow cooker / instant pot, covered, on medium.
SERVE IT WITH: To make this a complete meal, serve the beef taco soup with avocado guacamole on the side.
PER SERVING
calories: 205 | fat: 13.3g | total carbs: 4.4g | fiber: 0.8g | protein: 8.0g

CHEESY ZUCCHINI SOUP

Macros: Fat: 82% | Protein: 10% | Carbs: 8%
Prep time: 2 hours | Cook time: 10 minutes | Serves 5

This quick and easy soup is perfect for busy weekdays and nights. With ingredients you already have in your kitchen, each bite of this delicious low-carb soup helps you feel relaxed and comfortable in your home.

4 cups chicken broth	cut into cubes
1 medium zucchini, cut into	½ teaspoon ground cumin
½-inch pieces	Salt and black pepper, to taste
8 ounces (227 g) cream cheese	

SPECIAL EQUIPMENT:
Immersion blender

1. Pour the chicken broth into a large pot and add the zucchini. Boil for 5 minutes then reduce the heat and simmer for 10 minutes.
2. Mix in the cream cheese, then remove the pot from the heat. Blend the soup with an immersion blender until it is smooth, then add the cumin, salt, and pepper.
3. Put it in the refrigerator for 2 hours to chill.
4. Serve the soup into bowls.

STORAGE: Store in an airtight container in the fridge for up to 4 days or in the freezer for up to 1 month.
REHEAT: Microwave, covered, until the desired temperature is reached or reheat in a frying pan or instant pot, covered, on medium.
PER SERVING
calories: 178 | fat: 16.1g | total carbs: 4.1g | fiber: 0.4g | protein: 4.5g

CREAMY TOMATO SOUP

Macros: Fat 78% | Protein 15% | Carbs 7%
Prep time: 15 minutes | Cook time: 30 minutes | Serves 4

This tomato basil soup is an ultimate delight for a low-carb healthy menu. If you have tomatoes available at home, then put them to good use and make this soup by cooking them with a combination of water and heavy cream along with basic spices.

2 cups of water
4 cups tomato juice
3 tomatoes, peeled, seeded and diced

14 leaves fresh basil
2 tablespoons butter
1 cup heavy whipping cream
Salt and black pepper, to taste

1. Take a suitable cooking pot and place it over medium heat.
2. Add water, tomato juice, and tomatoes, then simmer for 30 minutes.
3. Transfer the soup to a blender, then add basil leaves.
4. Press the pulse button and blend the soup until smooth.
5. Return this tomato soup to the cooking pot and place it over medium heat.
6. Add butter, heavy cream, salt, and black pepper. Cook and mix until the butter melts.
7. Serve warm and fresh.

STORAGE: Store in an airtight container in the fridge for up to 4 days or in the freezer for up to 1 month.
REHEAT: Microwave, covered, until the desired temperature is reached or reheat in a saucepan or slow cooker / instant pot, covered, on medium.
SERVE IT WITH: To make this a complete meal, serve the creamy tomato soup with cauliflower mash on the side.
PER SERVING
calories: 203 | fat: 17.7g | total carbs: 13.0g | fiber: 5.6g | protein: 3.7g

CREAMY BACON AND TILAPIA CHOWDER

Macros: Fat: 69% | Protein: 23% | Carbs: 8%
Prep time: 5 minutes | Cook time: 40 minutes | Serves 6

This bacon and tilapia soup is a very healthy way to add fish to your soup diet. Whip up this delicious soup dish for your family and weekdays or nights at the table will never become boring.

2 tablespoons butter
4 bacon slices chopped
1 medium onion chopped
3 cups daikon radish, chopped
2½ cups chicken stock

½ teaspoon dried thyme
Salt and black pepper, to taste
2 cups heavy whipping cream
1 pound (454 g) tilapia, chopped

1. Heat the butter in a pan over medium heat and add the bacon to cook until it is crispy.
2. Mix in the onions and radish and cook it for 5 minutes. Pour in the chicken stock and cook on low heat for 10 minutes.
3. Season with thyme, salt, and pepper, then add the heavy cream and tilapia and cook for 4 minutes.
4. Serve into bowls while hot.

STORAGE: Store in an airtight container in the fridge for up to 4 days or in the freezer for up to 1 month.
REHEAT: Microwave, covered, until the desired temperature is reached or reheat in a frying pan or instant pot, covered, on medium.
SERVE IT WITH: To make this a complete meal, serve it with a bowl of salad.
PER SERVING
calories: 366 | fat: 28.0g | total carbs: 8.6g | fiber: 1.3g | protein: 21.3g

ZESTY DOUBLE BEEF STEW

Macros: Fat 27% | Protein 65% | Carbs 8%
Prep time: 10 minutes | Cook time: 8 hours | Serves 6

A few simple ingredients make this a sumptuous stew. It has the perfect combination of tender beef and spicy seasonings that is so full of flavor. You are sure to be blown away by the taste. And if you are ready to up the spice level still more, you can even add a spoon of red pepper flakes to the stew.

1½ pounds (680 g) stew beef
1 tablespoon Lea & Perrins Worcestershire sauce
1 (14½-ounce / 411-g) can chili-ready diced tomatoes

2 teaspoons Sriracha hot sauce
1 tablespoon chili mix
1 cup beef broth
Salt, to taste

1. In the crockpot, place the stew beef, Worcestershire sauce, diced tomatoes, hot sauce, chili mix, beef broth, and salt. Mix well.
2. Turn the crockpot on high power for 6 hours. Then pull apart the meat in the crockpot with a fork.
3. Sprinkle with more salt if needed and cook for further 2 hours on low heat.
4. Transfer the stew from the crockpot to the serving bowl. Enjoy it hot.

STORAGE: Store in an airtight container in the refrigerator for up to 3 days or the freezer for up to 3 months.
REHEAT: Microwave, covered, until the desired temperature is reached or reheat in a pan / instant pot, covered, on low.
SERVE IT WITH: To make this a complete meal, you can pair it with cauliflower rice.
PER SERVING
calories: 161 | fat: 4.9g | total carbs: 3.8g | fiber: 0.5g | protein: 26.0g

CREAMY MINTY SPINACH SOUP

Macros: Fat: 68% | Protein: 15% | Carbs: 17%
Prep time: 5 minutes | Cook time: 10 minutes | Serves 3

This creamy minty spinach soup is filling and healthy. It is delicious and nutritious and perfect for any time of the year. It is quick and easy and is great for lunch or dinner. Kick back and let your taste buds run wild.

1 tablespoon olive oil
4 spring onions, chopped
2 garlic cloves
12 ounces (340 g) spinach leaves

1½ cups chicken stock
½ cup mint leaves
4 tablespoons heavy cream
Salt and black pepper, to taste

1. Heat the oil in a pot over medium heat and add the onions and garlic. Cook for 3 minutes then add the spinach leaves.
2. Let it cook for 4 minutes, then add the stock and mint leaves, then pour it into a blender.
3. Pulse until it is smooth, then mix in the heavy cream, salt, and pepper.
4. Put it in the refrigerator to chill until ready to serve.
5. Serve chilled.

STORAGE: Store in an airtight container in the fridge for up to 4 days or in the freezer for up to 1 month.
REHEAT: Microwave, covered, until the desired temperature is reached or reheat in a frying pan or instant pot, covered, on medium.
SERVE IT WITH: To make this a complete meal, serve it with some warm keto bread.
PER SERVING
calories: 184 | fat: 13.9g | total carbs: 10.8g | fiber: 3.1g | protein: 7.1g

LETTUCE SOUP WITH POACHED EGG

Macros: Fat 58% | Protein 24% | Carbs 18%
Prep time: 10 minutes | Cook time: 14 minutes | Serves 2

You must not have tried a soup that simple yet so delicious as this lettuce soup. Just by using broth, lettuce, eggs, and salt, you can make a complete serving filled with protein, fibers, and other essential nutrients.

2 pounds (907 g) vegetable broth	1 head romaine lettuce, chopped
2 eggs	Salt, to taste

1. Take a large-sized cooking pot and place it over high heat.
2. Pour the vegetable broth into the cooking pot and bring to a boil.
3. Reduce pot's heat to low then use a wooden spoon to make a whirlpool in hot water by stirring it for a minute or two.
4. Crack the eggs into the broth and cook for 5 minutes to get the poached eggs.
5. Divide the poached eggs into 2 serving bowls.
6. Add lettuce and salt to the hot broth and let it cook for 4 minutes.
7. Divide the broth with lettuce in the serving bowls.
8. Serve warm and fresh.

STORAGE: Store in an airtight container in the fridge for up to 2 days.
REHEAT: Microwave, covered, until the desired temperature is reached or reheat in a saucepan or slow cooker / instant pot, covered, on medium.
SERVE IT WITH: To make this a complete meal, serve the lettuce soup with roasted or grilled mushrooms on the side.
PER SERVING
calories: 167 | fat: 10.6g | total carbs: 17.1g | fiber: 6.7g | protein: 12.8g

SWEET AND SOUR CHICKEN SOUP WITH CELERY

Macros: Fat: 37% | Protein: 57% | Carbs: 6%
Prep time: 5 minutes | Cook time: 30 minutes | Serves 10

This sweet and sour chicken soup dish is quick and easy to make and is perfect for busy weekdays. Made with delicious ingredients, this low-carb chicken soup is hearty and healthy and is perfect for all ages.

10 cups chicken broth	1½ tablespoons curry powder
2 tablespoons butter	2 tablespoons Swerve
5 cups chicken, chopped and cooked	½ cup sour cream
¼ cup apple cider	¼ cup fresh parsley, chopped
3 cups celery root, diced	Salt and freshly ground black pepper to taste

1. In a large pot, mix the broth, butter, chicken, celery root, apple cider, and curry powder together. Let it boil for 30 minutes.
2. Fold in the Swerve, sour cream, parsley, salt, and pepper.
3. Serve into bowls while it is hot.

STORAGE: Store in an airtight container in the fridge for up to 4 days or in the freezer for up to 1 month.
REHEAT: Microwave, covered, until the desired temperature is reached or reheat in a frying pan or instant pot, covered, on medium.
SERVE IT WITH: To make this a complete meal, serve it with some parmesan roasted zucchini.
PER SERVING
calories: 178 | fat: 7.3g | total carbs: 3.6g | fiber: 1.1g | protein: 25.5g

ZUCCHINI SOUP

Macros: Fat 74% | Protein 8% | Carbs 18%
Prep time: 15 minutes | Cook time: 1 hour 45 minutes | Serves 4

A delicious and smooth bowl of tempting zucchini soup is just the thing you need to complete your menu. This recipe calls for no complicated cooked steps or several ingredients, instead of by using just the zucchini, onion, broth, and some spice, you can cook it well.

3 tablespoons coconut oil	4 cups chicken broth
1 small onion, chopped	½ cup nutmeg, or as needed
1 large zucchini	Salt and black pepper, to taste

1. Take a large-sized pot and place it over medium heat.
2. Add oil and onion, then sauté for 3 minutes or until onion is soft.
3. Add zucchini and chicken broth. Cover the soup with a lid and simmer for 1 hour.
4. Transfer the cooked soup to a blender. Press the pulse button and blend the soup until smooth.
5. Add nutmeg, salt, and black pepper. Return the soup to medium heat and cook for 30 minutes.
6. Serve warm and fresh.

STORAGE: Store in an airtight container in the fridge for up to 4 days or in the freezer for up to 1 month.
REHEAT: Microwave, covered, until the desired temperature is reached or reheat in a saucepan or slow cooker / instant pot, covered, on medium.
SERVE IT WITH: To make this a complete meal, serve the zucchini soup with grilled bacon strips on the side.
PER SERVING
calories: 197 | fat: 16.1g | total carbs: 13.3g | fiber: 4.2g | protein: 3.8g

BUTTERY SALMON AND LEEK SOUP

Macros: Fat: 64% | Protein: 27% | Carbs: 9%
Prep time: 7 minutes | Cook time: 23 minutes | Serves 4

This buttery salmon and leek soup is a delicious low-carb dish for everyone. Packed with keto-friendly leeks, this creamy soup tastes like comfort with every bite. It is also quick and easy to make, which makes it perfect for busy weekdays.

2 tablespoons butter	Salt and freshly ground black pepper, to taste
2 leeks, rinsed, trimmed and sliced	1 pound (454 g) salmon, in bite-size pieces
3 garlic cloves, minced	1½ cups unsweetened coconut milk
6 cups seafood broth	
2 teaspoons dried thyme leaves	

1. Heat the butter in a pan over medium heat and add the leeks and garlic. Cook for 3 minutes.
2. Mix in the broth and thyme to cook on low heat for 15 minutes, then season with salt and pepper.
3. Add the salmon and the coconut milk to the pot. Cook on low heat for 5 minutes.
4. Remove the pot from the heat and serve the soup into bowls while hot.

STORAGE: Store in an airtight container in the fridge for up to 4 days or in the freezer for up to 1 month.
REHEAT: Microwave, covered, until the desired temperature is reached or reheat in a frying pan or instant pot, covered, on medium.
SERVE IT WITH: To make this a complete meal, serve it with Parmesan roasted zucchini.
PER SERVING
calories: 506 | fat: 36.0g | total carbs: 13.9g | fiber: 3.0g | protein: 34.5g

BROCCOLI CHEDDAR SOUP

Macros: Fat 79% | Protein 11% | Carbs 10%
Prep time: 15 minutes | Cook time: 10 minutes | Serves 2

You will love this broccoli Cheddar soup because of its mouth-pleasing flavors. Here you can get to enjoy all the flavors of nutmeg, garlic, mustard, and onion in a single bowl. The great part is that the soup can be easily cooked in your microwave in just a few minutes.

1 cup broccoli, cut into florets
¾ cup vegetable stock
¼ teaspoon garlic powder
¼ teaspoon mustard powder
Salt and black pepper, to taste
⅛ cup butter

⅓ cup sharp Cheddar cheese, shredded
¼ teaspoon onion powder
1 pinch nutmeg
¼ cup heavy whipping cream

1. Take a large-sized bowl and add broccoli florets to this bowl.
2. Place this bowl in the microwave and microwave for 4 minutes on high heat.
3. Transfer the broccoli florets to the blender.
4. Add vegetable stock, garlic powder, mustard powder, salt, black pepper, butter, Cheddar cheese, onion powder, nutmeg, and cream.
5. Press the pulse button and blend until smooth.
6. Pour this soup into a microwave-safe bowl and microwave for 2 minutes on high heat.
7. Mix it well, then microwave for 4 minutes.
8. Serve warm and fresh.

STORAGE: Store in an airtight container in the fridge for up to 4 days or in the freezer for up to 1 month.
REHEAT: Microwave, covered, until the desired temperature is reached or reheat in a saucepan or slow cooker / instant pot, covered, on medium.
SERVE IT WITH: To make this a complete meal, serve the broccoli Cheddar soup with roasted nuts and seeds on the side.
PER SERVING
calories: 296 | fat: 25.9g | total carbs: 9.6g | fiber: 2.1g | protein: 8.4g

NEW ENGLAND CLAM CHOWDER

Macros: Fat 57% | Protein 30% | Carbs 13%
Prep time: 10 minutes | Cook time: 30 minutes | Serves 8

This classic comfort food comes your way through this easy-to-make recipe which can be made in less than 40 minutes. Jam-packed with delectable clams, salty bacon, and hearty celery, this creamy, rich clam chowder will become your new family favorite fare. If you want to make the chowder thicker and indulgent, you can substitute the heavy cream with mascarpone cheese.

4 ounces (113 g) uncured bacon, chopped
2 tablespoons grass-fed butter
½ finely chopped onion
2 teaspoons minced garlic
1 celery stalk, chopped
2 tablespoons arrowroot powder
4 cups fish or chicken stock
2 bay leaves

1 teaspoon chopped fresh thyme
1½ cups heavy whipping cream
3 (6½-ounce / 185-g) cans clams, drained
Sea salt, for seasoning
Freshly ground black pepper, for seasoning
2 tablespoons chopped fresh parsley

1. Fry bacon in a medium stockpot over medium heat till crispy. With a slotted spoon, transfer the bacon to a plate. Keep it aside.
2. Spoon in butter to sauté the onion, garlic, and celery for 3 minutes.
3. Add the arrowroot powder and sauté for a minute.
4. Pour the fish stock, bay leaves, and thyme over it. Bring the mixture to just before it boils.
5. Lower the heat to medium-low and simmer for 9 minutes or until thickened.
6. Add the heavy cream and clams. Stir and simmer for further 4 minutes or till heated through.
7. Discard the bay leaves and sprinkle with salt and pepper.
8. Transfer to a serving bowl and top it with parsley and crumbled bacon. Serve hot.

STORAGE: Store in an airtight container in the refrigerator for up to 3days. If you need to freeze, then stop the cooking process at step 5. When you need to serve the chowder, take it out and stir the clams and heavy cream to it.
REHEAT: Microwave, covered with a plastic wrap, for 3 to 4 minutes at high power while stirring it once halfway or reheat in a pan, covered, on medium.
SERVE IT WITH: To make this a complete meal, serve the soup along with oyster crackers or with cauliflower rice.
PER SERVING
calories: 225 | fat: 14.3g | fiber: 8.1g | fiber: 0.7g | protein: 16.7g

SPICY SHRIMP AND CHORIZO SOUP WITH TOMATOES AND AVOCADO

Macros: Fat: 65% | Protein: 29% | Carbs: 6%
Prep time: 5 minutes | Cook time: 40 minutes | Serves 8

This Shrimp and chorizo soup packs the right amount of crunch and flavor with every spoonful. Made from the richest ingredients, it guarantees a fun family time and makes every experience a new journey.

2 tablespoons butter
3 medium celery stalks, diced
1 medium onion, diced
12 ounces (340 g) chorizo, diced
4 garlic cloves, sliced
1 teaspoon ground coriander
1½ teaspoons smoked paprika
1 teaspoon of sea salt
4 cups chicken broth

2 tomatoes, diced
1 pound (454 g) shrimp, peeled, deveined and chopped
2 tablespoons fresh cilantro, minced
1 avocado, diced
Chopped fresh cilantro, for garnish

1. Heat half of the butter in a large pot over medium heat. Add the celery and onions to cook for 8 minutes.
2. Mix in the chorizo, garlic, coriander, half of the paprika, and salt, then let it cook for 1 minute.
3. Pour in the broth and the tomatoes and cook for 20 minutes and set aside
4. Heat the rest of the butter in a small pan over medium heat. Remove the chorizo from the broth and put it in the pan. Cook for 5 minutes until it is crispy.
5. Mix in the rest of the paprika and shrimp and let it cook for 4 minutes, then remove it from the heat and sprinkle with the cilantro.
6. Serve into bowls topped with the chorizo, avocado, and chopped cilantro.

STORAGE: Store in an airtight container in the fridge for up to 4 days or in the freezer for up to 1 month.
REHEAT: Microwave, covered, until the desired temperature is reached or reheat in a frying pan or instant pot, covered, on medium.
SERVE IT WITH: To make this a complete meal, serve it with a bowl of salad.
PER SERVING
calories: 325 | fat: 23.6g | total carbs: 7.2g | fiber: 2.7g | protein: 23.7g

GREEN GARLIC AND CAULIFLOWER SOUP

Macros: Fat: 56% | Protein: 14% | Carbs: 30%
Prep time: 7 minutes | Cook time: 13 minutes | Serves 5

This garlic and cauliflower soup is a delicious, healthy substitute for potato soup. It is quick and easy to make, but that does not affect the delicious taste of the soup. Comfort your loved ones with this green garlic and cauliflower soup to remind them of all the love that comes from your kitchen. The carbs in this recipe is relatively high, but you can control the content of the carbs by using homemade low-carb vegetable soup.

2 teaspoons thyme powder
3 cups vegetable soup
½ teaspoon matcha green tea powder
1 head cauliflower

3 tablespoons olive oil
5 garlic cloves chopped
Salt and freshly ground black pepper, to taste

SPECIAL EQUIPMENT:
Immersion blender

1. Pour the thyme powder, vegetable soup, and the matcha green tea powder into a large pot over medium-high heat. Let it boil for 1 minute.
2. Add the cauliflower and let it cook for 10 minutes.
3. Meanwhile, in a small saucepan, add the olive oil and the garlic, then let it cook for 1 minute. Pour it into the pot with the cauliflower. Season with salt and pepper and cook for another 2 minutes.
4. Put an immersion blender into the pot and purée it until it is smooth.
5. Remove from the heat and serve while it still warm.

STORAGE: Store in an airtight container in the fridge for up to 4 days or in the freezer for up to 1 month.
REHEAT: Microwave, covered, until the desired temperature is reached or reheat in a frying pan or instant pot, covered, on medium.
SERVE IT WITH: To make this a complete meal, serve it with a bowl of salad.
PER SERVING
calories: 156 | fat: 9.7g | total carbs: 16.1g | fiber: 4.3g | protein: 5.3g

BAY SCALLOP AND BACON CHOWDER

Macros: Fat 69% | Protein 20% | Carbs 11%
Prep time: 35 minutes | Cook time: 25 minutes | Serves 6

With only a handful of ingredients, this soup is simple to throw together, and the flavors shine on their own, especially the bay scallops, which have a magical way of transforming any dish it is in. The fare is a tasty way to enjoy the sweet, tender, and creamy bay scallops. And the daikon radish is a delicious and perfect vegetable in making a keto-friendly soup. So if you want something comforting, yet light and quick, then this bay scallop chowder is the one for you.

1 tablespoon butter
4 slices bacon chopped
3 cups chopped daikon radish
1 medium onion chopped
2½ cups chicken stock

½ teaspoon dried thyme
Salt and freshly ground black pepper, to taste
1 pound (454 g) bay scallops
2 cups heavy cream

1. Heat a large saucepan over medium heat and melt the butter.
2. Add the bacon and fry until crisp. Then add the daikon radish and onion to it and cook for 4 minutes.
3. Pour the chicken stock and allow it to simmer for 7 minutes.
4. Sprinkle with thyme, pepper, and salt. Mix to combine well.
5. Add bay scallops and heavy cream to the soup and simmer for further 5 minutes. Stir to combine well.

6. Remove the saucepan from the heat and serve the chowder hot in serving bowls.

STORAGE: Store in an airtight container in the refrigerator for up to 4 days.
REHEAT: Microwave, covered, until the desired temperature is reached or reheat in an instant pot, covered, on medium.
SERVE IT WITH: To make this a complete meal, serve the soup along with baked beef rolls. If you prefer a healthier side dish, then have it with kale Caesar salad.
PER SERVING
calories: 400 | fat: 30.9g | total carbs: 11.5g | sugars: 1.4g | protein: 20.5g

KETO BEEF STEW

Macros: Fat 58% | Protein 37% | Carbs 5%
Prep time: 10 minutes | Cook time: 1 hour | Serves 4

Have you ever made something so rich, so savory, that it makes you go weak in the knees? This stew with fork-tender beef does that to me. It is that kind of comfort food which you would want to have all winter long. On top, the stew is thick, hearty and full of amazing classic flavor which tastes so better the next day.

1 tablespoon coconut oil
1 pound (454 g) beef short rib
¼ teaspoon pink salt
¼ teaspoon freshly ground black pepper
4 cloves garlic, minced

1 tablespoon butter
¾ cup sliced onions
2 cups beef broth
½ teaspoon xanthan gum
¾ cup radishes

1. Take a large saucepan and heat it over medium-high heat. Add the coconut oil and beef short ribs to it.
2. Apply pink salt and pepper over the ribs. Sear the meat for 3 minutes per side or until browned.
3. Then stir in the garlic, butter, and onion. Continue cooking for a further 3 minutes.
4. Pour the beef broth along with the xanthan gum and bring the mixture to a boil.
5. Allow it to simmer for 25 minutes and stir in the radishes.
6. Cook for further 25 minutes while stirring it continuously.
7. Transfer the stew from the saucepan to the serving bowl. Enjoy it hot.

STORAGE: Store in an airtight container in the refrigerator for up to 3 days or the freezer for up to 3 months.
REHEAT: Microwave, covered, until the desired temperature is reached or reheat in a pan / instant pot, covered, on low.
SERVE IT WITH: To make this a complete meal, you can serve it along with mashed cauliflower or roasted Brussels sprouts.
PER SERVING
calories: 262 | fat: 16.8g | total carbs: 3.9g | fiber: 0.1g | protein: 24.8g

LAMB SOUP

Macros: Fat 72% | Protein 19% | Carbs 9%
Prep time: 5 minutes | Cook time: 25 minutes | Serves 6

This soup has an abundance of flavor. Between the red chili paste, coconut milk, lime juice, and garlic, your taste buds are sure to tingle. What's more, the soup is super-quick, easy to make. And all these makes it a fantastic, comforting lunch or dinner.

1 tablespoon coconut oil
12 ounces (340 g) ground lamb
½ chopped onion
2 teaspoons minced garlic
2 cups shredded cabbage
4 cups chicken broth

1½ tablespoons red chili paste
2 cups unsweetened coconut milk
Zest and juice of 1 lime
1 cup shredded kale

1. Heat coconut oil in a medium stockpot over medium-high heat and then stir in the lamb.
2. Cook for 5 minutes or until browned while stirring the lamb continuously.
3. Stir in onion, garlic, and cabbage to it and sauté for 4 minutes or until softened.
4. Pour the chicken broth, red chili paste, coconut milk, lime juice, and lime zest. Mix to combine well.
5. Then, bring them to a boil and turn the heat to low. Simmer for further 8 minutes until the cabbage is tender.
6. Add the kale and stir for 3 minutes until wilted.
7. Transfer to a serving bowl and serve it hot.

STORAGE: Store in an airtight container in the refrigerator for up to 3 days or the freezer for up to 3 months.
REHEAT: Microwave, covered, until the desired temperature is reached or reheat in a pan / instant pot, covered, on low.
SERVE IT WITH: To make this a complete meal, serve the soup along with cauliflower rice or roasted Brussels sprouts.
PER SERVING
calories: 326 | fat: 26.1g | total carbs: 9.3g | fiber: 1.7g | protein: 15.2g

EASY BRAZILIAN SHRIMP STEW (MOQUECA DE CAMAROES)

Macros: Fat 60% | Protein 33% | Carbs 7%
Prep time: 25 minutes | Cook time: 20 minutes | Serves 6

Indulge in this simple yet outrageously scrumptious stew, and you will find yourself in heaven. Spiked with the flavors of lime, cilantro, and coconut, the soup is light and full of fresh taste. The soup has a luxurious texture from the coconut milk while having a fiery heat and tropical tang from the seasonings. If possible, try to get hold of red palm oil, which can give the soup a distinctive signature floral note. In Brazil, the stew is a must-have at any Latin table, especially on Easter.

¼ cup olive oil
1 garlic clove, minced
¼ cup onions, diced
1 (14-ounce / 397-g) can diced tomatoes with chilies
¼ cup red pepper, roasted and diced
¼ cup fresh cilantro, chopped plus extra for garnish

1½ pounds (680 g) raw shrimp, peeled and deveined
1 cup unsweetened coconut milk
2 tablespoons Sriracha hot sauce
Salt and freshly ground black pepper, to taste
2 tablespoons lemon juice
Fresh cilantro, for garnish

1. Start by adding olive oil to a heated medium saucepan and then spoon in the garlic and onion.
2. Sauté the onion-garlic mixture for 2 minutes and stir in tomatoes, pepper, cilantro, and shrimp.
3. Sauté for 4 minutes or until the shrimp is opaque. Pour coconut milk and Sriracha sauce over it.
4. Simmer the soup for 4 minutes and add pepper, salt, and lime juice. Do not bring the soup to a boil.
5. Top it with the fresh cilantro and transfer to soup bowls to serve.

STORAGE: Store in an airtight container in the refrigerator for up to 3 days or the freezer for up to 2 months.
REHEAT: Microwave, covered, until the desired temperature is reached or reheat in an instant pot, covered, on medium.
SERVE IT WITH: To make this a complete meal, you can spoon the delicious stew over hot steamed cauliflower rice. Or you can serve it with gluten-free bread of your choice.
PER SERVING
calories: 305 | fat: 20.2g | total carbs: 7.0g | fiber: 1.2g | protein: 24.9g

SPICY HALIBUT IN TOMATO SOUP

Macros: Fat: 32% | Protein: 58% | Carbs: 10%
Prep time: 5 minutes | Cook time: 30 minutes | Serves 10

This halibut in tomato soup dish is super easy to make and is a healthy fish soup. This delicious halibut soup is slow-cooked with garlic, tomatoes, and spices, which makes it a mouthwatering experience with every taste. It is a perfect dish for busy weekdays.

1 tablespoon olive oil
2 garlic cloves, minced
¼ cup fresh parsley, chopped
10 anchovies canned in oil, minced
1 teaspoon red chili flakes

6 cups vegetable broth
1 teaspoon black pepper
3 tomatoes, peeled and diced
1 teaspoon salt
1 pound (454 g) halibut fillets, chopped

1. In a large stockpot, heat the olive oil over medium heat. Add the garlic and half of the parsley and cook for 1 minute.
2. Mix in the anchovies, red chili flakes, vegetable broth, black pepper, tomatoes, and salt.
3. Reduce the heat to medium-low and let it cook for 20 minutes.
4. Put the halibut fillets into the pot and simmer for 10 minutes. Remove the halibut from the pot and put on a plate, then shred it with a fork.
5. Put the shredded fish back into the pot and let it cook for 2 minutes or until it is heated through.
6. Serve the soup with remaining parsley sprinkled on top.

STORAGE: Store in an airtight container in the fridge for up to 4 days or in the freezer for up to 1 month.
REHEAT: Microwave, covered, until the desired temperature is reached or reheat in a frying pan or instant pot, covered, on medium.
SERVE IT WITH: To make this a complete meal, serve it with some spinach salad.
PER SERVING
calories: 71 | fat: 2.5g | total carbs: 2.7g | fiber: 0.8g | protein: 10.2g

SOUR GARLIC ZUCCHINI SOUP

Macros: Fat: 79% | Protein: 5% | Carbs: 16%
Prep time: 13 minutes | Cook time: 27 minutes | Serves 2

This sour garlic zucchini soup dish perfectly combines delicious bone broth and that tasty zucchini. It is quick and easy to make and is perfect for cold nights or if you just have the flu. Grab a spoon and get cooking!

2 small zucchini, chopped
2 tablespoons olive oil
1 small onion peeled and grated.
2 garlic cloves, minced
½ teaspoon of sea salt

¼ teaspoon black pepper
¼ teaspoon poultry seasoning
1½ cups beef bone broth
1 small lemon, juiced
5 tablespoons sour cream

1. Pour some water into a medium-sized pan, then add the zucchini and bring it to a boil over medium heat.
2. Reduce the heat to low and let it simmer for 20 minutes, then drain the zucchini and set aside.
3. In a small saucepan, put the olive oil, onions, garlic, salt, black pepper, and poultry seasoning, then let it cook for 2 minutes. Pour the beef bone broth into the pan and simmer on low heat for 5 minutes.
4. Add the lemon juice, then pour the mixture into a blender and blend until it is smooth.
5. Top the soup with sour cream and serve hot.

STORAGE: Store in an airtight container in the fridge for up to 4 days or in the freezer for up to 1 month.
REHEAT: Microwave, covered, until the desired temperature is reached or reheat in a frying pan or instant pot, covered, on medium.
SERVE IT WITH: To make this a complete meal, serve it with garlicky roasted broccoli.
PER SERVING
calories: 199 | fat: 17.0g | total carbs: 9.1g | fiber: 1.0g | protein: 2.5g

CREAMY BEEF AND BROCCOLI SOUP

Macros: Fat: 59% | Protein: 26% | Carbs: 15%
Prep time: 4 minutes | Cook time: 46 minutes | Serves 6

The appeal of one-hour dishes cannot be overemphasized. This creamy beef and broccoli soup is the perfect soup for beef lovers. Made with an array of ingredients, the beef softly breaks down in your mouth while you enjoy the flavor-rich soup. This low-carb alternative helps cleanse the body while delivering great taste.

2 tablespoons avocado oil	1 pound (454 g) ground beef
1 onion, chopped	2 teaspoons fish sauce
2 garlic cloves, minced	½ teaspoon black pepper
2 tablespoons Thai green curry paste	4 cups beef bone broth
2-inch ginger, minced	1 cup unsweetened coconut milk
1 Serrano pepper, minced	2 large broccoli stalks, cut into florets
3 tablespoons coconut amino	Cilantro, garnish
½ teaspoon salt	

1. In a large pot, heat the oil and add the onions. Cook for 4 minutes then add the garlic, curry paste, ginger, and Serrano pepper to cook for 1 minute.
2. Add the coconut aminos, salt, ground beef, fish sauce, and black pepper and cook for 6 minutes.
3. Pour in the bone broth, then reduce the heat and cover the pot. Cook for 20 minutes.
4. Mix in the coconut milk and the broccoli florets. Cover the pot and cook for 10 minutes on high heat.
5. Reduce the heat and let it cook for another 5 minutes, then turn off the heat.
6. Serve the soup into bowls garnished with cilantro.

STORAGE: Store in an airtight container in the fridge for up to 4 days or in the freezer for up to 1 month.
REHEAT: Microwave, covered, until the desired temperature is reached or reheat in a frying pan or instant pot, covered, on medium.
SERVE IT WITH: To make this a complete meal, serve it with Parmesan roasted zucchini.
PER SERVING
calories: 424 | fat: 27.7g | total carbs: 18.0g | fiber: 1.4g | protein: 27.1g

CAULIFLOWER LEEK SOUP

Macros: Fat 69% | Protein 17% | Carbs 14%
Prep time: 15 minutes | Cook time: 1 hour 31 minutes | Serves 4

The crunchy leeks with cauliflower make a nutritious combination that can be cooked into a delicious soup. Once the veggies are cooked and blended together, crispy bacon is added to give this soup a chunky texture and an irresistible flavor.

1 leek, chopped	5 bacon strips
½ cauliflower head, chopped	Salt and black pepper, to taste
4 cups chicken broth	

1. Take a large-sized cooking pot and place it over medium heat.
2. Add leek, cauliflower, and chicken broth to the pot. Cook this soup mixture on medium heat for 1 hour.
3. Transfer the soup to a blender. Press the pulse button and blend the soup until smooth.
4. Return the blended soup to the cooking pot and place it over low heat.
5. Place bacon strips in a microwave-safe bowl and microwave for 1 minute.

6. Chop the bacon strips into small pieces and add them to the soup.
7. Continue cooking the soup for 30 minutes on low heat.
8. Add salt and black pepper for seasoning, then mix well.
9. Serve warm and fresh.

STORAGE: Store in an airtight container in the fridge for up to 4 days or in the freezer for up to 1 month.
REHEAT: Microwave, covered, until the desired temperature is reached or reheat in a saucepan or slow cooker / instant pot, covered, on medium.
SERVE IT WITH: To make this a complete meal, serve the cauliflower leek soup with roasted Brussels sprouts on the side.
PER SERVING
calories: 177 | fat: 13.6g | total carbs: 5.7g | fiber: 1.9g | protein: 7.4g

CHICKEN AND MUSHROOM SOUP

Macros: Fat 67% | Protein 27% | Carbs 6%
Prep time: 15 minutes | Cook time: 10 minutes | Serves 4

Chicken and mushrooms are the basic ingredients in this recipe. Measure the ingredients and follow the steps provided. A taste of this soup will leave you craving for more.

6 chicken thighs, cut into bite-sized pieces	1 tablespoon sesame oil
2 tablespoons melted butter	2 medium finely grated ginger
3 minced garlic cloves	2 cups flat mushrooms
4 thinly sliced spring onions	4 cups chicken stock
	Sea salt, to taste

1. In a bowl, lightly season the chicken strips with sea salt.
2. Melt the butter in a frying pan over medium heat.
3. Add the seasoned chicken strips and sauté for about 2 minutes until they are almost cooked through, then put aside.
4. In the same pan, add the garlic, onion, sesame oil, and ginger. Stir well and reduce the heat to low. Cook for 2 minutes until tender.
5. Stir in the mushrooms and stir-fry on medium heat for 2 minutes.
6. Return the chicken strips to the pan and mix well. Transfer the mixture to four serving bowls and keep warm.
7. Bring the chicken stock to a boil in a large saucepan until warmed through.
8. Pour the stock over the chicken and mushroom mixture in the serving bowls.

STORAGE: Store in an airtight container in the fridge for up to 1 week.
REHEAT: Microwave, covered, until the desired temperature is reached or reheat in a frying pan or instant pot, covered, on medium heat.
SERVE IT WITH: To make this a complete meal, serve the chicken and mushroom soup with cheese strips.
PER SERVING
calories: 357 | fat: 39.6g | total carbs: 8.7g | fiber: 0.7g | protein: 36.7g

STEWED MEAT AND PUMPKIN

Macros: Fat 59% | Protein 26% | Carbs 15%
Prep time: 15 minutes | Cook time: 44 minutes | Serves 6

Satisfy your meat desires while on a keto diet with the delicious stewed meat and pumpkin. The recipe is enriched with a variety of ingredients for body nourishment. You can prepare this meal for lunch or dinner.

1 tablespoon olive oil
½ cup chopped onion
1 minced garlic clove
2 pounds (907 g) chopped pork stew meat
½ cup dry white wine
1 cup pumpkin purée
1 tablespoon butter
¼ cup stevia
¼ teaspoon cardamom powder
2 cups water
2 cups chicken stock
Salt and freshly ground black pepper, to taste
1 teaspoon lemon juice

1. In a large saucepan, melt the olive oil then fry the onions until translucent, for about 3 minutes.
2. Add the garlic and cook until soft, about 1 minute.
3. Add the pork and cook for about 6 minutes until browned.
4. Pour in the white wine and cook for 1 minute more.
5. Add the pumpkin purée, butter, stevia, cardamom powder, water, and chicken stock. Allow to boil for 5 minutes.
6. Cover and reduce the heat to low. Simmer for 30 minutes. Season as needed with salt and pepper to taste.
7. Mix in the lemon juice, then transfer to serving bowls and serve.

STORAGE: Store in an airtight container in the fridge for up to 1 week
REHEAT: Microwave, covered, until the desired temperature is reached or reheat in a frying pan or instant pot, covered, on medium.
SERVE IT WITH: To make this a complete meal, serve the stewed meat and pumpkin with Mexican-style cauliflower rice.
PER SERVING
calories: 315 | fat: 11.3g | total carbs: 6.6g | fiber: 0.3g | protein: 47.1g

CREAMY CROCKPOT CHICKEN STEW

Macros: Fat 50% | Protein 40% | Carbs 10%
Prep time: 5 minutes | Cook time: 4 hours | Serves 6

Here is an excellent chicken stew recipe that is so hearty and healthy, which is ideal for chilly nights. In fact, there is nothing more cozy and comforting than this crockpot chicken stew. And the radish is a delicious and perfect vegetable in making a keto-friendly soup. With just a few minutes of prep, you can make this satisfying classic comfort food dinner that is a meal unto itself as it is loaded with protein and vegetables. For a depth of flavor, you can pour over some dry red wine.

1.75 pounds (794 g) skinless and deboned chicken thighs, diced into 1-inch pieces
½ teaspoon dried oregano
½ onion, diced
½ teaspoon dried rosemary
2 cups chicken stock
½ cup radish, peeled and finely diced
2 celery sticks, diced
3 garlic cloves, minced
¼ teaspoon dried thyme
Salt and black pepper, to taste
½ cup heavy cream
½ teaspoon xanthan gum
1 cup fresh spinach

1. In the crockpot, add the chicken thighs, oregano, onion, rosemary, chicken stock, radish, celery, garlic, and thyme. Stir to combine well.

2. Press the 'low' heat button and cook for 4 hours.
3. Sprinkle salt and pepper over the chicken mixture and then add heavy cream, xanthan gum, and spinach.
4. Cook further for 9 minutes while stirring it continuously.
5. Transfer the stew from the crockpot to the serving bowl and serve it hot.

STORAGE: Store in an airtight container in the refrigerator for up to 3 days or the freezer for up to 3 months.
REHEAT: Microwave, covered, until the desired temperature is reached or reheat in a crockpot or instant pot, covered, on low.
SERVE IT WITH: To make this a complete meal, you can have the stew along with a veggie salad and roasted chicken thighs.
PER SERVING
calories: 227 | fat: 10.2g | total carbs: 5.8g | fiber: 0.6g | protein: 28.8g

EASY GREEN SOUP

Macros: Fat 67% | Protein 8% | Carbs 25%
Prep time: 10 minutes | Cook time: 12 minutes | Serves 4

A taste of grated Gruyere cheese on minestrone soup makes the soup more delicious. If you want to enjoy the goodness of minestrone soup, making sure you use the fresh keto-friendly vegetables. The carbs in this recipe is relatively high, but it mainly depend on the vegetable soup you use, you can make your own low-carb vegetable soup to control the intake of the carbs.

2 tablespoons butter
2 tablespoons onion-garlic purée
2 chopped celery stalks
2 heads broccoli, cut into florets
5 cups vegetable soup
Salt and freshly ground black pepper, to taste
1 cup baby spinach
2 tablespoons grated Gruyere cheese

1. In a saucepan, melt the butter over medium heat.
2. Add the onion-garlic purée and sauté for about 3 minutes until tender.
3. Add the celery and broccoli, then cook until slightly tender, for about 4 minutes.
4. Add the vegetable soup and season with salt and black pepper. Reduce the heat to medium-low, and cook for 5 minutes while covered.
5. Add the spinach and cook until it wilts for about 4 minutes.
6. Transfer the soup to serving bowls and sprinkle with Gruyere cheese before serving.

STORAGE: Store in an airtight container in the fridge for up to 1 week
REHEAT: Microwave, covered, until the desired temperature is reached or reheat in a frying pan or instant pot, covered, on medium.
SERVE IT WITH: You can spread the Parmesan cheese on top of this green soup and serve it with roasted chicken thighs and asparagus salad.
PER SERVING
calories: 195 | fat: 14.5g | total carbs: 12.7g | fiber: 1.5g | protein: 4.1g

CREAMY VEGGIE SOUP

Prep time: 20 minutes | Cook time: 10 minutes | Serves 7
Macros: Fat: 69% | Protein: 11% | Carbs: 20%

This creamy veggie dish is the perfect low-carb soup for everyone. Made with a variety of healthy ingredients and spices, this dish is quick and easy to make and will give you enough energy to stay on top of your daily activities.

¼ cup butter
1 medium white onion, diced
2 garlic cloves
1 medium head cauliflower
1 bay leaf, crumbled
7 ounces (198 g) fresh spinach

5 ounces (142 g) watercress
4 cups vegetable stock
1 cup coconut cream
Salt and freshly ground black pepper, to taste

SPECIAL EQUIPMENT:
Immersion blender

1. Heat the butter in a pot over medium heat and add the onions and garlic. Cook until it is golden brown.
2. Mix in the cauliflower and the bay leaf, then let it cook for 5 minutes.
3. Add the spinach and the watercress. Cook for another 3 minutes, then pour in the stock and let it boil.
4. Add the coconut cream and sprinkle it with salt and pepper. Remove the pot from the heat.
5. Puree with an immersion blender until it is smooth, then put it in the refrigerator to chill for 1 hour.
6. Serve chilled.

STORAGE: Store in an airtight container in the fridge for up to 4 days or in the freezer for up to 1 month.
REHEAT: Microwave, covered, until the desired temperature is reached or reheat in a frying pan or instant pot, covered, on medium.
SERVE IT WITH: To make this a complete meal, serve it with some warm keto bread.
PER SERVING
calories: 259 | fat: 20.0g | total carbs: 18.0g | fiber: 5.1g | protein: 6.9g

SOUR CHICKEN AND KALE SOUP

Macros: Fat: 51% | Protein: 42% | Carbs: 7%
Prep time: 7 minutes | Cook time: 13 minutes | Serves 6

This is the chicken soup that satisfies all cravings. This delicious chicken kale soup has the perfect tanginess that keeps you awake when eating with the delicious juiciness of the chicken and kale. It is a perfect leftover dish and helps with cleansing your body and boosting your immune system.

2 pounds (907 g) chicken breast, skinless
Salt and freshly ground black pepper, to taste
1 tablespoon olive oil
⅓ cup onion

14 ounces (397 g) chicken bone broth
½ cup olive oil
4 cups chicken stock
¼ cup lemon juice
5 ounces (142 g) baby kale leaves

1. Sprinkle the chicken with salt and pepper and set aside.
2. Pour the olive oil and onion into a pan over medium heat and lay the chicken on the pan. Reduce the temperature and let it fry for 15 minutes on both sides.
3. Remove the chicken from pan and put on a plate, then use a fork to shred the chicken and put it in a blender.
4. Pour the chicken bone broth into the blender and pulse until it is smooth.

5. Pour the puréed chicken into the crockpot and add the remaining olive oil, chicken stock, lemon juice, and baby kale leaves.
6. Allow to simmer on low, covered, for 6 hours stirring once in a while until the soup has thickened.
7. Remove from the heat and serve hot.

STORAGE: Store in an airtight container in the fridge for up to 4 days or in the freezer for up to 1 month.
REHEAT: Microwave, covered, until the desired temperature is reached or reheat in a frying pan or instant pot, covered, on medium.
SERVE IT WITH: To make this a complete meal, serve it with some Parmesan roasted zucchini.
PER SERVING
calories: 496 | fat: 28.0g | total carbs: 9.4g | fiber: 1.0g | protein: 52.5g

SPICY SHRIMP AND VEGGIES CREAM SOUP

Macros: Fat: 64% | Protein: 27% | Carbs: 9%
Prep time: 5 minutes | Cook time: 40 minutes | Serves 8

This creamy shrimp and veggie soup are for seafood lovers who enjoy that spicy flavor on their tongues when they eat their favorite seafood soup. This delicious soup is perfect for all ages and serves easily as a lunch or dinner meal.

2 tablespoons avocado oil
¼ cup onions, diced
Salt and freshly ground black pepper, to taste
2 celery stalks chopped
1 jalapeño, seeded and diced
2 tablespoons green Thai curry paste
1 (15-ounce / 425-g) can unsweetened coconut milk

3 cups chicken broth
½ head cabbage, roughly chopped
½ pound (227 g) raw shrimp peeled and deveined
1 pound (454 g) wild Pacific cod cut into 1-inch chunks
2 tablespoons fresh lime juice
2 tablespoons fish sauce
¼ cup fresh cilantro, chopped

1. Heat the oil in a pan over medium heat and add the onion, salt, and pepper. Cook for 4 minutes then add the celery and jalapeño.
2. Cook for 3 minutes then add the curry paste and cook for 30 seconds. Pour in the coconut milk and the broth.
3. Add the cabbage and cook on low heat for 10 minutes.
4. Mix in the shrimp and cod chunks. Cook for 10 minutes again.
5. Remove from the heat and mix in the lime juice and fish sauce.
6. Serve the soup into bowls topped with fresh cilantro.

STORAGE: Store in an airtight container in the fridge for up to 4 days or in the freezer for up to 1 month.
REHEAT: Microwave, covered, until the desired temperature is reached or reheat in a frying pan or instant pot, covered, on medium.
SERVE IT WITH: To make this a complete meal, serve it with a bowl of salad.**PER SERVING**
calories: 250 | fat: 17.6g | total carbs: 8.0g | fiber: 2.2g | protein: 17.1g

SPICY PORK AND SPINACH STEW

Macros: Fat 44% | Protein 46% | Carbs 10%
Prep time: 5 minutes | Cook time: 40 minutes | Serves 4

Everyone will surprise once you make this quick and hearty weeknight dinner fare, loaded to the brim with tender pork stew, spinach and Cajun seasoning along with the onion. I think everyone will ask for seconds. Since it is made in a pressure cooker, you can make it with minimal effort but still have so much flavour.

4 garlic cloves	2 teaspoons Cajun seasoning
1 large onion	blend
1 pound (454 g) pork butt meat	½ cup heavy whipping cream
cut into 2-inch chunks	4 cups baby spinach, chopped
1 teaspoon dried thyme	

1. Place garlic and onion in the blender and process until smooth. Pour the purée to the pressure cooker.
2. Then, add the pork, thyme, and the Cajun seasoning to it. Mix and seal the lid.
3. Press the 'manual' or 'pressure button' and set the timer to 20 minutes.
4. Once the time is up, allow the pressure to release naturally for 10 minutes.
5. Carefully open the lid and stir in the cream and spinach.
6. Select the 'sauté' button and cook for 5 minutes until the spinach is wilted.
7. Transfer to a serving bowl and enjoy it hot.

STORAGE: Store in an airtight container in the refrigerator for up to 3 days or the freezer for up to 3 months.
REHEAT: Microwave, covered, until the desired temperature is reached or reheat in a pan / instant pot, covered, on low.
SERVE IT WITH: To make this a complete meal, serve the soup along with a broccoli salad, or riced cauliflower.
PER SERVING
calories: 230 | fat: 11.2g | total carbs: 6.9g | fiber: 1.2g | protein: 31.4g

CREAMY SPINACH SOUP

Macros: Fat 83% | Protein 4% | Carbs 13%
Prep time: 5 minutes | Cook time: 15 minutes | Serves 2

Wonderfully nutritious and delicious, this vibrant green soup is the perfect evening snack or as the starter for your dinner. Furthermore, the soup is a never-fail recipe. If you love crispy bacon and Parmesan cheese, go wild and add those as toppings to make it more flavorful.

1 tablespoon butter	1½ cups water
1 (2-ounce / 57-g) small onion, sliced	⅔ cup chopped spinach
2 (½-ounce / 14-g) medium garlic cloves, finely minced	1 chicken stock cube
	½ cup heavy whipping cream

1. Heat a saucepan and melt the butter over medium heat.
2. Add onion to it and cook till softened. Stir in the garlic and keep cooking.
3. Once the onion is browned, pour half the water along with spinach and stock cube.
4. Cover and continue cooking until the spinach has wilted.
5. Transfer the mixture in the saucepan to a blender and pulse until smooth and silky.
6. Pass it through a fine sieve and add the remaining water according to your desired consistency.

7. Return to the saucepan and heat it through. Off the heat and stir in the cream.
8. Pour the soup to the bowl and serve warm.

STORAGE: Store in an airtight container in the refrigerator for up to 3 days or the freezer for up to 3 months.
REHEAT: Microwave, covered, until the desired temperature is reached or reheat in a pan / instant pot, covered, on low.
SERVE IT WITH: To make this a complete meal, you can top it with pepper slices and toasted nuts, then pair it with grilled chicken or fish.
PER SERVING
calories: 185 | fat: 19.1g | total carb: 6.0g | fiber: 6.7g | protein: 1.9g

CREAMY GARLIC PORK WITH CAULIFLOWER SOUP

Macros: Fat: 68% | Protein: 21% | Carbs: 11%
Prep time: 10 minutes | Cook time: 39 minutes | Serves 6

This creamy garlic pork and cauliflower soup is the mouthwatering soup dish for all pork lovers. It is a low-carb alternative to having a creamy pork soup. It has a tangy taste from the garlic and the sour cream which would have you reaching for the next bite.

½ cup butter	1 teaspoon of sea salt
1 medium onion	2 teaspoons dried oregano
8 garlic cloves	1½ cups pulled pork
1 pound (454 g) cauliflower	3 tablespoons sour cream
7 cups chicken broth	

SPECIAL EQUIPMENT:
Immersion blender

1. Heat the butter in a pan over medium heat and add the onions and garlic. Cook for 3 minutes.
2. Add the cauliflower, broth, and salt and let it cook for 20 minutes. Remove it from the heat. Use an immersion blender to purée until it is smooth.
3. Mix in the oregano, then put it back on the heat and let it cook for 5 minutes.
4. Mix in the pork and the sour cream and let it cook for 15 minutes.
5. Serve into bowls, hot.

STORAGE: Store in an airtight container in the fridge for up to 4 days or in the freezer for up to 1 month.
REHEAT: Microwave, covered, until the desired temperature is reached or reheat in a frying pan or instant pot, covered, on medium.
SERVE IT WITH: To make this a complete meal, serve it with some spinach salad.
PER SERVING
calories: 247 | fat: 18.7g | total carbs: 8.9g | fiber: 2.0g | protein: 12.7g

CHEESY SAUSAGE SOUP WITH TOMATOES AND SPINACH

Macros: Fat: 69% | Protein: 22% | Carbs: 9%
Prep time: 2 minutes | Cook time: 6 hours 6 minutes | Serves 10

This delicious cheesy sausage soup is packed with delicious spices and ingredients, which makes it a perfect dish for everyone. Made with tomatoes and spinach, this soup bursts with a delicious flavor that delights your taste buds.

2 tablespoons extra virgin olive oil
2 pounds (907 g) hot Italian sausage cut into bite-size pieces
2 sweet bell peppers, chopped
2 cups chicken broth low sodium
4 garlic cloves, minced
1 onion, chopped
2 tablespoons red wine vinegar

2 cups of water
1 (28-ounce / 794-g) can diced tomatoes with juice
4 ounces (113 g) fresh spinach leaves
1 teaspoon dried basil
1 teaspoon dried parsley
½ cup Parmesan cheese, grated

SPECIAL EQUIPMENT:
Slow cooker

1. Heat the olive oil in a pan over medium heat, then add the sausages. Cook for 5 minutes or until it is brown.
2. Put the cooked sausages into the slow cooker, then add the bell peppers, broth, garlic, onion, vinegar, water, and the tomatoes and its juice into the slow cooker. Cook on low for 6 hours.
3. Mix in the fresh spinach, basil, and parsley.
4. Serve into bowls topped with the grated Parmesan cheese.

STORAGE: Store in an airtight container in the fridge for up to 4 days or in the freezer for up to 1 month.
REHEAT: Microwave, covered, until the desired temperature is reached or reheat in a frying pan or instant pot, covered, on medium.
PER SERVING
calories: 387 | fat: 29.5g | total carbs: 11.9g | fiber: 2.9g | protein: 21.3g

GARLICKY PORK SOUP WITH CAULIFLOWER AND TOMATOES

Macros: Fat: 45% | Protein: 48% | Carbs: 7%
Prep time: 20 minutes | Cook time: 45 minutes | Serves 8

This garlicky pork soup dish is a comforting, hearty, flavorful dish for everyone. Made under an hour, it is a quick and easy no-fuss soup perfect for everyday cooking.

2 pounds (907 g) boneless pork ribs, cut into 1-inch pieces
2 tablespoons olive oil
1 tablespoon garlic, chopped
½ cup onions, chopped
½ cup dry white wine
1 cup chicken stock
1 cup of water

2 cups fresh tomatoes, chopped
2 cups cauliflower, finely chopped
2 tablespoons fresh oregano, chopped
Salt and freshly ground black pepper, to taste

1. Generously sprinkle the pork with salt and pepper.
2. Heat the olive oil in a pan over medium heat and add the pork. Cook for 3 minutes on each side until it is brown, then add the garlic and the onions.

3. Cook for 2 minutes then add the wine, chicken stock, water, and tomatoes.
4. Let it boil, then pour it into a crockpot to cook on high for 4 hours.
5. Mix in the cauliflower and the oregano, then let it cook for 20 minutes more.
6. Serve immediately.

STORAGE: Store in an airtight container in the fridge for up to 4 days or in the freezer for up to 1 month.
REHEAT: Microwave, covered, until the desired temperature is reached or reheat in a frying pan or instant pot, covered, on medium.
SERVE IT WITH: To make this a complete meal, serve it with Parmesan roasted zucchini.
PER SERVING
calories: 210 | fat: 10.4g | total carbs: 6.5g | fiber: 1.8g | protein: 25.5g

CREAMY AND CHEESY SPICY AVOCADO SOUP

Macros: Fat: 80% | Protein: 10% | Carbs: 10%
Prep time: 5 minutes | Cook time: 10 minutes | Serves 6

What dish is better than guacamole? This creamy and cheesy guacamole soup is the right answer. This avocado soup dish is the perfect soup dish for all guacamole lovers, made with spicy and creamy ingredients, this soup dish will take you on a gooey ride your taste buds will not want to return from.

2 avocados, peeled and pitted
¼ cup red onion, chopped
1 tablespoon fresh cilantro, chopped
2½ cups low-sodium chicken broth, divided
2 garlic cloves, coarsely chopped
1 jalapeño, seeded and coarsely chopped

1 tablespoon lime juice
¼ teaspoon black pepper
½ teaspoon salt
¼ teaspoon cayenne
¼ cup whipping cream
2 tablespoons sour cream
6 tablespoons Cheddar cheese, shredded

1. Put the avocado, onion, cilantro, 1 cup of the chicken broth, garlic, jalapeño, and lime juice into a food processor and pulse until it is smooth.
2. Add the rest of the broth, black pepper, salt, cayenne, and whipping cream to the food processor and pulse again until it is creamy, then pour it into a bowl.
3. Put the bowl in the refrigerator to chill for 1 hour.
4. Serve the soup into bowls topped with sour cream and Cheddar cheese.

STORAGE: Store in an airtight container in the fridge for up to 4 days or in the freezer for up to 1 month.
REHEAT: Microwave, covered, until the desired temperature is reached or reheat in a frying pan or instant pot, covered, on medium.
SERVE IT WITH: To make this a complete meal, serve it with roasted zucchini sticks.
PER SERVING
calories: 185 | fat: 16.4g | total carbs: 9.4g | fiber: 4.7g | protein: 4.6g

CHEESY TURKEY AND BACON SOUP WITH CELERY AND PARSLEY

Macros: Fat: 50% | Protein: 41% | Carbs: 9%
Prep time: 7 minutes | Cook time: 33 minutes | Serves 8

This mouthwatering turkey and bacon soup with celery and parsley is the perfect soup combination for all poultry and meat lovers. This delicious soup is quick and easy to make, especially during busy weekdays and nights. It can be eaten whether during lunch or dinner and stores perfectly to be eaten at a later date.

1 tablespoon olive oil
8 ounces (227 g) bacon, crumbled
1 large shallot, peeled and chopped
½ cup celery, chopped
4 cups cooked turkey meat, shredded or chopped
8 cups turkey (or chicken) stock

½ cup heavy whipping cream
½ cup extra sharp Cheddar cheese, shredded
1 teaspoon dried parsley
½ teaspoon liquid smoke
1 teaspoon xanthan gum
1 tablespoon fresh thyme leaves
Salt and freshly ground black pepper, to taste

1. Heat the olive oil in a pot over medium heat, then add the bacon, shallots, and celery. Cook for 5 minutes.
2. Pour in the turkey meat, turkey stock, whipping cream, and add the Cheddar cheese. Cook for 3 minutes.
3. Mix in the parsley and liquid smoke, then let it cook on low heat for 20 minutes.
4. Add the xanthan gum and whisk it well, then let it cook for 5 minutes.
5. Mix in the fresh thyme, then season with salt and black pepper.
6. Serve into bowls while it is hot.

STORAGE: Store in an airtight container in the fridge for up to 4 days or in the freezer for up to 1 month.
REHEAT: Microwave, covered, until the desired temperature is reached or reheat in a frying pan or instant pot, covered, on medium.
PER SERVING
calories: 461 | fat: 25.7g | total carbs: 10.2g | fiber: 0.2g | protein: 47.5g

CURRIED SHRIMP AND GREEN BEANS SOUP

Macros: Fat 67% | Protein 30% | Carbs 3%
Prep time: 10 minutes | Cook time: 12 minutes | Serves 4

You will enjoy the coconut-flavored soup containing shrimp and tasty spices. To enjoy curried shrimp and green beans soup, serve it while still hot. You can take this soup during any time of the day.

2 tablespoons butter
1 pound (454 g) jumbo shrimp, peeled and deveined
Chili pepper, to taste
Salt, to taste

2 tablespoons red curry paste
2 teaspoons ginger-garlic purée
6 ounces (170 g) unsweetened coconut milk
1 bunch green beans, halved

1. In a medium saucepan, melt the butter over medium heat.
2. Add the shrimp, chili pepper, and salt. Cook for about 3 minutes until the shrimps are opaque. Transfer the shrimps to a plate and set aside.
3. Add the red curry paste and ginger-garlic purée to the saucepan, then cook until fragrant, for about 2 minutes.
4. Pour in the shrimp, coconut milk, green beans, then season with salt and cook for 4 minutes as you stir.
5. Reduce the heat to medium low, and simmer for 3 minutes more, stirring occasionally.
6. Remove from the heat and serve warm.

STORAGE: Store in an airtight container in the fridge for up to 1 week.
REHEAT: Microwave, covered, until the desired temperature is reached or reheat in a frying pan or instant pot, covered, on medium heat
SERVE IT WITH: To make this a complete meal, serve the curried shrimp and green beans soup with zucchini noodles.
PER SERVING
calories: 325 | fat: 35.5g | total carbs: 3.0g | fiber: 1.2g | protein: 9.0g

Chapter 10
Appetizers and Snacks

EASY ENCHILADA CHICKEN DIP

Macros: Fat 82% | Protein 15% | Carbs 3%
Prep time: 15 minutes | Cook time: 50 minutes | Serves 30

If you are looking for an amazing appetizer to please your crowd, this Enchilada chicken dip is a solid choice. It's delicious and super easy to prepare. It's perfect when served with some baked keto vegetable chips or raw veggies.

1 pound (454 g) chicken breasts, skin and bones removed
1 (8-ounce / 227-g) jar mayonnaise, keto-friendly
1 (8-ounce / 227-g) package cream cheese, softened
1 (4-ounce / 114-g) can diced red chile peppers
1 (8-ounce / 227-g) package shredded Cheddar cheese
1 jalapeño pepper, diced finely

1. Preheat your oven to 350°F (180°C). Line a baking sheet with parchment paper and set aside.
2. Place the chicken on the prepared baking sheet. Bake for 20 minutes or until the chicken is cooked through.
3. Remove from the oven and let the chicken cool, then shed it using forks on a clean work surface.
4. Transfer the shredded chicken to a medium mixing bowl and add the remaining ingredients. Stir to combine well.
5. Arrange the chicken mixture on the baking sheet and bake uncovered for 30 minutes, or until the edges are browned.
6. Remove from the oven and let it cool for 5 minutes to serve.

STORAGE: Store in an airtight container in the fridge for up to 3 days.
REHEAT: Microwave, covered, until it reaches the desired temperature.
SERVE IT WITH: To make this a delicious and complete meal, serve the dip with some baked keto vegetables or raw veggies.
PER SERVING
calories: 113 | fat: 10.6g | total carbs: 0.9g | fiber: 0.1g | protein: 3.9g

KETO BAKED EGGS

Macros: Fat 60% | Protein 35% | Carbs 4%
Prep time: 5 minutes | Cook time: 10 minutes | Serves 1

The combination of ingredients in this meal makes it perfect whether it is breakfast, lunch, or dinner. Make this recipe with your preferred meat. It can be beef, pork, or lamb. If you have some leftovers, then you can use them.

3 ounces (85 g) cooked ground meat (beef, pork, or lamb)
2 eggs
2 ounces (57 g) shredded cheese

1. Start by preheating the oven to 400°F (205°C).
2. In a greased baking dish, put the cooked ground meat. Using a spoon to make two holes, then crack the eggs into the holes.
3. Top with a sprinkle of shredded cheese.
4. Bake in the oven for 15 minutes until the eggs are set.
5. Remove from the oven and cool for about 5 minutes before serving.

STORAGE: Store in an airtight container in the fridge for up to 4 days.
REHEAT: Microwave, covered, until the desired temperature is reached or reheat in a frying pan or air fryer, covered, on medium.
SERVE IT WITH: To make this a complete meal, serve the eggs with avocados and fresh herbs. The baked eggs also taste better with crunchy and crispy green salad.
PER SERVING
calories: 606 | fat: 40.8g | total carbs: 7.0g | fiber: 0g | protein: 41.0g

BUTTERED LOBSTER AND CREAM CHEESE DIP

Macros: Fat 83% | Protein 15% | Carbs 2%
Prep time: 10 minutes | Cook time: 0 minutes | Serves 16

A delicious meal that is suitable when you prepare it a day before eating it. It is creamy and sweet to the taste buds. Why not try this simple recipe?

1 (7-ounce / 198-g) can drained and flaked lobster meat
1 tablespoon lemon juice
1 tablespoon minced onion
4 tablespoons softened butter
1 (8-ounce / 227-g) package softened cream cheese
Salt and freshly ground black pepper, to taste

1. In a bowl, add the lobster meat, lemon juice, onion, butter, cream cheese, pepper, and salt. Mix well until the mixture is smooth.
2. Cover the mixture with plastic wrap, then transfer to the refrigerator and chill until ready to serve.

STORAGE: Store in an airtight container in the fridge for up to 4 days.
SERVE IT WITH: To make this a complete meal, serve it with Bacon Cauliflower Chowder.
PER SERVING
calories: 85 | fat: 7.8g | total carbs: 0.7g | fiber: 0g | protein: 3.0g

DEVILED MAYONNAISE EGGS

Macros: Fat 69% | Protein 25% | Carbs 6%
Prep time: 10 minutes | Cook time: 20 minutes | Serves 8

The meal is perfect for gatherings such as holidays and the Easter. The ingredients are simple and easy to prepare. The paprika pops the flavor of the meal. It is a healthy appetizer or a snack.

8 eggs
⅓ cup keto-friendly mayonnaise
2 tablespoons horseradish sauce
2 tablespoons low-carb Worcestershire sauce
1 teaspoon hot pepper sauce
Salt and pepper to taste
1 teaspoon paprika, for garnish
1 teaspoon dried parsley flakes, for garnish

1. Put the eggs in a saucepan of water and allow to boil for 7 minutes. Remove the eggs from the hot water with a slotted spoon. Let them cool under running cold water in the sink. Peel the eggs and place them on a plate.
2. Halve the eggs and put the yolks in a bowl. Reserve the egg whites on the plate. Using a fork, mash the egg yolks until finely smooth.
3. Add the mayonnaise, horseradish sauce, Worcestershire sauce, hot sauce, pepper, and salt. Stir to combine well.
4. Using a plastic bag, spoon in the yolk mixture. Snip off one corner to make a ½-inch opening and pipe the yolk filling into each halved egg white. Garnish with paprika and parsley before serving.

STORAGE: Store in an airtight container in the fridge for up to 4 days.
REHEAT: Microwave, covered, until it reaches the desired temperature.
SERVE IT WITH: To make this a complete meal, serve the dish with keto chicken soup.
PER SERVING
calories: 164 | fat: 12.9g | total carbs: 2.2g | fiber: 0.2g | protein: 9.2g

TASTY ARTICHOKE DIP

Macros: Fat 86% | Protein 9% | Carbs 5%
Prep time: 10 minutes | Cook time: 25 minutes | Serves 30

This is one of the easiest and delicious chafing-dish dips you can make in your home. It's the best baked dip and a huge hit to serve your family and friends.

1 (6½-ounce / 184-g) jar marinated artichoke hearts, drained and quartered
1½ cups grated Parmesan cheese, divided

1 cup keto-friendly mayonnaise
1 (4-ounce / 113-g) can chopped green chile pepper
1 (8-ounce / 227-g) package cream cheese, softened

1. Preheat your oven to 350°F (180°C).
2. Combine the artichoke hearts, 1 cup Parmesan cheese, mayonnaise, chile pepper, and cream cheese in a mixing bowl. Stir to incorporate.
3. Spoon the artichoke mixture into a greased baking pan, and sprinkle with the remaining Parmesan cheese.
4. Bake in the oven for 25 minutes, or until the top is lightly browned.
5. Remove from the oven and serve warm.

STORAGE: Store in an airtight container in the fridge up to 4 to 5 days.
REHEAT: Microwave, covered, until it reaches the desired temperature.
SERVE IT WITH: To make this a complete meal, serve it with cucumber pieces or celery sticks.
PER SERVING
Calories: 73 | Fat: 6.3g | Total Carbs: 2.0g | Fiber: 0.4g | Protein: 2.2g

GRILLED PORTOBELLO MUSHROOMS

Macros: Fat 80% | Protein 3% | Carbs 17%
Prep time: 10 minutes | Cook time: 10 minutes | Serves 3

This is a delicious snack food that you can easily make on your grill. Everybody in your family or friends coming over will rave on about how wonderful it is. It's also insanely irresistible, so you will want to make it repeatedly.

3 portobello mushrooms
¼ cup olive oil
4 tablespoons balsamic vinegar

4 garlic cloves, minced
3 tablespoons onions, chopped

1. Thoroughly clean the mushrooms and cut off the stems on your cutting board. Reserve the stems for other use.
2. Place the mushroom caps on a platter, grills facing up. Set aside.
3. Mix the oil, vinegar, garlic, and onions in a small bowl, then pour the mixture evenly over the mushroom caps. Let them rest in the marinade for about 1 hour.
4. Preheat the grill to medium-high heat.
5. Grill the mushrooms for 10 minutes, flipping them halfway through, or until the mushrooms are lightly browned.
6. Transfer to a plate and let cool for 5 minutes before serving.

STORAGE: Store in an airtight container in the fridge for up to 3 days.
REHEAT: Microwave, covered, until it reaches the desired temperature.
SERVE IT WITH: To make this a delicious complete meal, serve the grilled mushrooms with a hearty topping.
PER SERVING
calories: 206 | fat: 18.3g | total carbs: 9.1g | fiber: 1.3g | protein: 2.2g

BACON-WRAPPED JALAPENO POPPERS

Macros: Fat 81% | Protein 15% | Carbs 5%
Prep time: 30 minutes | Cook time: 30 minutes | Serves 30

If you are looking for a snack that is packed with a bit of punch, look no further. These mouth-watering party favorite bites will please your taste buds and everyone in your family or party will love them.

2 (12-ounce / 340-g) packages ground sausage
2 (8-ounce / 227-g) packages cream cheese, softened

30 jalapeño chile peppers
1 pound (454 g) sliced bacon, halved

SPECIAL EQUIPMENT:
Toothpicks, soaked for at least 30 minutes

1. Preheat your oven to 375°F (190°C). Line a baking sheet with parchment paper and set aside.
2. Meanwhile, cook the sausages in a large skillet over medium-high heat until it's evenly browned, for about 12 minutes.
3. Drain the cooked sausages and transfer them to a mixing bowl. Add the cream cheese and stir until well combined. Set aside.
4. On a flat work surface, slice the jalapeños lengthwise and remove the seeds. Using a spoon to stuff the jalapeño halves with uniform sausage and cream cheese filling. Wrap each stuffed jalapeño half with a half slice of bacon, then secure with a toothpick.
5. Arrange the stuffed jalapeños on the baking sheet and bake in the oven for 20 minutes, or until the bacon is crispy.
6. Remove from the oven and cool for about 5 minutes before serving.

STORAGE: Store in an airtight container in the fridge for up to 4 days or in the freezer for up to 1 month.
REHEAT: Microwave, covered, until it reaches the desired temperature.
SERVE IT WITH: To make this a complete meal, serve it with ranch dressing for dipping.
PER SERVING
calories: 197 | fat: 18.4g | total carbs: 1.8g | fiber: 0.4g | protein: 6.2g

TOMATOES AND JALAPEÑO SALSA

Macros: Fat 8% | Protein 11% | Carbs 81%
Prep time: 10 minutes | Cook time: 0 minutes | Serves 4

It is an easy to make a recipe that takes only 10 minutes to prepare. The ingredients you use are fresh with lots of nutrients. Best when served immediately after preparation.

4 chopped large tomatoes
½ cup chopped fresh cilantro
1 chopped onion
3 cloves minced garlic

1 diced tomatillo
Salt, to taste
1 tablespoon lime juice
1 minced jalapeño pepper

1. Using a bowl, mix the tomatoes, cilantro, onion, garlic, tomatillo, salt, lime juice and jalapeño pepper. Stir to incorporate.
2. Cover the salsa with plastic wrap. Allow to chill until ready to serve or up to 24 hours.

STORAGE: Store in an airtight container in the fridge for up to 4 days. It is not recommended to freeze.
SERVE IT WITH: To make this a complete meal, serve the dish with zucchini chips.
PER SERVING
calories: 56 | fat: 0.5g | total carbs: 12.3g | fiber: 3.1g | protein: 2.4g

KETO BACON-WRAPPED BARBECUE SHRIMP

Macros: Fat 79% | Protein 18% | Carbs 3%
Prep time: 20 minutes | Cook time: 10 minutes | Serves 4

This keto bacon-wrapped barbecue shrimp is a hit when served as an appetizer or for dinner. Use large shrimps for a most satisfaction. Kick up its flavors by serving it with spicy sriracha mayo dip.

16 large shrimps, peeled and deveined
8 bacon slices, halved lengthwise
Barbecue seasoning to taste, keto-friendly

SPECIAL EQUIPMENT:
Toothpicks, soaked for at least 30 minutes

1. Preheat your oven to 450°F (235°C).
2. On a clean work surface, tightly wrap each shrimp with half slice of bacon, then secure with a toothpick.
3. Line your jelly roll pan with foil and position a baking rack in it.
4. Arrange the bacon-wrapped shrimp on a wire rack and generously sprinkle the barbecue seasoning on both sides. The rack prevents the shrimp from sitting on draining bacon fat when baking.
5. Allow to rest for 15 minutes, or until the bacon turns a little opaque after soaking in the seasoning.
6. Bake in the oven for 10 to 15 minutes, or until the shrimp is opaque and bacon is crispy.
7. Remove from the oven and cool for 5 minutes before serving.

STORAGE: Store in an airtight container in the fridge for up to 4 days. It is not recommended to freeze.
REHEAT: Microwave, covered, until it reaches the desired temperature.
SERVE IT WITH: To make this a complete meal, serve it with some keto veggies.
PER SERVING
calories: 238 | fat: 20.7g | total carbs: 1.1g | fiber: 0.1g | protein: 10.4g

BALSAMIC MUSHROOMS

Macros: Fat 73% | Protein 8% | Carbs 19%
Prep time: 15 minutes | Cook time: 10 minutes | Serves 8

Balsamic mushrooms are yummy and a brilliant way to kick off your dinner party. The mushrooms are equally mouth watering whether you serve them warm or cold. This means you can prepare them ahead of appetizer time.

3 tablespoons olive oil
3 minced garlic cloves
1 pound (454 g) mushrooms,
freshly sliced
3 tablespoons balsamic vinegar
Salt and pepper, to taste

1. Heat the olive oil in a skillet and sauté the garlic for about 2 minutes. Make sure you do not brown the garlic.
2. Fold in the mushrooms and continue to cook as you stir for 3 minutes. Add the vinegar and cook for 2 minutes more. Lightly season with salt and pepper.
3. Remove from the heat and serve on a plate.

STORAGE: Store in an airtight container in the fridge up to 3 to 5 days.
REHEAT: Microwave, covered, until it reaches the desired temperature.
SERVE IT WITH: To make this a complete meal, serve it with a grilled steak or pork chops.
PER SERVING
calories: 64 | fat: 5.3g | total carbs: 3.25g | fiber: 0.6g | protein: 1.89g

KETO CHEDDAR AND BACON MUSHROOMS

Macros: Fat 79% | Protein 17% | Carbs 4%
Prep time: 15 minutes | Cook time: 30 minutes | Serves 8

Make your next family gathering hosting opportunity a breeze with this cheese and bacon stuffed mushrooms. They are deceptively simple, fast to prepare and tastier than you can imagine.

3 bacon slices
8 cremini mushrooms
1 tablespoon butter
1 tablespoon onions, chopped
¾ cup shredded Cheddar cheese, divided

1. Cook the bacon in a large skillet over medium-high heat until evenly browned, for about 12 minutes.
2. Transfer to a plate lined with paper towels to drain the excess grease. When cool enough to handle, crumble and set it aside.
3. Preheat your oven to 400°F(205°C).
4. Remove the mushrooms stems and chop them on your cutting board. Reserve the caps on a platter and set aside.
5. Melt the butter in the skillet over medium-high heat. Add the chopped mushroom stems and onions, then cook until the onions are tender.
6. Remove from the heat to a mixing bowl.
7. Put the crumbled bacon and ½ cup of Cheddar cheese in the mixing bowl. Stir to combine well.
8. Use a spoon to scoop the bacon filling to the mushroom caps.
9. Bake the stuffed caps in the oven for 15 minutes, or until the cheese melts.
10. Remove from the oven and sprinkle the remaining cheese on top for garnish and serve.

STORAGE: Store in an airtight container in the fridge for up to 4 days or in the freezer for up to 1 month.
REHEAT: Microwave, covered, until the desired temperature is reached or reheat in a frying pan or instant pot, covered, on medium.
SERVE IT WITH: To make this a complete meal, serve it with a cup of coffee.
PER SERVING
calories: 107 | fat: 8.9g | total carbs: 0.95g | fiber: 0.2g | protein: 4.3g

RED PEPPER ROASTED DIP

Macros: Fat 86% | Protein 11% | Carbs 3%
Prep time: 10 minutes | Cook time: 20 minutes | Serves 30

Enjoy the amazing snack after a busy day. You can change the recipe by adding some walnuts to improve the taste and flavors. Try out this recipe and your cool evenings will never be the same.

1 tablespoon onion, minced
1 (7-ounce / 198-g) jar roasted red peppers, drained and diced
2 tablespoons Dijon mustard
1 (8-ounce / 227-g) package
cream cheese, softened
¾ pound (340 g) shredded Monterey Jack cheese
1 garlic clove, minced
1 cup keto-friendly mayonnaise

1. Start by preheating the oven to 350°F (180°C)
2. Mix the onion, roasted red peppers, Dijon mustard, cream cheese, Monterey Jack cheese, garlic, and mayonnaise in a baking dish
3. Place in the prepared oven and bake for 20 minutes until lightly browned.
4. Remove from the oven and serve while still warm.

STORAGE: Store in an airtight container in the fridge for up to 1 week or in the freezer for up to 1 month.
REHEAT: Microwave, covered, until the desired temperature is reached or reheat in a frying pan or instant pot, covered, on medium.
SERVE IT WITH: To make this a complete meal, serve the dip with keto veggies.
PER SERVING
calories: 123 | fat: 12.2g | total carbs: 0.9g | fiber: 0.1g | protein: 3.1g

EASILY BAKED BUFFALO CHICKEN DIP

Macros: Fat 80% | Protein 17% | Carbs 3%
Prep time: 15 minutes | Cook time: 20 minutes | Serves 8

If you are tired of showing up at every super bowl party with a large bag of chips, then this is buffalo chicken dip will get you from snack shrub to an all-star appetizer. It's immensely delicious and very easy to put together.

3 cups rotisserie chicken, diced and cooked
2 (8-ounce / 227-g) packages cream cheese, softened
½ cup blue cheese dressing
¾ cup hot pepper sauce

½ tablespoon seafood seasoning
½ cup plus 2 tablespoons shredded pepper Jack cheese
½ cup crumbled blue cheese
Cayenne pepper, to taste

1. Preheat your oven to 400°F (205°C).
2. In a large bowl, mix the chicken, cream cheese, blue cheese dressing, hot pepper sauce, seafood seasoning, ½ cup of pepper Jack cheese, crumbled blue cheese, and cayenne pepper.
3. Transfer the mixture to a greased baking dish and top with 2 tablespoons pepper Jack cheese.
4. Bake for 15 to 20 minutes or until the dip is lightly browned.
5. Remove from the oven and garnish with cayenne pepper to serve.

STORAGE: Store in an airtight container in the fridge for 3 days.
REHEAT: Microwave, covered, until it reaches the desired temperature.
SERVE IT WITH: To make this a complete meal, serve it with some zucchini crisps.
PER SERVING
calories: 450 | fat: 37.2g | total carbs: 5.3g | fiber:0.2g | protein: 23.3g

KETO SMOKED SALMON FAT BOMBS

Macros: Fat 90% | Protein 10% | Carbs 0%
Prep time: 10 minutes | Cook time: 0 minutes | Serves 12 Fat Bombs

Salmon fat bombs are a combination of healthy fat like grass-fed butter, coconut oil, nut and the protein salmon. It provides an excellent keto diet with the low-carb content.

½ cup goat cheese, at room temperature
2 teaspoons freshly squeezed lemon juice
2 ounces (57 g) smoked salmon

Freshly ground black pepper, to taste
½ cup butter, at room temperature

1. Line a baking sheet with parchment paper and set aside.
2. Make the fat bombs: In a bowl, add cheese, lemon juice, smoked salmon, pepper, and butter, then stir well to blend.
3. Scoop 1 tablespoon of the butter mixture onto the baking sheet until you make 12 equally sized mounds.
4. Transfer the sheet into the refrigerator for about 3 hours until fat bombs become firm.
5. Remove from the refrigerator and let stand under room temperature for a few minutes before serving.

STORAGE: Store in an airtight container in the fridge for up to 4 days or in the freezer for up to 1 month.
SERVE IT WITH: To make this a complete meal, you can serve it with plain Greek yogurt.
PER SERVING
calories: 88 | fat: 9.0g | total carbs: 0g | fiber: 0g | protein: 1.9g

BABA GHANOUSH

Macros: Fat 66% | Protein 9% | Carbs 25%
Prep time: 5 minutes | Cook time: 40 minutes | Serves 12

This Baba Ghanoush is a creamy and flavorful dip that you can make at your home with very few preparations. It highly complements keto diet and can even be served as vegan, Whole30, and gluten-free diets.

1 eggplant
¼ cup tahini
¼ cup lemon juice
2 garlic cloves, minced

2 tablespoons sesame seeds
Salt and pepper, to taste
1 ½ tablespoon olive oil
Cooking spray

1. Preheat your oven to 400°F (205°C) and lightly grease the baking sheet with cooking spray.
2. Arrange the eggplant on the greased baking sheet and use a fork to poke holes in the skin.
3. Roast the eggplant for 40 minutes until tender, turning it over occasionally.
4. Remove from the oven to a bowl with cold water. Drain the water and peel off the skin.
5. Process the eggplant, tahini, lemon juice, garlic, and sesame seeds in a food processor until smooth. Sprinkle the salt and pepper to season.
6. Place the mixture in a serving bowl, then add the olive oil. Mix well.
7. Chill in the refrigerator for about 3 hours before serving.

STORAGE: Store in an airtight container in the fridge up to 4 days.
SERVE IT WITH: To make this a complete meal, serve it with spinach or kale crisps.
PER SERVING
calories: 72 | fat: 5.3g | total carbs: 4.5g | fiber: 2.0g | protein: 1.6g

MEXICAN-STYLE SCRAMBLED EGGS

Macros: Fat 68% | Protein 24% | Carbs 7%
Prep time: 5 minutes | Cook time: 10 minutes | Serves 4

Prepare this dish for your breakfast. Filled with the flavorful eggs, tomatoes, jalapeños, and scallions, you will have wonderful breakfast moments to spice up your day.

1 ounce (28 g) butter
1 chopped tomato
1 chopped scallion
2 chopped pickled jalapeños pepper

6 eggs
Salt and freshly ground black pepper, to taste
3 ounces (85 g) shredded cheese

1. Put the butter in a medium pan over medium-high heat to melt.
2. Add the tomatoes, scallions, and jalapeños, then cook for 4 minutes until tender.
3. Beat the eggs in a small bowl, then add to the pan. Cook as you scramble for 2 minutes.
4. Sprinkle with the pepper, cheese, and salt. Stir well and serve warm.

STORAGE: Store in an airtight container in the fridge for up to 4 days.
REHEAT: Microwave, covered, until the desired temperature is reached or reheat in a frying pan, covered, on medium.
SERVE IT WITH: To make this a complete meal, serve the eggs with crisp lettuce, avocados, and a dressing to add taste.
PER SERVING
calories: 216 | fat: 16.7g | total carbs: 4.3g | fiber: 0.7g | protein: 12.2g

CHEESY CAULIFLOWER CRACKERS

Macros: Fat 63% | Protein 28% | Carbs 9%
Prep time: 20 minutes | Cook time: 25 minutes | Serves 18

It is a keto cracker that is spicy. It is perfect since it is a low-carb meal. It's delicious and a must-try recipe. It is also cheesy and sweet as it is enriched with the salad dressing and pepper.

1 (12-ounce / 340-g) package frozen riced cauliflower	dressing mix
1/2 teaspoon cayenne pepper	1 egg, whisked
1 tablespoon dry ranch salad	1 cup shredded Parmesan cheese

1. Preheat the oven to 425°F (220°C). Line a baking sheet with parchment paper and set aside.
2. In a microwave-safe bowl, put the riced cauliflower. Microwave it for about 4 minutes. Set aside to cool for 15 minutes.
3. In a separate bowl, mix the riced cauliflower, cayenne pepper, ranch mix, and whisked egg. Stir well. Add the Parmesan cheese, then mix well until it is incorporated.
4. Make the crackers: Scoop about 2 tablespoons of the mixture onto the prepared baking sheet one at a time and flatten each to about 1/8-inch thickness with a rolling pin.
5. Transfer to the oven and bake for about 10 minutes. Flip the crackers over and bake for 10 minutes more, then place them on a wire rack to cool. Serve warm.

STORAGE: Store in an airtight container in the fridge for up to 4 days or in the freezer for up to 1 month.
REHEAT: Microwave, covered, until it reaches the desired temperature.
SERVE IT WITH: To make this a complete meal, serve the dish with Keto Broccoli Cheddar Soup.
PER SERVING
calories: 80 | fat: 3.0g | total carbs: 9.8g | fiber: 4.4g | protein: 5.9g

CRAB–STUFFED AVOCADO

Macros: Fat 72% | Protein 17% | Carbs 11%
Prep time: 20 minutes | Cook time: 0 minutes | Serves 2

Crab-stuffed avocado salad is an amazingly delicious dish suitable for a light lunch. The meal is healthy, scrumptious, and filing. The stuffed crab goes well with the nutritive avocado.

1 halved lengthwise avocado, peeled and pitted	and chopped
1/2 teaspoon freshly squeezed lemon juice	1/4 cup red bell pepper, chopped
4 1/2 ounces (127 g) Dungeness crab meat	1/2 cup cream cheese
1/4 cup English cucumber, peeled	1 teaspoon cilantro, chopped
	1/2 scallion, chopped
	Sea salt and freshly ground black pepper, to taste

1. Brush the avocado edges with lemon juice, then set in a bowl.
2. In a bowl, add the crab meat, cucumber, red pepper, cream cheese, cilantro, scallion, salt, and pepper then stir to mix.
3. Divide the crab meat mixture in the avocado halves before serving.

STORAGE: Store in an airtight container in the fridge for up to 4 days or in the freezer for up to 1 month.
SERVE IT WITH: To make this a complete meal, serve the dish on a bed of greens.
PER SERVING
calories: 420 | fat: 32.0g | total carbs: 12.6g | fiber: 7.0g | protein: 16.8g

PROSCIUTTO AND ASPARAGUS WRAPS

Macros: Fat 21% | Protein 51% | Carbs 28%
Prep time: 15 minutes | Cook time: 15 minutes | Serves 4

It is a special and easy to make a meal. It is suitable for Mother's Day, Easter or any special occasion. When served, the meal is fancy and appealing to the eyes. The salty flavor complements the sweet asparagus flavor.

1/2 pound (227 g) sliced prosciutto	softened Parmesan cheese
1/2 (8-ounce / 227-g) package	12 spears trimmed fresh asparagus

1. Preheat the oven to 450°F (235°C).
2. On a flat work surface, spread the prosciutto slices with the cheese. Tightly wrap the slices around 3 asparagus spears. Repeat with the remaining slices and asparagus spears.
3. Arrange the wrapped spears on a greased baking sheet in a single layer.
4. Transfer to the oven and bake for about 15 minutes until the asparagus spears become tender.
5. Transfer to four serving plates and cool for a few minutes before serving.

STORAGE: Store in an airtight container in the fridge for up to 4 days.
REHEAT: Microwave the sliced prosciutto, covered, until it reaches the desired temperature.
SERVE IT WITH: To make this a complete meal, serve the dish with Creamy Broccoli Cheddar Soup.
PER SERVING
calories: 178 | fat: 4.3g | total carbs: 12.6g | fiber: 0.2g | protein: 22.1g

HEARTY BACON AND MUSHROOM PLATTER

Macros: Fat: 49% | Protein: 19% | Carbs: 33%
Prep time: 15minutes | Cook time: 15 minutes | Serves 4

A one-pan family favorite recipe of bacon and mushrooms... This easy to cook but richly delicious dish is prepared with only 5 ingredients.

6 uncured bacon strips, chopped	2 tablespoons homemade chicken stock
4 cups fresh wild mushrooms, sliced	1 tablespoon fresh thyme, chopped
2 teaspoons garlic, minced	

1. Heat a large nonstick skillet over medium-high heat and cook the bacon for about 7 minutes or until crispy, stirring frequently. Add the mushrooms and garlic and sauté for about 7 minutes. Add the chicken stock and with the wooden spoon, stir to scrape up any browned bits from the bottom of skillet.
2. Remove from the heat and serve hot with fresh thyme sprinkled on top.

STORAGE: Store in an airtight container in the fridge for up to 4 days or in the freezer for up to 1 month.
REHEAT: Microwave, covered, until the desired temperature is reached or reheat in a frying pan or air fryer / instant pot, covered, on medium.
SERVE IT WITH: Serve this dish with your favorite greens.
TIP: Topping of Parmesan cheese will enhance the flavor of bacon and mushrooms.
PER SERVING
calories: 67 | fat: 3.9g | total carbs: 6.0g | fiber: 2.6g | protein: 3.9g

LOW-CARB CHEESY ALMOND BISCUITS

Macros: Fat 72% | Protein 25% | Carbs 3%
Prep time: 20 minutes | **Cook time:** 20 minutes | **Serves 8**

The biscuits are delicious. For cheese lovers, you won't miss out your favorite cheese. It can make individual biscuits or a large loaf. The biscuits are perfect for both keto and non-keto diet individuals.

1 tablespoon baking powder
2 cups almond flour
2½ cups shredded Cheddar
cheese
4 eggs
⅛ cup heavy cream

1. Preheat the oven to 350°F (180°C) and line a baking sheet with parchment paper. Set aside.
2. In a bowl, add the baking powder, almond flour and Cheddar cheese. Stir well to mix. In a separate bowl, whisk the eggs until frothy.
3. Make a well in the center of the almond mixture bowl, then gently pour in the whisked eggs and heavy cream. Using a fork, stir the mixture until it forms a sticky batter.
4. Make the biscuits: Divide the batter into 9 equal portions and transfer to the baking sheet, then form into a rounded biscuit shape. Bake for 20 minutes until a toothpick inserted in the center comes out clean.
5. Divide the biscuits among serving plates and allow to cool for 5 minutes before serving.

STORAGE: Store in an airtight container in the fridge for up to 4 days.
REHEAT: Microwave, covered, until it reaches the desired temperature.
SERVE IT WITH: To make this a complete meal, serve the biscuits with a cup of coffee.
PER SERVING
calories: 243 | fat: 19.7g | total carbs: 2.1g | fiber: 0.1g | protein: 14.5g

CHEESY CAULIFLOWER BAKE

Macros: Fat 82% | Protein 9% | Carbs 9%
Prep time: 5 minutes | **Cook time:** 30 minutes | **Serves 6**

The cheesy cauliflower recipe takes a quick time to prepare. The cheesy cauliflower is a delicious way to make a low-carb and keto-friendly side dish that's packed with vegetables.

2 tablespoons olive oil
2 teaspoons avocado
mayonnaise, keto-friendly
2 tablespoons mustard
2 chopped cauliflower heads
½ cup butter, chopped into
½-inch pieces
1 cup grated Parmesan cheese

1. Preheat the oven to 400°F (205°C) and grease a baking dish with olive oil.
2. In a bowl, add the avocado mayonnaise and mustard and mix well. Coat cauliflower heads with this mixture before placing in the baking dish.
3. Top with butter and Parmesan cheese and bake in the preheated oven until the cauliflower heads are soft for 25 minutes.
4. Transfer to serving plates to cool before serving.

STORAGE: Store in an airtight container in the fridge for up to 4 days or in the freezer for up to 1 month.
REHEAT: Microwave, covered, until it reaches the desired temperature.
SERVE IT WITH: To make this a complete meal, serve with Turmeric Beef Bone Broth.
PER SERVING
calories: 282 | fat: 26.2g | total carbs: 7.0g | fiber: 2.0g | protein: 6.8g

BUTTERED COCONUT PUFFS

Macros: Fat 87% | Protein 10% | Carbs 3%
Prep time: 0 minutes | **Cook time:** 40 minutes | **Serves 2**

It has simple ingredients that can be prepared in no time. They are basic and sweet. The meal is versatile as it can complement a number of different foods. It can be taken as breakfast or dinner.

1 tablespoon olive oil, for
greasing the cookie sheet
¼ cup butter
½ cup water
½ cup coconut flour
2 eggs
A handful of spiced fennel, for
filling

1. Preheat the oven to 375°F (190°C) and grease the cookie sheet with olive oil. Set aside.
2. Heat the butter and water in a saucepan over medium heat until the butter melts. Pour the flour into the saucepan all at once. Vigorously stir until it forms a ball in the middle of the pan. Set aside.
3. Add the eggs, one at a time, then beat the mixture until fully blended and stiff. Drop about ¾ teaspoon portions onto the cookie sheet. Gently smooth the pointed peaks with a moistened finger, and round the tops to ensure even rising.
4. Bake for about 40 minutes until puffs rise and are golden brown on top. Transfer to a wire rack to cool completely.
5. Slit an opening on one side, then stuff with the filling before serving.

STORAGE: Store in an airtight container in the fridge for up to 3 days.
SERVE IT WITH: To add more flavors to this meal, you can serve sprinkled with coconut flakes.
PER SERVING
calories: 404 | fat: 39.5g | total carbs: 3.3g | fiber: 0.7g | protein: 9.6g

DEVILED EGGS WITH BACON AND CHEESE

Macros: Fat 80% | Protein 16% | Carbs 4%
Prep time: 15 minutes | **Cook time:** 0 minutes | **Serves 12**

The deviled eggs contain finely shredded Swiss cheese and bacon. They are nutritionally better than ordinary eggs. The recipe is easy and takes a short duration of time to cook.

6 large hard-boiled eggs, peeled
¼ cup keto-friendly mayonnaise
¼ cup finely shredded Swiss
cheese
½ teaspoon Dijon mustard
¼ chopped avocado
Ground black pepper, to taste
6 cooked and chopped bacon
slices

1. Cut the eggs in halves. Spoon the yolk out carefully and put in a bowl. Arrange the whites, hollow side facing up, on a plate.
2. Crumble the yolks with a fork. Add the mayonnaise, cheese, mustard, and avocado. Stir well to mix. Add the pepper to season.
3. Fill the hollow egg whites with the yolk mixture.
4. Top every egg half with the bacon before serving.

STORAGE: Store in an airtight container in the fridge for up to 4 days or in the freezer for up to 1 month.
REHEAT: Microwave, covered, until it reaches the desired temperature.
SERVE IT WITH: To make this a complete meal, serve with broccoli Cheddar soup.
PER SERVING
calories: 134 | fat: 11.9g | total carbs: 1.45g | fiber: 0.3g | protein: 5.2g

BAKED BEEF, PORK AND VEAL MEATBALLS

Macros: Fat 74% | Protein 24% | Carbs 2%
Prep time: 30 minutes | Cook time: 30 minutes | Serves 8

The combination of the beef, veal, and pork sound perfect, right? The mixture makes the meal very delicious. A perfect snack for all times.

1 pound (454 g) ground beef	Salt and ground black pepper, to
½ pound (227 g) ground pork	taste
½ pound (227 g) ground veal	1½ tablespoons chopped Italian
1 cup freshly grated Romano	flat leaf parsley
cheese, plus more Romano for	2 cups shredded coconut
garnish	1½ cups lukewarm water
2 minced cloves garlic	1 cup olive oil
2 eggs, whisked	

1. In a large bowl, add the beef, pork, and veal. Stir to mix well. Add the cheese, whisked eggs, garlic, pepper, salt, and parsley. Blend well.
2. Add the coconut, then slowly add ½ cup water as you stir until the mixture is moist but still able to hold its shape when rolled into meatballs. Form the mixture into 2-inch meatballs with your wet hands.
3. In a nonstick skillet, heat the olive oil, then fry the meatballs for about 15 minutes (in batches), turning occasionally, until evenly browned and slightly crispy.
4. Remove from the heat and sprinkle with Romano cheese on top for garnish, if desired.

STORAGE: Store in an airtight container in the fridge for up to 4 days or in the freezer for up to 1 month.
REHEAT: Microwave, covered, until the desired temperature is reached or reheat in a frying pan or air fryer / instant pot, covered, on medium.
SERVE IT WITH: To make this a complete meal, serve with Turmeric Beef Bone Broth.
PER SERVING
calories: 591 | fat: 49g | total carbs: 3.2g | fiber: 0.7g | protein: 33.1g

ALMOND SAUSAGE BALLS

Macros: Fat 74% | Proteins 19% | Carbs 7%
Prep time: 30 minutes | Cook time: 25 minutes | Serves 6

With only five ingredients, get into the kitchen and prepare almond sausage balls within a few minutes. Take the keto balls anytime you feel hungry. Prepare in advance to save time. If you have kids, do not miss out on these tasty balls.

1 cup almond flour, blanched	shredded
3 ounces bulk Italian sausage	2 teaspoons baking powder
1¼ cups sharp Cheddar cheese,	1 large egg

1. Start by preheating the oven to 350°F (180°C) then grease a baking tray.
2. In a mixing bowl, mix the almond flour, Italian sausage, Cheddar cheese, baking powder, and the egg until mixed evenly.
3. Make equal-sized balls out of the mixture, then put them on the baking tray.
4. Put in the oven and bake for 20 minutes or until golden brown.
5. Remove from the oven and serve.

STORAGE: Store in an airtight container in the fridge for up to 1 week.
REHEAT: Microwave, covered, until it reaches the desired temperature.
PER SERVING
calories: 266 | fat: 22.5g | total carbs: 4.7g | fiber: 2.0g | protein: 13.0g

MEDITERRANEAN BAKED SPINACH

Macros: Fat 75% | Protein 13% | Carbs 11%
Prep time: 5 minutes | Cook time: 25 minutes | Serves 6

Spinach gets a Mediterranean touch when baked in a casserole with a mixture of feta cheese with pitted black olives and butter. The recipe is easy to follow and takes a short time to prepare.

2 tablespoons olive oil	1½ cups grated feta cheese
2 cups water	½ cup halved and pitted black
2 pounds (907 g) chopped	olives
spinach	4 teaspoons grated fresh lemon
4 tablespoons butter	zest
Salt and black pepper, to taste	

1. Preheat the air fryer to 400°F (205°C) and grease the air fryer basket with olive oil.
2. In a pan, add water and bring to a boil. Add the spinach and blanch for about 4 minutes. Drain the excess water.
3. In a bowl, add the spinach, butter, salt, and black pepper and mix. Transfer to the air fryer basket and cook for 15 minutes. Stir once halfway through the cooking time.
4. Transfer to serving bowls and add the cheese, olives, and lemon zest. Stir well before serving.

STORAGE: Store in an airtight container in the fridge for up to 3 days.
SERVE IT WITH: If you are a meat lover, you can enjoy this dish with roast chicken breasts or garlicky shrimp skewers; if you are a vegan, then you can serve it with a cup of green smoothie or a green salad.
PER SERVING
calories: 254 | fat: 21.9g | total carbs: 7.9g | fiber: 3.7g | protein: 9.8g

EASY PARMESAN ROASTED BAMBOO SPROUTS

Macros: Fat 67% | Protein 17% | Carbs 16%
Prep time: 8 minutes | Cook time: 15 minutes | Serves 6

Parmesan roasted bamboo sprouts are vegetarian-friendly and gluten-free. Pepper is added to the treat to spice it up. It takes a short time to prepare.

2 tablespoons olive oil	Salt and black pepper, to taste
2 pounds (907 g) bamboo shoots	4 tablespoons butter
½ teaspoon paprika	2 cups grated Parmesan cheese

1. Preheat the oven to 375°F (190°C) and grease a baking dish with olive oil.
2. Combine the bamboo shoots with paprika, salt, black pepper, and butter in a large bowl. Wrap the bowl in plastic and refrigerate to marinate for at least 1 hour.
3. Discard the marinade and transfer the bamboo sprouts to the baking dish and bake in the preheated oven for 15 minutes.
4. Transfer to serving plates to cool and top with cheese before serving.

STORAGE: Store in an airtight container in the fridge for up to 4 days or in the freezer for up to 1 month.
REHEAT: Microwave, covered, until it reaches the desired temperature.
SERVE IT WITH: To make this a complete meal, serve with chicken stuffed avocados.
PER SERVING
calories: 289 | fat: 21.9g | total carbs: 12.6g | fiber: 3.4g | protein: 13.5g

STUFFED CHEESY MUSHROOMS

Macros: Fat 76% | Protein 9% | Carbs 16%
Prep time: 25 minutes | Cook time: 20 minutes | Serves 3

Are you a mushroom lover? This is a delicious meal tailored just for you. The meal can turn to be your favorite as it is rich in flavors. It is a keto-friendly meal you will always enjoy.

12 whole fresh mushrooms	pepper
1 tablespoon olive oil	¼ teaspoon ground black
1 tablespoon minced garlic	pepper
1 (8-ounce / 227-g) package	¼ teaspoon onion powder
softened cream cheese	¼ cup grated Parmesan cheese
¼ teaspoon ground cayenne	Cooking spray

1. Preheat the oven to 350°F (180°C) and spray a baking sheet with cooking spray. Set aside.
2. On a flat work surface, remove the mushroom stems, and finely chop them as you discard the tough stem endings. Reserve the mushroom caps on a plate.
3. In a nonstick skillet, heat the olive oil over medium heat. Add the chopped mushroom stems and garlic. Fry them until all the moisture disappears, then transfer to a bowl to cool for 5 minutes.
4. Add the cream cheese, cayenne pepper, black pepper, onion powder and Parmesan cheese into the bowl of mushroom mixture. Stir thoroughly until well combined.
5. Using a spoon, stuff every mushroom cap with a considerable amount of the filling, then arrange the stuffed mushroom caps on the baking sheet.
6. Bake for about 20 minutes until the liquid starts to form under the caps and caps are piping hot.
7. Remove from the oven and serve warm on a plate.

STORAGE: Store in an airtight container in the fridge for up to 3 days.
REHEAT: Microwave, covered, until it reaches the desired temperature.
SERVE IT WITH: To make this a complete meal, serve with fresh salad greens or a side dish of your choice.
PER SERVING
calories: 361 | fat: 29.9g | total carbs: 16.6g | fiber: 2.0g | protein: 9.8g

GRILLED SPICY SHRIMP

Macros: Fat 75% | Protein 22% | Carbs 3%
Prep time: 30 minutes | Cook time: 10 minutes | Serves 6

This is a great recipe to enjoy. The oregano adds color and taste to the food. It takes a few minutes to cook. It is also spicy because of the hot pepper sauce.

1 cup plus 1 tablespoon olive oil	2 teaspoons dried oregano
1 juiced lemon	1 teaspoon ground black pepper
¼ cup chopped fresh parsley	1 teaspoon salt
3 minced cloves garlic	2 pounds (907 g) peeled and
2 tablespoons hot pepper sauce	deveined large shrimp, tail-on

SPECIAL EQUIPMENT:
6 bamboo skewers (about 10 inches (25 cm) long), soaked for at least 30 minutes

1. Make the marinade: Combine 1 cup of olive oil, lemon juice, parsley, garlic, hot sauce, oregano, black pepper, and salt in a bowl. Stir well to incorporate.
2. Reserve some of the marinade for basting in a separate bowl. Pour the remaining marinade into a resealable plastic bag containing the shrimp. Shake and seal the bag, then transfer to the refrigerator and marinate for approximately 2 hours.
3. Preheat the grill to medium-low heat.
4. Thread the marinated shrimp onto the skewers, then discard the marinade.
5. Slightly oil the grill grates with 1 tablespoon of olive oil, then grill each side of the shrimp for about 5 minutes until the flesh is totally pink and opaque, basting frequently with the marinade you have reserved.
6. Cool for 5 minutes before serving.

STORAGE: Store in an airtight container in the fridge for up to 4 days or in the freezer for up to 1 month.
REHEAT: Microwave, covered, until it reaches the desired temperature.
SERVE IT WITH: To make this a complete meal, enjoy the grilled shrimp on a bed of greens.
PER SERVING
calories: 436 | fat: 37.6g | total carbs: 3.9g | fiber: 0.6g | protein: 21.0g

SPINACH AND CHEESE STUFFED MUSHROOMS

Macros: Fat 85% | Protein 9% | Carbs 6%
Prep time: 15 minutes | Cook time: 55 minutes | Serves 12

Spinach and cheese stuffed mushrooms are flavor packed keto appetizer. The mushrooms are stuffed with cheese, spinach and vibrant garlic to make a recipe that for sure will impress.

5 tablespoons melted butter, divided	2 garlic cloves, minced
5 bacon slices	2 tablespoons chopped onion
1 (10-ounce / 284-g) package	4 cups heavy cream
frozen spinach, chopped	½ cup grated Parmesan cheese
¼ cup water	Salt and freshly ground pepper,
12 large mushrooms	to taste

1. Preheat your oven to 400°F (205°C). Grease a baking dish with 2 tablespoons of melted butter and set aside.
2. In a large skillet, cook the bacon over medium-high heat for 12 minutes until evenly browned, flipping occasionally.
3. Transfer to a plate lined with paper towels to absorb the excess grease. When cool enough to handle, crumble it and set aside.
4. Add the spinach in a saucepan, then add ¼ cup of water. Bring the water to a boil, then cook the spinach over medium heat for about 10 minutes.
5. Remove the spinach from the heat and drain the water. Set aside.
6. On a flat work surface, remove stems from the mushrooms and chop them. Reserve the chopped stems in a bowl, then arrange the caps on the prepared baking dish.
7. Heat the remaining butter in the saucepan over medium heat. Add the garlic and onions, then cook for 3 to 5 minutes, or until the onions are tender.
8. Stir in the cooked bacon, spinach, mushroom stems, and heavy cream, then bring them to a boil. Remove from the heat to another bowl.
9. Add the cheese, salt, and pepper. Stir with a fork until well combined. Using a spoon, scoop the mixture into the mushroom caps.
10. Bake in the oven for 30 minutes or until the cheese melts.
11. Remove from the oven and serve on a plate.

STORAGE: Store in an airtight container in the fridge up to 3 days. It is not recommended to freeze.
REHEAT: Microwave, covered, until the desired temperature is reached or reheat in an air fryer, covered, on medium.
SERVE IT WITH: The leftovers can be served with baked chicken as a side dish.
PER SERVING
calories: 239 | fat: 23.6g | Total carbs: 3.63g | fiber: 0.8g | protein: 4.76g

SIMPLE BROCCOLI CASSEROLE

Macros: Fat 83% | Protein 6% | Carbs 11%
Prep time: 20 minutes | Cook time: 45 minutes | Serves 8

This is an easy-to-prepare recipe, filled with tasty flavors, creamy, and savory makes it stand out delicious. The touch of mushroom soup, cheese, and eggs makes the recipe perfect for dinner needs.

5 tablespoons butter, divided	cheese
1 chopped onion	1 cup mayonnaise, keto-friendly
2 (10-ounce / 284-g) packages chopped frozen broccoli, thawed	2 beaten eggs
	½ teaspoon garlic salt
1 (11-ounce / 312-g) can condensed cream of mushroom soup	¼ teaspoon ground black pepper
	½ teaspoon seasoned salt
1 cup shredded sharp Cheddar	1½ teaspoons lemon juice

1. Start by preheating the oven at 350°F (180°C).
2. Put a medium saucepan over medium-high heat.
3. Melt 3 tablespoons of butter, then fry the onion to a gold brown color.
4. Mix the broccoli, eggs, lemon juice, onion, pepper, garlic salt, soup, seasoned salt, and cheese, mayonnaise in a mixing bowl. Top with the remaining 2 tablespoons of butter.
5. Place in the prepared oven and bake uncovered until the top starts to brown, for 45 minutes.
6. Remove from the oven and serve warm.

STORAGE: Store in an airtight container in the fridge for up to 3 days or in the freezer for up to three months.
REHEAT: Microwave, covered, until it reaches the desired temperature.
SERVE IT WITH: To make this a complete meal, serve the snack with pork tenderloins or chicken breast.
PER SERVING
calories: 606 | fat: 42.5g | total carbs: 42.5g | fiber: 21.9g | protein: 28.9g

LOW CARB KETO SAUSAGE BALLS

Macros: Fat 80% | Protein 17% | Carbs 4%
Prep time: 30 minutes | Cook time: 20 minutes | Serves 6

The keto sausage balls are the ideal low-carb snacks for various occasions. These sausage balls offer the best appetizers. The recipe has easy steps that make the snack simple to prepare.

2 tablespoons olive oil	1¼ cups shredded sharp Cheddar cheese
1 cup almond flour, blanched	
1 pound (454 g) bulk Italian sausage	2 teaspoons baking powder
	1 large beaten egg

1. Preheat the oven to 350°F (180°C) and grease a baking sheet with olive oil.
2. In a bowl, mix the flour, sausage, cheese, baking powder, and the egg.
3. Divide the mixture into 6 equal portions and roll to form into balls.
4. Transfer to the baking sheet and bake in the preheated oven until golden brown for about 20 minutes.
5. Transfer to a platter to cool before serving.

STORAGE: Store in an airtight container in the fridge for up to 4 days or in the freezer for up to 1 month.
REHEAT: Microwave, covered, until it reaches the desired temperature.
SERVE IT WITH: To make this a complete meal, serve with a cup of plain yogurt and a green salad.
PER SERVING
calories: 515 | fat: 46.2g | total carbs: 5.2g | fiber: 2.0g | protein: 21.2g

BUFFALO CHICKEN AND CHEESE DIP

Macros: Fat 79% | Protein 17% | Carbs 4%
Prep time: 20 minutes | Cook time: 50 minutes | Serves 8

Enjoy the tasty buffalo chicken and cheese dip snack at any time of the day. The meal is filled with rich cheese flavors that improve the texture and taste. You can prepare such snack and enjoy with family together or when friends visit.

2 bone-in chicken breast halves	softened cream cheese
1 teaspoon olive oil	¾ cup blue cheese dressing
1 stalk celery, finely diced	⅓ cup hot pepper sauce
¾ cup ranch dressing	1 cup shredded Cheddar cheese
1 (8-ounce / 227-g) package	

1. In a large saucepan, put the halved breasts and cover with water. Boil for 20 minutes until cooked through.
2. Remove the breasts from the pan. When cooled enough to handle, shred the meat and reserve them in a bowl.
3. Start by preheating the oven to 350°F (180°C)
4. In a large skillet, heat the olive oil until sizzling, then add the celery and fry until tender,
5. Add the ranch dressing, cream cheese, and blue cheese dressing.
6. Cook while stirring gently until creamy and smooth.
7. Add the shredded chicken and hot sauce. Stir to combine well.
8. Pour the mixture in a greased baking tray, then top with the shredded cheese.
9. Bake in the prepared oven until golden brown, for about 30 minutes.
10. Remove from the oven and serve hot.

STORAGE: Store in an airtight container in the fridge for up to 5 days or in the freezer for up to 1 month.
REHEAT: Microwave, covered, until it reaches the desired temperature. Do not overheat because it will look greasy.
SERVE IT WITH: To make this a complete meal, serve the buffalo chicken dip with celery sticks.
PER SERVING
calories: 430 | fat: 38.0g | total carbs: 3.9g | fiber: 0.2g | protein: 18.5g

ALMOND FRITTERS WITH MAYO SAUCE

Macros: Fat 67% | Protein 18% | Carbs 15%
Prep time: 5 minutes | Cook time: 15 minutes | Serves 2

I know you do fancy fritters. You will realize that the ingredients reveal how nutritious the dish is. You will enjoy the flavors and the cheesy nature of the recipe. You will take less than 20 minutes to prepare the recipe.

FRITTERS:

1 ounce (28 g) fresh broccoli	4 tablespoons almond flour
1 small whisked egg	¼ teaspoon baking powder
1 ounce (28 g) Mozzarella cheese	Salt and freshly ground black pepper, to taste
2 tablespoons plus 1 tablespoon flaxseed meal, divided	

SAUCE:

4 tablespoons fresh dill, chopped	½ teaspoon lemon juice
4 tablespoons mayonnaise, keto-friendly	Salt and freshly ground black pepper, to taste

1. Make the fritters: In a food processor, add the broccoli and process until chopped thoroughly.
2. In a bowl, add the processed broccoli, whisked egg, Mozzarella cheese, 2 tablespoons of flaxseed meal, almond flour, baking powder, black pepper and salt. Mix well to form batter. Divide and roll into 4 equal balls.
3. In a bowl, add the remaining 1 tablespoon of flaxseed meal. Dip the balls in this bowl to coat well.
4. Preheat an air fryer to 375°F (190°C) and place balls in the basket.
5. Fry fritters until golden brown for 5 minutes. Transfer to a serving plate.
6. Make the sauce: In a bowl, add the dill, mayonnaise, lemon juice, salt, and pepper and mix well.
7. Dip the fritters into the sauce and serve.

STORAGE: Store in an airtight container in the fridge for up to 4 days or in the freezer for up to 1 month.
REHEAT: Microwave, covered, until it reaches the desired temperature.
SERVE IT WITH: To make this a complete meal, serve with keto tropical smoothie.
PER SERVING
calories: 381 | fat: 29.5g | total carbs: 17.7g | fiber: 9.6g | protein: 18.2g

KETO BROILED BELL PEPPER

Macros: Fat 66% | Proteins: 26% | Carbs 8%
Prep time: 15 | Cook time: 10 minutes | Serves 4

Enjoy this tasty appetizer during any time of the day. You can add your favorite spices to taste even better.

2 medium bell peppers (a mix of colors)	4 ounces (113 g) ground beef
Kosher salt, to taste	1 cup shredded Mexican blend cheese
1 tablespoon olive oil	¼ cup guacamole
¼ teaspoon ground cumin	¼ cup salsa
¼ teaspoon chili powder	2 tablespoons sour cream

1. Cut the bell peppers through the stem into six equal parts. Remove the seeds and the stem.
2. Put the bell peppers in a microwave-approved dish, then add a splash of water and some salt.
3. Microwave while covered until the pepper pieces are pliable, for about 4 minutes.
4. Allow the bell peppers to cool slightly, then arrange on a baking tray lined with a foil with the cut side facing up.
5. In the meantime, heat the olive oil in a skillet over medium-high heat.
6. Add cumin and chili powder, then cook for 30 seconds while stirring.
7. Add ¼ teaspoon of salt, and ground beef. Sauté until the beef turns brown, for about 4 minutes.
8. Preheat the broiler, then spoon the beef mixture into each piece of bell pepper.
9. Add the cheese on top and then broil until the cheese melts, about 1 minute.
10. Put the guacamole and salsa on top.
11. Thin the sour cream out with some water and sprinkle over the peppers, then serve.

STORAGE: Store in an airtight container in the fridge for up to 3 days.
REHEAT: Microwave, covered, until the desired temperature is reached or reheat in an air fryer, covered, on medium.
PER SERVING
calories: 243 | fat: 18.1g | total carbs: 5.6g | fiber: 1.7g | protein: 15.4g

CHEDDAR CHEESE JALAPEÑO POPPERS

Macros: Fat 83% | Protein 13% | Carbs 4%
Prep time: 15 minutes | Cook time: 20 minutes | Serves 3

Jalapeño poppers require few ingredients mainly bacon, jalapeño peppers and shredded Cheddar cheese. The yummy treat takes a short time to prepare.

5 slices bacon	¼ teaspoon garlic powder
6 jalapeño peppers	¼ cup Cheddar cheese, shredded
3 ounces (85 g) softened cream cheese	

1. In a skillet over medium-high heat, add the bacon and fry for 3 to 4 minutes on each side until crispy. Allow the bacon to cool on a paper towel-lined plate.
2. Chop the bacon into ½-inch pieces.
3. Preheat the oven to 400°F (205°C) and line a rimmed baking sheet with parchment paper.
4. Slice the jalapeño peppers into halves. Using a spoon, scrap out the membranes and seeds.
5. In a bowl, use a fork to mix the cream cheese, garlic powder, Cheddar cheese, and bacon bits. Spoon the mixture into every jalapeño half, then arrange them on the lined baking sheet.
6. Bake in the preheated oven until the cheese melts for about 20 minutes and slightly crispy on top.
7. Transfer to serving plates to cool before serving.

STORAGE: Store in an airtight container in the fridge for up to 4 days or in the freezer for up to 1 month.
REHEAT: Microwave, covered, until it reaches the desired temperature.
SERVE IT WITH: To make this a complete meal, serve with a cup of zoodles or kelp pasta.
PER SERVING
calories: 314 | fat: 16.2g | total carbs: 3.5g | fiber: 0.8g | protein: 10.4g

FLUFFY WESTERN OMELET

Macros: Fat 73% | Protein 23% | Carbs 4%
Prep time: 5 minutes | Cook time: 25 minutes | Serves 2

Enjoy the fluffy filled with cheesy egg goodness omelet. This keto meal will fulfill our choices for dinner, lunch, or even breakfast. Filled with tasty flavors from bell pepper, ham, and onion, you will love it.

2 tablespoons heavy whipping cream or sour cream	2 ounces (57 g) butter
6 eggs	½ chopped green bell pepper
Salt and freshly ground pepper, to taste	5 ounces (142 g) diced smoked deli ham
3 ounces (85 g) shredded cheese	½ chopped yellow onion

1. Whisk the cream and eggs in a bowl until fluffy, then add the pepper and salt. Stir well.
2. Mix in half of the shredded cheese and set aside.
3. In a large pan, melt the butter over medium heat. Add the peppers, ham, and onions and fry for 5 minutes. Pour in the egg mixture and cook until it is almost firm, making sure not to burn the edges.
4. Reduce the heat to low, then top with the remaining cheese.
5. Transfer to a plate and slice in half before serving.

STORAGE: Store in an airtight container in the fridge for up to 4 days. It is not recommended to freeze.
REHEAT: Microwave, covered, until the desired temperature is reached or reheat in a frying pan, covered, on medium.
PER SERVING
calories: 872 | fat: 71.3g | total carbs: 10.7g | fiber: 0.5g | protein: 46.9g

CHEESY BAKED JALAPEÑO PEPPERS

Macros: Fat 73% | **Protein** 14% | **Carbs** 13%
Prep time: 30 minutes | Cook time: 30 minutes | Serves 15

Baked jalapeños taste better than fried ones. The recipe is rich in nutritional value and flavors from the eggs, cheese, milk, and mayonnaise. Enjoy this meal anytime you feel hungry.

1 cup Cheddar cheese
¼ cup keto-friendly mayonnaise
1 cup cream cheese
15 jalapeño peppers, halved lengthwise and seeded

½ tablespoon unsweetened almond milk
2 beaten eggs
1½ cups crushed almond
Cooking spray

1. Start by preheating the oven to 350°F (180°C) and spray a baking tray lightly with cooking spray. Set aside.
2. Mix the Cheddar cheese, mayonnaise, and cream cheese in a mixing bowl.
3. Fill the jalapeño halves with the cheese mixture.
4. In a small bowl, whisk together the milk and eggs, then put the crushed almonds in another bowl.
5. Dredge the stuffed jalapeño halves in the egg mixture completely, then roll in the crushed almonds for a good coating.
6. Arrange the coated jalapeños on the prepared baking tray.
7. Bake in the preheated oven until browned lightly, for about 30 minutes.
8. Remove from the oven and serve while still warm

STORAGE: Store in a wrapped plastic paper in the fridge for up to 4 days.
REHEAT: Microwave, covered, until the desired temperature is reached or reheat in an air fryer / instant pot, covered, on medium.
SERVE IT WITH: To make this a complete meal, serve the jalapeño peppers with blue cheese dressing.
PER SERVING
calories: 147 | fat: 12.1g | total carbs: 5.2g | fiber: 0.7g | protein: 5.4g

CRISPY CHICKEN

Macros: Fat 67% | **Protein** 32% | **Carbs** 2%
Prep time: 2 minutes | Cook time: 20 minutes | Serves 12

Chicken crisps are naturally crunchy dish that can be served for dinner. The meal is protein packed and takes a very short time to prepare. Everyone in the family will love it.

12 (9-ounces / 255-g) chicken thigh skins

SEASONING:

3 tablespoons coriander, ground
2 tablespoons gray sea salt, finely ground
1¼ teaspoons turmeric powder
¾ teaspoon celery seed, ground
¾ teaspoon parsley, dried

2 teaspoons mustard, ground
2 tablespoons onion powder
2 teaspoons paprika
½ teaspoon black pepper, ground

1. Preheat the oven to 325°F (160°C) and line a rimmed baking sheet with parchment paper.
2. Cut another parchment paper similar in size to the above and have a separate smaller baking sheet so you can nestle the smaller baking sheet inside the bigger baking sheet.
3. Make the seasoning: In a ½-cup glass jar, add the coriander, salt, turmeric, celery, parsley, mustard, onion powder, paprika, and black pepper. Cover the jar, then shake.
4. In a bowl, transfer the chicken skins, then sprinkle 1 tablespoon of the seasoning. Toss until the skins are coated evenly.

5. On the larger baking sheet, arrange the skins evenly by placing them close.
6. Set the second parchment paper on the skins, then top with the smaller baking sheet to force the skins to remain in flattened state throughout the baking process.
7. Bake in the preheated oven until crispy for 20 minutes. Flip the chicken thigh skins halfway through.
8. Transfer the crisp chicken skins to serving plates to cool before serving.

STORAGE: Store in an airtight container in the fridge for up to 5 days or in the freezer for up to 1 month.
REHEAT: You can remove them from the freezer and enjoy immediately, or microwave, covered, until it reaches the desired temperature.
SERVE IT WITH: To make this a complete meal, serve with broccoli chowder soup.
PER SERVING
calories: 434 | fat: 32.2g | total carbs: 2.0g | fiber: 0.5g | protein: 32.2g

EASY PARMESAN CHIVE AND GARLIC CRACKERS

Prep time: 40 minutes | Cook time: 15 minutes| Serves 4
Macros: Fat 72% | **Protein** 16% | **Carbs** 12%

Parmesan chive and garlic crackers are perfect for holiday nights and weekday dinners. They are also perfect low-carb snacks for keto diet. The recipe is super easy and produces amazing results.

1 tablespoon olive oil
1 cup Parmesan cheese, finely grated
¼ cup chives, chopped

1 cup almond flour, blanched
½ teaspoon garlic powder
1 large egg, whisked
1 tablespoon butter, melted

SPECIAL EQUIPMENT:
A pastry cutter

1. Preheat the oven to 350°F (180°C) and grease 2 large baking sheets with 1 tablespoon olive oil each.
2. In a bowl, add the cheese, chives, almond flour, and garlic powder and mix well to combine.
3. In another bowl, add the eggs and butter, then whisk them well.
4. Pour the egg mixture into the cheese mixture and blend well until you form a dough.
5. Divide dough into two equal portions and press well until they are ¼ inch thick.
6. Use a pastry cutter to slice each dough sheet into 25 equally sized crackers.
7. Lay the crackers onto the prepared baking sheets.
8. Bake in the preheated oven for 15 minutes until crispy. Turn off the oven and let the crackers rest for a few minutes before serving.

STORAGE: Store in an airtight container in the fridge for up to 4 days or in the freezer for up to 1 month.
REHEAT: Microwave, covered, until it reaches the desired temperature.
SERVE IT WITH: To make this a complete meal, serve with a cup of plain Greek yogurt.
PER SERVING
calories: 313 | fat: 26.4g | total carbs: 9.0g | fiber: 3.0g | protein: 12.9g

CHEESY CRAB STUFFED MUSHROOMS

Macros: Fat: 75% | Protein: 21% | Carbs: 4%
Prep time: 15 minutes | Cook time: 17 minutes | Serves 6

Aparty favorite appetizer of stuffed mushrooms with a flavorsome filling... These mushrooms are stuffed with a flavorsome combination of crab meat, cream cheese, parmesan, almonds and herbs.

12 large button mushrooms, cleaned and stemmed	1 scallion, chopped
1 cup cooked crab meat, chopped	1 tablespoon fresh parsley, chopped
1 cup cream cheese, softened	1 teaspoon garlic, minced
½ cup Parmesan cheese, grated	Olive oil spray
¼ cup ground almonds	

1. Preheat the oven to 375°F (190°C) and line a baking sheet with parchment paper.
2. Arrange the mushrooms onto the prepared baking sheet, stem-side up. Lightly spray them with olive oil spray. Bake in the preheated oven for about 2 minutes. Remove from the oven to a plate lined with paper towels to drain the grease.
3. Meanwhile, make the filling: In a large bowl, place the remaining ingredients and mix until well combined. Stuff each mushroom with about 1½ tablespoons of the filling mixture. Arrange the stuffed mushrooms onto the same baking sheet. Bake for about 14 to 15 minutes or until the mushrooms become bubbly and golden brown.
4. Remove the baking sheet from oven and serve warm.

STORAGE: You can store the filling in a container in the refrigerator for 1 to 2 days.
REHEAT: Microwave, covered, until the desired temperature is reached or reheat in a frying pan or air fryer / instant pot, covered, on medium.
SERVE IT WITH: Serve the stuffed mushrooms with the mashed broccoli or cauliflower.
PER SERVING
calories: 198 | fat: 15.9g | total carbs: 4.6g | fiber: 0.6g | protein: 10.2g

SWEET AND ZESTY CHICKEN WINGS

Macros: Fat: 49% | Protein: 45% | Carbs: 6%
Prep time: 15 minutes | Cook time: 40 minutes | Serves 4

Alip-smacking recipe of sticky wings is ideal for a snack party! These chicken wings are baked in the oven until crispy and then coated with a sweet and zesty sauce.

WINGS:
2 pounds (907 g) chicken wings
2 tablespoons coconut oil, melted

SAUCES:

4 tablespoons butter	3 to 4 tablespoons fresh lime juice
2 teaspoons garlic, minced	
2 teaspoons fresh ginger, grated	2 to 3 teaspoons lime zest, grated
2 to 3 tablespoons granulated monk fruit sweetener	

1. Preheat the oven to 400°F (205°C) and line a baking sheet with parchment paper.
2. For the wings: In a large bowl, place the wings and coconut oil. Toss to coat well. Arrange the wings onto the prepared baking sheet in a single layer. Bake for about 40 minutes, flipping once halfway through.

3. Meanwhile, make the sauce: In a small saucepan, melt the butter over medium-high heat and sauté the garlic and ginger for about 3 minutes. Stir in the monk fruit sweetener, lime juice and zest, then bring to a gentle boil. Reduce the heat to medium and cook for about 10 to 15 minutes or until it reaches the desired thickness, stirring frequently. Remove the saucepan from heat.
4. Remove the wings from the oven to a large bowl. Pour the sauce over the wings and serve warm.

STORAGE: In a resealable plastic bag, place the baked and then cooled chicken wings. Seal the bag and refrigerate for about 3 to 4 days.
REHEAT: Microwave, covered, until the desired temperature is reached or reheat in a frying pan or air fryer / instant pot, covered, on medium.**PER SERVING**
calories: 474 | fat: 26.4g | total carbs: 6.9g | protein: 50.1g | fiber: 0.1g

HOMEMADE CHEDDAR CRACKERS

Macros: Fat: 67% | Protein: 29% | Carbs: 4%
Prep time: 15 minutes | Cook time: 20 minutes | Serves 4

One of the easy to make crackers that are totally addicting! These homemade crackers are super cheesy with a delicious kick.

1 cup almond flour	¼ teaspoon garlic powder
½ cup Cheddar cheese, shredded finely	¼ teaspoon sea salt
	2 teaspoons olive oil
1 tablespoon nutritional yeast	1 egg
¼ teaspoon baking soda	Olive oil spray

1. Preheat your oven to 350°F (180°C) and line a baking sheet with parchment paper. Lightly grease two parchment papers with olive oil spray and set them aside.
2. In a large mixing bowl, add the almond flour, Cheddar cheese, nutritional yeast, baking soda, garlic powder, and salt and mix well. In a separate bowl, place the oil and egg, then beat until well combined. Add the egg mixture into the bowl of flour mixture and with a wooden spoon, mix well until a dough ball forms.
3. On a flat work surface, knead the dough for 1 to 2 minutes with your hands. Arrange 1 greased parchment paper onto the work surface. Place the dough ball onto the greased parchment paper and with your hands, then press into a disk. Arrange another greased parchment paper on top of dough, then roll it into a 9×12-inch (⅛-inch thick) rectangle with a rolling pin. With a pizza cutter, cut the edges of the dough into an even rectangle. Now, cut the dough into 1½×1½-inch columns and rows. Arrange the crackers onto the prepared baking sheet. Bake for about 15 to 20 minutes or until crispy.
4. Remove from the oven to a wire rack to cool completely before serving.

STORAGE: Place the crackers in an airtight container and store at room temperature for up to 1 week.
SERVE IT WITH: Spread a thin layer of cream cheese over crackers and top with crispy bacon bits before serving.
PER SERVING
calories: 184 | fat: 13.8g | total carbs: 1.8g | fiber: 0.3g | protein: 7.2g

CAULIFLOWER BREAD STICKS WITH CHEESE

Macros: Fat 76% | Protein 21% | Carbs 3%
Prep time: 10 minutes | Cook time: 20minutes | Serves 2

The delicacy is gluten-free, low-carb and very simple to make. The treat has a very direct recipe that takes a short time to prepare. The crust can also be used for making pizza.

1 tablespoon olive oil	1 small beaten egg
½ cup riced cauliflower	½ cup freshly grated Monterey
⅛ teaspoon ground oregano	jack cheese
⅛ teaspoon ground sage	Salt and ground black pepper, to
⅛ teaspoon ground mustard	taste
⅛ teaspoon thyme, dried	Minced fresh parsley, for garnish

1. In a toaster oven, add the cauliflower and cook for 8 minutes or until soft.
2. In a bowl, add the cooked cauliflower. Add the oregano, sage, mustard, and thyme for seasoning.
3. Add the egg, ½ of cheese, salt and black pepper.
4. Preheat the oven to 450ºF (235ºC) and grease a baking sheet with olive oil.
5. Arrange the cauliflower mixture on the greased baking sheet.
6. Bake in the preheated oven for 8 minutes. Top with remaining cheese and bake for an additional 5 minutes or until the cheese melts.
7. Remove from oven, garnish with parsley, and slice into sticks before serving

STORAGE: Store in an airtight container in the fridge for up to 4 days or in the freezer for up to 1 month.
REHEAT: Microwave, covered, until it reaches the desired temperature.
SERVE IT WITH: To make this a complete meal, serve with blackberry chocolate shake.
PER SERVING
calories: 218 | fat: 18.7g | total carbs: 1.8g | fiber: 0.6g | protein: 11.0g

CHEESY KETO CUPCAKES

Macros: Fat 85% | Proteins 9% | Carbs 6%
Prep time: 10 minutes | Cook: 20 minutes | Serves 12

It requires few ingredients when preparing this recipe. Only six ingredients and you have your cupcakes ready. They are soft, tasty and delicious. Good, especially for kids.

¼ cup melted butter	cream cheese, softened
½ cup almond meal	¾ cup Swerve
1 teaspoon vanilla extract	2 beaten eggs
2 (8-ounce / 227-g) packages	

SPECIAL EQUIPMENT:
A 12-cup muffin pan

1. Start by preheating the oven at 350ºF (180ºC) then line a muffin pan with 12 paper liners.
2. In a mixing bowl, mix the butter and almond meal until smooth, then spoon the mixture into the bottom of the muffin cups. Press into a flat crust.
3. In a mixing bowl, combine vanilla extract, cream cheese, Swerve, and eggs.
4. Set the electric mixer to medium, then beat the mixture until smooth.
5. Spoon the mixture on top of the muffin cups.

6. Bake in the oven until the cream cheese is nearly set in the middle, for about 17 minutes.
7. Remove from the oven and let the cupcakes cool.
8. Once cooled, refrigerate for 8 hours to overnight before serving.

STORAGE: Store in an airtight container in the fridge for up to 1 days or in the freezer for up to 1 month.
REHEAT: Microwave, covered, until the desired temperature is reached or reheat in a frying pan or air fryer / instant pot, covered, on medium.
PER SERVING
calories: 169 | fat: 16.0g | total carbs: 2.7g | fiber: 0g | protein: 3.8g

CHIVE DEVILED EGGS AND SAVORY CHORIZO

Macros: Fat 72% | Protein 24% | Carbs 4%
Prep time: 15 minutes | Cook time: 12 minutes | Serves 8

This recipe is nearly in every way superior. It is ideal for holidays, and they can be a common thing for your oven during the holidays. This recipe takes more time, but it is worth the wait as you will enjoy it! It is also keto-friendly!

2 tablespoons olive oil	1 tablespoon lemon juice
4 ounces (113 g) Spanish chorizo	8 hard-boiled eggs, halved and
½ teaspoon garlic powder	yolks reserved
¼ cup Greek yogurt	½ teaspoon kosher salt
1 teaspoon lemon zest	1 tablespoon chives chopped
½ teaspoon chili powder	

1. In a skillet over medium heat, heat the olive oil for 2 minutes. Add Spanish chorizo and cook for 3 minutes, or until crispy. Remove the chorizo and pat dry with a clean kitchen towel. Reserve a tablespoon of the cooking oil.
2. Whisk reserved oil, garlic powder, yogurt, zest, chili powder, lemon juice, yolks and salt together in a bowl until well combined.
3. Scoop the yolk mixture into every egg white. Place chorizo and chives on top and serve.

STORAGE: Store in an airtight container in the fridge for up to 2 days. It is not recommended to keep in a freezer.
REHEAT: Microwave, covered, until the desired temperature is reached or reheat in a frying pan or air fryer / instant pot, covered, on medium.
SERVE IT WITH: To make this recipe complete meal, serve with veggie salad.
PER SERVING
calories: 166 | fat: 13.2g | total carbs: 1.7g | fiber: 0.1g | protein: 10.2g

Chapter 11
Desserts

ALMOND MEAL CUPCAKES

Macros: Fat 86% | Protein 10% | Carbs 4%
Prep time: 15 minutes | Cook time: 15 minutes | Serves 12

These low-carb almond meal cupcakes make a perfect dessert for a ketogenic menu. The simple and easy recipe allows you to bake them in no time, and you can serve with quickly with a variety of cream topping of your choice.

½ cup almond meal	2 eggs
¼ cup butter, melted	¾ teaspoon liquid stevia
2 (8-ounce / 227-g) packages cream cheese, softened	1 teaspoon vanilla extract

SPECIAL EQUIPMENT:
A 12-cup muffin pan

1. Preheat your oven to 350°F (180°C). Line a muffin pan with 12 paper liners.
2. Thoroughly mix the almond meal with butter in a bowl, then spoon this mixture into the bottoms of each paper liner and press it into a thin crust.
3. Make the cupcakes: Whisk the cream cheese with liquid stevia, eggs, and vanilla extract in a medium bowl. Beat with an electric beater until the mixture is fluffy, creamy and smooth. Spoon this filling over the crust layer in the muffin pan.
4. Bake in the preheated oven until the cream cheese mixture is cooked from the center, for 15 to 17 minutes.
5. Leave the cupcakes to cool at room temperature. Serve immediately or refrigerate to chill for 8 hours, preferably overnight.

STORAGE: Store in an airtight container in the fridge for up to 4 days or in the freezer for up to 1 month.
SERVE IT WITH: To make this a complete meal, serve the cupcakes with a creamy topping.
PER SERVING
calories: 199 | fat: 19.1g | total carbs: 2.6g | fiber: 0.5g | protein: 4.7g

KETO VANILLA ICE CREAM

Macros: Fat 93% | Protein 2% | Carbs 5%
Prep time:10 minutes | Cook time:0 minutes | Serves 3

This no-churn vanilla ice cream is a perfect delight for all the keto dieters who don't own an ice cream machine. Now you can enjoy refreshing flavors of vanilla ice cream in dazzling summers with the help of this recipe.

1 cup heavy whipping cream	1 teaspoon vanilla extract
2 tablespoons Swerve confectioners' style sweetener	¼ teaspoon xanthan gum
1 tablespoon vodka	1 pinch salt

1. Add the cream, vodka, xanthan gum, Swerve, vanilla extract, and salt in a large jar.
2. Beat the cream mixture with a hand blender until the cream has thickened, and it makes soft peaks, after 60 to 75 seconds.
3. Cover this cream jar and place in your freezer for 3 to 4 hours, stirring occasionally.
4. Serve the vanilla ice cream in scoops and enjoy.

STORAGE: Store in an airtight container in your freezer for 1 month.
SERVE IT WITH: To make this a complete meal, serve the ice cream with toasted nuts.
PER SERVING
calories: 143 | fat: 14.8g | total carbs: 1.6g | fiber: 0g | protein: 0.8g

ALMOND CINNAMON COOKIES

Macros: Fat 73% | Protein 15% | Carbs 12%
Prep time: 10 minutes | Cook time: 15 minutes | Serves 12

The rich and strong cinnamon flavor makes these cookies special. Prepare out of blanched almond flour; the cookies have a distinct taste and aroma, which is enhanced by the use of vanilla in the recipe. Serve them warm and fresh for the best culinary experience.

2 cups blanched almond flour	1 teaspoon sugar-free vanilla extract
½ cup butter, softened	1 teaspoon ground cinnamon
1 egg	
½ cup Swerve	

1. Preheat your oven to 350°F (180°C). Layer a baking sheet with parchment paper.
2. Whisk the almond flour with butter, vanilla extract, Swerve, egg, and cinnamon in a bowl. Mix well until these ingredients form a smooth dough.
3. Make the cookies: Divide the dough and roll it into 1-inch balls on a lightly floured surface. Arrange these balls on the prepared baking sheet and press each ball lightly with a fork to make a criss-cross pattern.
4. Bake these cinnamon cookies in the preheated oven for 12 to 15 minutes, or until their edges turn golden.
5. Allow the cinnamon cookies to cool on the baking sheet for 5 minutes, then transfer them to a wire rack to cool completely before serving.

STORAGE: Store in an airtight container in the fridge for up to 4 days or in the freezer for up to 1 month.
SERVE IT WITH: To make this a complete meal, serve the cookies with blueberry smoothies or coffee.
PER SERVING
calories: 92 | fat: 7.4g | total carbs: 3.0g | fiber: 0.1g | protein: 3.4g

EGG AVOCADO CUPS

Macros: Fat 79% | Protein 18% | Carbs 3%
Prep time: 10 minutes | Cook time: 20 minutes | Serves 2

Here comes a hearty meal for your dinner table. These protein and fat-rich avocado cups can be served of the day. By using just a few basic ingredients, you can use these cups in no time. If you have avocados at home, a few eggs, and cheese, then you can enjoy them in just a few minutes with minimum efforts.

1 avocado, halved and pitted	Salt and ground black pepper to taste
2 eggs	1 tablespoon fresh parsley, chopped
¼ cup Cheddar cheese, shredded	

1. Preheat your oven to 425°F (220°C).
2. Using a large spoon to scoop the avocado flesh out of the skin on a flat work surface.
3. Place the avocado halves on a greased baking sheet, then crack an egg into each of the halves.
4. Bake in the preheated oven for 15 to 20 minutes until the eggs are completely set.
5. When ready to serve, top with the Cheddar cheese. Season the cups lightly with salt and black pepper.
6. Sprinkle the fresh parsley on top for garnish to serve.

STORAGE: Store in an airtight container in the fridge for up to 1 day. It is not recommended to freeze.
SERVE IT WITH: To make this a complete meal, serve with crispy bacon slices or sautéed sausages.
PER SERVING
calories: 342 | fat: 30.0g | total carbs: 9.9g | fiber: 6.8g | protein: 15.0g

CREAM CHEESE CHOCOLATE MOUSSE

Macros: Fat 88% | Protein 6% | Carbs 6%
Prep time:10 minutes | Cook time: 0 minutes | Serves 2

Creamy, soft, and smooth chocolate mousse is a basic need of every dessert menu. You can serve it directly with fresh berries and low-carb fruits, or you can use this mousse in other recipes as well as chocolate mousse cake or mousse sandwiches, etc.

3 ounces (85 g) cream cheese, softened
½ cup heavy cream
1 teaspoon vanilla extract

¼ cup Swerve
2 tablespoons cocoa powder
1 pinch salt

1. Beat the cream cheese in a large mixing bowl with an electric beater until it makes fluffy mixture.
2. Switch the beater to low speed, and add the vanilla extract, heavy cream, salt, Swerve, and cocoa powder to beat for 2 minutes until it is completely smooth.
3. Chill in the refrigerator until ready to serve.

STORAGE: Store in an airtight container in the fridge for up to 4 days.
SERVE IT WITH: To make this a complete meal, serve the mousse with fresh berries.
PER SERVING
calories: 270 | fat: 26.4g | total carbs: 6.0g | fiber: 2.0g | protein: 4.2g

VANILLA MUG CAKE

Macros: Fat 72% | Protein 13% | Carbs 15%
Prep time:5 minutes | Cook time:5 minutes | Serves 1

This mug cake recipe provides instant relief to your cravings by providing a delicious cake in just a few minutes. No need of oven, as long as you have microwave oven at home, you can literally bake this cake in 1 to 2 minutes with minimum efforts.

1 tablespoon butter, melted
2 tablespoons cream cheese
2 tablespoons coconut flour
1 tablespoon Swerve confectioners' style sweetener

½ teaspoon baking powder
1 medium egg
¼ teaspoon liquid stevia
3 drops vanilla extract
6 frozen raspberries

1. Beat the butter with 2 tablespoons cream cheese in a mug, then place it in the microwave on high heat for about 1 minute until smooth.
2. Remove the mug from the microwave and let cool for 3 minutes.
3. Add the stevia, coconut flour, and baking powder, then mix again until the ingredients are well combined.
4. Add the Swerve, egg, and vanilla extract, and whisk while scraping down the sides of the mug. Put the frozen raspberries on top and press them into the mixture.
5. Again, bake in the microwave on high heat for 1 minute and 20 seconds until the top springs back lightly when gently pressed with your fingertip.
6. Remove from the microwave and cool for 5 minutes before serving.

STORAGE: Store in an airtight container in the fridge for up to 4 days or in the freezer for 1 month.
SERVE IT WITH: To make this a complete meal, serve the mug cake with a cup of coffee.
PER SERVING
calories: 300 | fat: 23.9g | total carbs: 12.1g | fiber: 0.8g | protein: 9.9g

CHEESECAKE STRAWBERRIES

Macros: Fat 79% | Protein 7% | Carbs 16%
Prep time: 20 minutes | Cook time: 0 minutes | Serves 6

Easy and quick, this zero-cooking recipe provides an instant serving for all. If you have the following ingredients at home, then simply beat them together to stuff fresh berries and serve. So many nutrients, all packed together in this simple mini treat.

1 pound (454 g) whole fresh strawberries
½ (8-ounce / 227-g) package cream cheese, softened

¼ cup heavy cream
⅓ cup powdered erythritol
1 teaspoon vanilla extract

1. Using a paring knife to core all the strawberries on a flat work surface, then place them on a baking sheet, cut side up.
2. Add the cream cheese, heavy cream, vanilla extract, and erythritol in a large mixing bowl, then beat this cream mixture well with an electric hand mixer until it is creamy and fluffy, and it makes stiff peaks.
3. Transfer this cream cheese mixture to a piping bag fitted with a suitable tip.
4. Pipe this mixture into the core of each strawberry and up to 1 inch above the core.
5. Arrange them on a plate and refrigerate for 1 hour or up to 2 days until chilled.

STORAGE: Store in an airtight container in the fridge for up to 1 to 2 days.
SERVE IT WITH: To make this a complete meal, serve the strawberry cups with coconut shreds.
PER SERVING
calories: 171 | fat: 15.0g | total carbs: 7.6g | fiber: 1.5g | protein: 2.9g

KETO PUMPKIN SPICE FAT BOMBS

Macros: Fat 94% | Protein 3% | Carbs 3%
Prep time: 10 minutes | Cook time: 0 minutes | Serves 16

If you love all things pumpkin spice, then you are going to love these fat bombs. Loaded with healthy fat, zero sugar, and tons of pumpkin spice flavor, these creamy keto treats are the perfect sweet treats idea! Even if you are a terrible cook, you can try making them as they take less than 15 minutes from start to finish to make and is utterly fail-proof since there isn't anything much to do other than whisking and freezing them with absolutely no baking.

½ cup butter, at room temperature
½ cup cream cheese, at room temperature
⅓ cup pumpkin purée

4 drops liquid stevia
¼ teaspoon ground nutmeg
½ teaspoon ground cinnamon
3 tablespoons chopped almonds

1. Take a baking pan and line it with parchment paper. Set aside.
2. Place the butter and cream cheese in a small mixing bowl, and whisk well until it becomes smooth.
3. Pour in the pumpkin purée and blend until combined.
4. Add the stevia, nutmeg, cinnamon, and almonds. Stir to incorporate.
5. Transfer the pumpkin mixture into the pan and smooth the top with a spatula or the back of a spoon.
6. Keep the pan in the freezer for about 60 minutes.
7. Remove from the freezer and slice into 16 pieces to serve. You can preserve the fat bombs in an airtight container in the freezer until ready to eat.

STORAGE: Store in an airtight container in the fridge for up to 4 days or in the freezer for up to 1 month.
PER SERVING
calories: 80 | fat: 8.4g | total carbs: 0.7g | fiber: 0.1g | protein: 0.6g

CHOCOLATE VANILLA CAKE

Macros: Fat 80% | Protein 8% | Carbs 12%
Prep time: 20 minutes | Cook time: 20 minutes | Serves 12

Now you can enjoy a chocolate-vanilla cake on your low-carb ketogenic menu by using this recipe. It requires no flour, and you can make it quick time by beating eggs with butter and chocolate.

1 tablespoon melted butter, for greasing the pan	5 ounces (142 g) butter
9 ounces (255 g) dark chocolate with a minimum of 70% cocoa solids	5 eggs
	1 pinch salt
	1 teaspoon vanilla extract

SPECIAL EQUIPMENT:
A springform pan

1. Preheat your oven to 325°F (160°C).
2. Grease a springform pan with melted butter, then layer a piece of parchment paper on the bottom of the pan.
3. On your cutting board, cut the chocolate into pieces and cut the butter into small cubes.
4. Mix them in a bowl, then melt together either in a double boiler or by heating in the microwave oven.
5. When the chocolate is melted, stir well until it is smooth and leave the mixture to cool. Set aside.
6. Separate the eggs and keep the egg yolks and egg whites in two separate bowls.
7. Add a pinch of salt to the bowl with egg whites and beat them together with an electric mixer until it forms stiff peaks. Keep this mixture aside.
8. Now add the vanilla to the egg yolks and beat them together until it forms a smooth mixture.
9. Add the melted chocolate and butter mixture into the egg yolks and stir well to mix.
10. Gently fold in the egg whites until thoroughly and evenly incorporated.
11. Pour this batter into the prepared springform pan and spread it all over. Bake for 15 minutes in the oven. Insert a toothpick to check its doneness, it must come out with a moist crumb stuck on its tip.
12. Remove from the oven and slice to enjoy.

STORAGE: Store in an airtight container in the fridge for up to 4 days or in the freezer for 1 month.
SERVE IT WITH: To make this a complete meal, serve the cake with whipped cream topping.
PER SERVING
calories: 263 | fat: 23.3g | total carbs: 10.2g | fiber: 2.3g | protein: 5.5g

CHOCOLATE PEANUT FUDGE

Macros: Fat 77% | Protein 9% | Carbs 14%
Prep time:10 minutes | Cook time: 35 minutes | Serves 12

This mouth-pleasing fudge is prepared without any cooking so that you will have to spend lesser time in the kitchen. Simply bring all the ingredients together in the perfect proportions and then freeze the mixture to prepare the fudges. Serve it in small-sized squares.

3½ ounces (99 g) dark chocolate with a minimum of 80% cocoa solids	¼ cup peanut butter
4 tablespoons butter	½ teaspoon vanilla extract
1 pinch salt	1 teaspoon ground cinnamon
	1½ ounces (43 g) salted peanuts, finely chopped

1. Mix the chocolate with butter in a microwave-safe bowl, and heat in the microwave oven or in a double boiler to melt.
2. When the chocolate is melted, stir well until it is smooth, and leave the mixture to cool.
3. Mix well and add the remaining ingredients except for nuts, then stir to combine.
4. Transfer this chocolate batter to a greased baking pan lined with parchment paper.
5. Top the batter with peanuts and chill in the refrigerator for 2 hours until firm.
6. Remove from the refrigerator and cut into squares to serve.

STORAGE: Store in an airtight container in the fridge for up to 5 to 6 days or in the freezer for 1 month.
SERVE IT WITH: To make this a complete meal, serve the fudge squares with a cup of hot coffee.
PER SERVING
calories: 124 | fat: 10.6g | total carbs: 5.9g | fiber: 1.6g | protein: 2.9g

MINI CHEESECAKES

Macros: Fat 84% | Protein 10% | Carbs 6%
Prep time: 15 minutes | Cook time: 17 minutes | Makes 8 cakes

Mini cheesecakes are the perfect dessert to turn to when you're in the mood for a cheesecake but not quite ready to bake a whole cake. They are great desserts for every meal.

CRUST:

1 tablespoon melted unsalted butter	½ cup and 2 tablespoons almond meal
1 tablespoon stevia	

FILLING:

1 (8-ounce / 227-g) package of softened cream cheese	1½ teaspoons fresh lemon juice
1 large egg	Sliced strawberries, for garnish (optional)
1½ teaspoons vanilla extract	
⅓ cup monk fruit sweetener	

1. Preheat the oven to 350°F (180°C) and set up 8 liners in a muffin pan.
2. Pour all the crust ingredients in a small bowl, and mix until smooth. Sprinkle a bit of your crust mix on the paper liner and spread them out evenly.
3. Slowly pour the ingredients for the fillings into a medium bowl, starting with the cream cheese and ending with the lemon juice. Mix them thoroughly with a hand mixer.
4. Pour the filling inside the muffin pan and stop when it fills ⅔ of the liner. Arrange the muffin pan in the preheated oven.
5. Bake for about 17 minutes or until the top of the cake springs back when gently pressed with your fingers.
6. Remove the cheesecakes from the oven, and allow to cool under room temperature before removing each mini cheesecake from the pan.
7. Garnish with sliced strawberries and serve warm.

STORAGE: Store the cheesecake by placing it in an airtight container, and store in a refrigerator. The cheesecake can be stored for 5 to 7 days.
SERVE IT WITH: To make this a complete meal, you can enjoy them as dessert and serve with nut-based snacks, or a full keto meals.
PER SERVING
calories 174 | fat: 16.3g | total carbs 4.1g | fiber: 1.4g | protein 4.2g

SPICY ALMOND FAT BOMBS

Macros: Fat 94% | Protein 4% | Carbs 2%
Prep time: 10 minutes | Cook time: 4 minutes | Serves 12

Often the simplest dishes are the most satisfying. And this is true about these spiced fat bombs. The mellow nutty flavor of the almond butter and the spices highlighted with chocolate gives these fat bombs a surprisingly delicious flavor with smoky spiciness that is sure to warm you up a little. On top, this is an easy recipe that is incredibly good for you.

¾ cup coconut oil
¼ cup almond butter
¼ cup cocoa powder

3 drops liquid stevia
⅛ teaspoon chili powder

SPECIAL EQUIPMENT:
A 12-cup muffin pan

1. Line a muffin pan with 12 paper liners. Keep aside.
2. Heat the oil in a small saucepan over low heat, then add the almond butter, cocoa powder, stevia, and chili powder. Stir to combine well.
3. Divide the mixture evenly among the muffin cups and keep the muffin pan in the refrigerator for 15 minutes, or until the bombs are set and firm.
4. Serve immediately or refrigerate to chill until ready to serve.

STORAGE: Store in an airtight container in the fridge for up to 4 days or in the freezer for up to 1 month.
PER SERVING
calories: 160 | fat: 16.8g | total carbs: 2.0g | fiber: 1.2g | protein: 1.5g

STRAWBERRIES IN CHOCOLATE

Macros: Fat 86% | Protein 1% | Carbs 13%
Prep time: 5 minutes | Cook time: 1 minute | Serves 2

Everything tastes absolutely divine when you smear a lot of chocolate over it. The sweet and salty chocolate crust makes this dessert perfect for all kinds of situations. Chocolate covered strawberries are, in fact, a delightful treat every dark chocolate lover should try out at least once.

¼ cup sugar-free dark chocolate chips
1½ teaspoons coconut oil

10 medium-sized fresh strawberries, rinsed and drained

1. Melt the chocolate chips by placing it in a small microwave-safe bowl and microwaving it for 1 minute or until it's completely melted.
2. Remove the bowl from the microwave, add chocolate chips into the bowl and mix until it completely dissolves.
3. Add the oil to the melted chocolate and mix thoroughly.
4. Line the parchment paper on a baking sheet. Dip ⅔ of each strawberry inside the melted chocolate and set it on the parchment paper.
5. Place the baking sheet inside a refrigerator for 15 minutes to allow the chocolate to set.
6. Remove them from the refrigerator and serve chill.

STORAGE: Store in an airtight container in the fridge for no more than 2 days
SERVE IT WITH: To make this a complete meal, you can enjoy them as dessert with your low-carb beverage or dry wines.
PER SERVING
calories: 133 | fat 12.6g | total carbs 5.6g | fiber: 1.2g | protein 0.4g

CHOCOLATE GRANOLA BARS

Macros: Fat 82% | Protein 10% | Carbs 8%
Prep time: 10 minutes | Cook time:20 minutes | Serves 20

Rich and healthy granola bars are an essential part of every ketogenic menu; that is why we bring you the best of the granola bar recipe. It is prepared out of a coarse mixture of all our favorite nuts, like almonds and walnuts, along with healthy seeds and chocolate melt.

3 ounces (85 g) almonds
3 ounces (85 g) walnuts
2 ounces (57 g) sesame seeds
2 ounces (57 g) pumpkin seeds
1 ounce (28 g) flaxseed
2 ounces (57 g) unsweetened coconut, shredded
2 ounces (57 g) dark chocolate

with a minimum of 70% cocoa solids
6 tablespoons coconut oil
4 tablespoons tahini
1 teaspoon vanilla extract
2 teaspoons ground cinnamon
1 pinch sea salt
2 eggs

1. Preheat your oven to 350°F (180°C).
2. Except for dark chocolate, process all the ingredients for granola in a food processor until they make a coarse and crumbly mixture.
3. Spread the granola mixture into a greased baking dish lined with parchment paper.
4. Bake the granola for 15 to 20 minutes in the oven until the cake turns golden brown.
5. Once baked, allow it to cool for 5 minutes, then remove from the baking dish.
6. Cut the granola cake into 24 bars using a sharp knife on a clean work surface. Set aside.
7. Melt the chocolate by heating in a double boiler or in the microwave. Let it cool for 5 minutes.
8. Serve the granola bars with the melted chocolate for dipping.

STORAGE: Store in an airtight container in the fridge for up to 4 days or in the freezer for 1 month.
SERVE IT WITH: To make this a complete meal, serve the granola bars with a glass of unsweetened almond milk.
PER SERVING
calories: 189 | fat: 17.2g | total carbs: 7.0g | fiber: 3.2g | protein: 4.7g

RASPBERRY AND CHOCOLATE FAT BOMBS

Macros: Fat 99% | Protein 0% | Carbs 1%
Prep time: 1 hour 5 minutes | Cook time: 0 minutes | Serves 12

The raspberry and chocolate fat bombs are sweet and are made with amazing ingredients that will satisfy all your sweet cravings!

½ cup coconut oil, melted
2 ounces (57 g) cacao butter

½ cup dried raspberries
¼ cup Swerve

SPECIAL EQUIPMENT:
A 12-cup muffin pan

1. Line a muffin pan with 12 paper liners and set it aside.
2. Combine the melted coconut oil and cocoa butter in a bowl.
3. Blend the raspberries in a blender until smooth and pour into the bowl of coconut oil mixture. Drizzle with the Swerve.
4. Divide the mixture equally among the muffin cups.
5. Refrigerate for at least 1 hour, or until steady and then serve.

STORAGE: Store in an airtight container in the fridge for up to 4 days or up to 2 months in a freezer.
SERVE IT WITH: To make this recipe complete meal, serve with strawberry smoothie or pumpkin almond pie.
PER SERVING
calories: 127 | fat: 13.9g | total carbs: 0.7g | fiber: 0.4g | protein: 0.1g

KETO LAVA CAKE

Macros: Fat 81% | Protein 11% | Carbs 8%
Prep time: 15 minutes | Cook time:10 minutes | Serves 6

Lava cake is that sweet delight that everyone longs for. Being on the ketogenic diet cannot stop you from having a lava cake as we are bringing you this carb-free recipe. Enjoy the classic lava cake at home after your favorite meal.

1 tablespoon melted butter, for greasing the ramekins
2 ounces (57 g) dark chocolate with a minimum of 70% cocoa

solids
2 ounces (57 g) butter
¼ teaspoon vanilla extract
3 eggs

SPECIAL EQUIPMENT:
4 to 6 small ramekins

1. Preheat your oven to 400°F (205°C) and lightly grease 4 to 6 small ramekins with 1 tablespoon melted butter.
2. Cut the chocolate into small pieces on your cutting board. Add the chocolate and butter to a double broiler, and heat until they are melted. Mix well.
3. Add the vanilla to the chocolate mixture, then allow the mixture to cool.
4. Beat all the eggs in a mixing bowl for 3 minutes until fluffy, then add the chocolate mixture. Stir to combine.
5. Divide the mixture among the greased ramekins. Bake all the ramekins in the preheated oven for 5 minutes.
6. Remove from the oven and cool for 5 minutes before enjoying.

STORAGE: Store in an airtight container in the fridge for up to 2 days or in the freezer for 1 month.
SERVE IT WITH: To make this a complete meal, serve the lava cake with a scoop of low-carb vanilla ice cream on the side.
PER SERVING
calories: 197 | fat: 17.8g | total carbs: 4.9g | fiber: 1.0g | protein: 5.4g

DOUBLE CHOCOLATE BROWNIES

Macros: Fat 87% | Protein 7% | Carbs 6%
Prep time: 15 minutes | Cook time:25 minutes | Serves 14

Brownies attract all due to their warming sweet flavors. This double chocolate brownie gives a unique and mouth-pleasing experience through its simple and basic chocolate flavors paired with a strong coffee flavor.

6 ounces (170 g) butter, softened
½ cup almond butter
2 eggs
¾ cup erythritol
½ cup cocoa powder
1 cup almond flour
½ teaspoon baking powder
¼ teaspoon salt

2 tablespoons water
1 tablespoon vanilla extract
½ teaspoon instant coffee powder (optional)
2 ounces (57 g) dark chocolate with a minimum of 80% cocoa solids, chopped

1. Preheat your oven to 350°F (180°C) and line a baking dish with parchment paper.
2. Use a hand mixer to beat the almond butter with the butter, eggs, and erythritol in a mixing bowl, or until it makes a smooth mixture.
3. Add the almond flour, cocoa powder, baking powder, water, salt, vanilla extract, and coffee powder, then mix them until it forms a smooth dough.
4. Gently pour the chopped chocolate into the mixture, and blend well.

5. Pour this chocolate mixture into the prepared baking dish and spread it with a spatula.
6. Bake for 25 to 28 minutes until the tops spring back lightly when gently pressed with a fingertip.
7. Leave it at room temperature to cool for 20 to 30 minutes before slicing.

STORAGE: Store in an airtight container in the fridge for up to 4 days or in the freezer for 1 month.
SERVE IT WITH: To make this a complete meal, serve the brownies with roasted nuts on top. They also taste great paired with a rich sugar-free chocolate sauce.
PER SERVING
calories: 230 | fat: 22.3g | total carbs: 5.7g | fiber: 2.5g | protein: 4.2g

FROSTED SNICKERDOODLE CUPCAKES

Macros: Fat: 83% | Protein 9% | Carbs 8%
Prep time: 10 minutes | Cook time: 13 minutes | Makes 6 cupcakes

Snickerdoodles have always been a family favourite. Something about its rich cinnamon and sugar tastes always leave you wanting more. Cookies have always been the traditional form that most baked snickerdoodles come in, but with this recipe, we attempt the unusual.

SNICKERDOODLE CUPCAKE BATTER:
1 large egg
½ cup blanched almond flour
1 tablespoon coconut flour
½ teaspoon baking powder

¼ cup stevia
3 ounces (85 g) softened cream cheese
1 teaspoon vanilla extract

FROSTING:
¼ teaspoon vanilla extract
2 tablespoons unsalted softened butter
2 ounces (57 g) softened cream

cheese
¼ teaspoon ground cinnamon, plus more for garnish
1½ tablespoons stevia

SPECIAL EQUIPMENT:
A 6-cup muffin pan

1. Preheat the oven to 350°F (180°C), and line the muffin pan with cupcake liners.
2. Whisk the eggs, almond flour, coconut flour, baking powder, and sweetener in a bowl.
3. Add cream cheese and the vanilla extract and mix it thoroughly with a hand mixer.
4. Pour the batter inside each cup of muffin pan. Stop filling when ¾ of the muffin container is filled.
5. Place the muffin pan in the preheated oven and bake for 10 to 12 minutes or until browned.
6. Let it cool down to room temperature before frosting.

FROSTING:
Pour all the frosting ingredients in a bowl and blend it with a hand mixer until it's smooth.
Apply frosting to each snickerdoodles cupcake and sprinkle a dash of cinnamon on top before serving.

STORAGE: Store the snickerdoodles by placing in an airtight container, and store in a refrigerator. They can be stored for 5 to 7 days.
SERVE IT WITH: To make this a complete meal, you can enjoy them as dessert and serve with nut-based snacks, or a full keto meal.
PER SERVING
calories: 161 | fat: 14.8g | total carbs: 3.5g | fiber: 0.1g | protein: 3.5g

KETO MOCHA ICE CREAM

Macros: Fat 84% | Protein 7% | Carbs 9%
Prep time: 15 minutes | Cook time: 0 minutes | Serves 6

Mocha lovers! Now you can enjoy the same flavors in your ice cream. This low-carb mocha ice cream is known for its distinctive peppermint taste and mild sweetness. By adding coffee and chocolate to the ice cream mixture, a delicious and healthy combination can be created.

2 cups heavy whipping cream
2 ounces (57 g) dark chocolate, chopped
6 large egg yolks, whisked
2 tablespoons instant coffee powder

⅔ cup powdered erythritol
1 to 2 drops peppermint extract
½ teaspoon salt
2 teaspoons vanilla extract
6 drops liquid stevia

1. Take a heavy saucepan and place it over low heat. Melt the heavy cream.
2. Add the chocolate and continue mixing until it is melted. Pour in the egg yolks and stir the mixture on low heat until it is warm.
3. Add the coffee powder and erythritol, then stir to cook for 10 minutes until it thickens.
4. Remove from the heat. Add the peppermint, salt, vanilla extract, and liquid stevia. Blend well.
5. Refrigerate it to chill for 30 minutes, then churn the mixture in the ice cream machine as per the machine's instructions. Serve immediately.

STORAGE: Store in an airtight container in the freezer for up to 1 months.
SERVE IT WITH: To make this a complete meal, serve the ice cream with sugar-free chocolate chip topping.
PER SERVING
calories: 252 | fat: 23.4g | total carbs: 7.0g | fiber: 1.0g | protein: 4.4g

KETO CHOCOLATE-COCONUT BITES

Macros: Fat 94% | Protein 3% | Carbs 3%
Prep time: 10 minutes | Cook time: 3 minutes | Serves 16

Not only does this naturally low-carb delicious chocolate coconut bites offer plenty of health benefits, but it also comes together with incredible ease and makes for a convenient snack. The bliss balls can satisfy your sweet tooth while being the perfect health snack that can keep you energized for a long time.

⅓ cup coconut oil
¼ cup unsweetened cocoa powder
4 drops liquid stevia

Pinch sea salt
¼ cup shredded unsweetened coconut

1. Line a baking dish with parchment paper. Keep it aside.
2. Add the coconut oil, cocoa powder, stevia, and salt in a small saucepan over low heat. Stir the mixture continuously for 2 to 3 minutes.
3. Once combined, stir in the shredded coconut, then transfer the mixture into the prepared baking dish.
4. Keep the baking dish in the refrigerator for about 30 minutes, or until the mixture is firm and set.
5. Slice into 16 pieces and serve immediately.

STORAGE: Store in an airtight container in the fridge for up to 4 days or in the freezer for up to 1 month.
PER SERVING
calories: 49 | fat: 5.1g | total carbs: 1.0g | fiber: 0.6g | protein: 0.3g

COCO AVOCADO TRUFFLES

Macros: Fat 77% | Protein 5% | Carbs 18%
Prep time: 35 minutes | Cook time:0 minutes | Serves 20

Truffles are excellent to serve as a dessert or on the snack table. These truffles are even better as they are made out of avocado mash, which is then mixed with chocolate and coated with cocoa powder, a double treat for all the chocolate lovers.

1 ripe avocado, chopped
½ teaspoon vanilla extract
½ lime zest
1 pinch salt
5 ounces (142 g) dark chocolate

with a minimum of 80% cocoa solids, finely chopped
1 tablespoon coconut oil
1 tablespoon unsweetened cocoa powder

1. In a bowl, thoroughly mix the avocado flesh with vanilla extract with an electric hand mixer until it forms a smooth mixture.
2. Add the lime zest and a pinch of salt, then mix well. Set aside.
3. Mix and melt the chocolate with coconut oil in a double broiler or by heating in the microwave.
4. Add the chocolate mixture to the avocado mash. Blend well until a smooth batter forms.
5. Refrigerate this batter for 30 minutes until firm.
6. Scoop portions of the batter (about 2 teaspoons in size) and shape into small truffle balls with your hands, then roll each truffle ball in the cocoa powder. Serve immediately.

STORAGE: Store in an airtight container in the fridge for up to 3 days or in the freezer for 1 month.
SERVE IT WITH: To make this a complete meal, serve the truffles with a hot cup of coffee.
PER SERVING
calories: 61 | fat: 5.2g | total carbs: 4.3g | fiber: 1.6g | protein: 0.8g

HEALTHY VANILLA-ALMOND ICE POPS

Macros: Fat 79% | Protein 8% | Carbs 13%
Prep time: 10 minutes | Cook time: 5 minutes | Serves 8

I feel like this recipe is a dream. Vanilla almond ice pops taste exactly how you imagine they would be. It should come as no surprise that these ice pops taste great, though, and are freaking delicious while being healthy and so easy to make. Just wait till you try it!

2 cups unsweetened almond milk
1 vanilla bean, halved lengthwise

1 cup heavy whipping cream
1 cup unsweetened coconut, shredded

1. Heat the almond milk in a saucepan over medium heat, then add the vanilla bean, and heavy cream. Mix well and bring the mixture to a simmer.
2. Reduce the heat to low and simmer for 5 minutes more.
3. Turn off the heat and allow the mixture to cool.
4. Remove the vanilla bean from the mixture, then scrape out the seeds out of the pod with a knife, throwing the seeds into the mixture.
5. Add the shredded coconut and pour the liquid between the ice pop molds evenly.
6. Place the ice molds in the refrigerator for 4 hours until ready to serve.

STORAGE: Store in an airtight container in the fridge for up to 4 days or in the freezer for up to 1 week.
PER SERVING (1 ICE POP)
calories: 125 | fat: 10.9g | total carbs: 5.0g | fiber: 0.9g | protein: 2.6g

ALMOND FLOUR SHORTBREAD COOKIES

Macros: Fat 83% | Protein 10% | Carbs 7%
Prep time: 10 minutes | Cook time: 10 minutes | Serves 18

I make these shortbread cookies when I want a light sweet treat which is rich and indulgent. They have a buttery and slightly crumbly texture similar to traditional shortbread but with a healthy twist. What's more, they are easy to make. And if you wish to make them chocolaty, you can even dip them in chocolate.

½ cup butter, at room temperature, plus more for greasing the baking sheet
1 teaspoon vanilla extract

½ cup Swerve
1½ cups almond flour
½ cup ground hazelnuts
1 pinch sea salt

1. Start by mixing the butter, vanilla extract, and Swerve in a medium mixing bowl until well combined.
2. Add the almond four, salt, and ground hazelnuts. Stir until you get a firm dough.
3. Shape the mixture into a 2-inch cylinder. Cover it with plastic wrap and let rest in the refrigerator for about 30 minutes until it's firm.
4. Preheat the oven to 350℉ (180°C) and grease a parchment paper-lined baking sheet with butter. Keep it aside.
5. Remove the almond flour dough from the refrigerator. On a clean work surface, slice it into 18 pieces and put them on the prepared baking sheet.
6. Bake for 8 to 10 minutes or until firm and lightly browned in color.
7. Transfer to a wire rack to cool completely before serving.

STORAGE: Store in an airtight container in the fridge for up to 4 days or in the freezer for up to 1 week.
SERVE IT WITH: To make this a complete meal, serve it with a cup of coffee.
PER SERVING (1 COOKIE)
calories: 116 | fat: 10.7g | total carbs: 2.6g | fiber: 0.4g | protein: 2.8g

KETO ALMOND BUTTER FUDGE SLICES

Macros: Fat 92% | Protein 6% | Carbs 2%
Prep time: 10 minutes | Cook time: 0 minutes | Serves 36

These almond butter fudges are silky smooth and creamy that it will literally melt in the mouth. On top, you can have them without an ounce of guilt as it is a healthy dessert with loads of healthy fat and added protein. What's more, they take less than 10 minutes to make while being deceptively filled. If you desire, you can even add chocolate chips to it.

1 cup coconut oil, at room temperature
10 drops liquid stevia

1 cup almond butter
1 pinch sea salt
¼ cup heavy whipping cream

1. Take a baking dish and line it with parchment paper. Set aside.
2. Whisk together the coconut oil, stevia, almond butter, salt, and heavy cream in a medium bowl until the mixture becomes smooth.
3. Transfer the mixture into the prepared baking dish. Smooth the top with the back of a spoon or spatula.
4. Keep the dish in the refrigerator for 2 hours or until the fudge is totally set and firm.
5. Remove from the refrigerator and slice into 36 pieces to serve.

STORAGE: Store in an airtight container in the fridge for up to 4 days or in the freezer for up to 2 weeks.
PER SERVING (2 PIECES OF FUDGE)
calories: 100 | fat: 10.2g | total carbs: 1.3g | fiber: 0.7g | protein: 1.5g

LOW-CARB RASPBERRY CHEESECAKE

Macros: Fat 87% | Protein 10% | Carbs 3%
Prep time: 10 minutes | Cook time: 30 minutes | Serves 12

This raspberry cheesecake keto dessert is a winning recipe for everyone since it is such a simple, easy recipe that anyone can make. Make it, eat it, and love it. I assure you it will be an instant, love-at-first bite reaction. The cheesecake can totally satisfy your sweet tooth craving and makes for a great low-carb dessert.

⅔ cup coconut oil, melted
½ cup cream cheese, at room temperature
6 eggs, whisked
3 tablespoons granulated

sweetener
½ teaspoon baking powder
1 teaspoon vanilla extract
¾ cup raspberries

1. Preheat the oven to 350℉ (180°C) and line a baking dish with parchment paper. Keep it aside.
2. Place the coconut oil and cream cheese in a large mixing bowl and whisk the mixture with an electric mixer until smooth.
3. Add the whisked eggs to the bowl, stopping once to scrape down the sides of the bowl with a spatula.
4. Fold in the sweetener, baking powder, and vanilla extract, and blend well.
5. Transfer the mixture into the lined baking dish and smooth the top with a spatula. Top with the raspberries.
6. Bake for 28 to 30 minutes or until the center is set and firm.
7. Once the cheesecake has cooled completely, slice them into 12 squares to serve.

STORAGE: Store in an airtight container in the fridge for up to 4 days or in the freezer for up to 1 month.
PER SERVING (1 SQUARE)
calories: 210 | fat: 20.4g | total carbs: 1.9g | fiber: 0.5g | protein: 5.2g

CARDAMOM ORANGE BARK

Macros: Fat 96% | Protein 3% | Carbs 1%
Prep time: 15 minutes | Cook time: 0 minutes | Serves 6

The Cardamom orange bark is a sweet, cold and savoury orange-flavored snack that can be incorporated into a variety of diets. They are often integrated into keto diets, and can even be enjoyed outside a serious diet. The orange extract in this recipe can also be substituted with chocolate, apple extract, or any unique flavor that you are interested in testing out.

⅛ teaspoon finely ground gray sea salt
½ teaspoon orange extract
½ teaspoon vanilla extract
¾ cup melted coconut oil
1¾ teaspoons ground

cardamom
2 teaspoons ginger powder
2 tablespoons erythritol
⅔ cup raw walnut pieces, roasted

1. Pour all the ingredients except for the walnuts in a food processor and pulse for 20 seconds or until smooth and creamy.
2. Add the crushed walnuts. Pulse the food processor until each walnut is about ¼ inch in size.
3. Pour the mixture into a parchment-lined square baking pan, and leave it in the freezer for about an hour.
4. Remove the frozen mixture from the pan and break it into six pieces to serve.

STORAGE: It will remain fresh for about two weeks in the refrigerator and up to 2 months in a freezer
SERVE IT WITH: You can enjoy the barks as a snack with plain Greek yogurt or unsweetened coffee.
PER SERVING
calories: 336 | fat: 35.8g | total carbs: 2.4g | fiber: 1.1g | protein: 2.1g

HEALTHY BLUEBERRY FAT BOMBS

Macros: Fat 94% | Protein 2% | Carbs 4%
Prep time: 10 minutes | Cook time: 0 minutes | Serves 12

You will be amazed at how much flavor these little purple bites have. You literally have to try to hide them from yourself as they are unspeakably addictive and incredibly delicious on their own. The blueberry fat bombs are a hearty and healthy way to start or end any day.

½ cup cream cheese, at room temperature
½ cup coconut oil, at room temperature

½ cup blueberries, mashed with a fork
Pinch ground nutmeg
6 drops liquid stevia

1. Use the silicone mold or line a mini-sized muffin tin with paper liners. Keep it aside.
2. Combine the cream cheese with coconut oil in a medium mixing bowl and stir to blend well.
3. Fold in the blueberries, nutmeg, and stevia, and mix well.
4. Spoon the mixture into the muffin cups evenly and keep the muffin tin or mold in the refrigerator for 3 hours or until firm.

STORAGE: Store in an airtight container in the fridge for up to 4 days or in the freezer for up to 1 month.
PER SERVING
calories: 119 | fat: 12.5g | total carbs: 1.3g | fiber: 0.2g | protein: 0.6g

LOW-CARB CHOCOLATE CHIP COOKIES

Macros: Fat 76% | Protein 9% | Carb 15%
Prep time: 5 minutes | Cook time: 15 minutes | Serves 2

Chocolate chip cookies can be eaten as snacks, desserts, or meals. They taste great with coffee, tea, and milk. They are incredibly tasty and are sometimes considered an independent meal.

1 large egg yolk
1 tablespoon melted and salted butter
¼ teaspoon of vanilla extract
⅓ cup blanched almond flour

1½ tablespoons stevia
⅛ teaspoon baking powder
A pinch of salt
2 tablespoons sugar-free dark chocolate chips

1. Preheat the oven to 350°F (180°C) and line a baking sheet with parchment paper.
2. Mix the egg yolk, butter, and vanilla extract with a whisk in a large bowl until smooth. Add the flour, sweetener, baking powder, and salt. Mix it thoroughly with a wooden spoon and fold in the chocolate chips until a dough forms.
3. Make the cookies: Divide and roll the dough out into two equally sized balls. Bash them into 3-inch thick cookies and place them on the lined baking sheet.
4. Bake them in the preheated oven for 12 to 15 minutes or until the cookies become golden brown.
5. Transfer the hot cookies to a kitchen table or wire rack and wait for them to cool down before serving.

STORAGE: Store your chocolate chip cookies by either placing them in a sealed airtight container or a Ziploc bag. You should only store them when they have completely cooled down; this will prevent condensation in the container of your choosing. You can also refrigerate them by placing them in an airtight container and keeping them in a freezer for up to 5 months.
SERVE IT WITH: Cookies are best served with unsweetened almond milk, hot cocoa, or tea.
PER SERVING
calories: 220 | fat: 18.5g | total carbs 9.9g | fiber: 1.6g | protein: 5.1g

CREAM CHEESE BROWNIES

Macros: Fat 74% | Protein 8% | Carbs 18%
Prep time: 10 minutes | Cook time: 40 minutes | Serves 16

Simple, quick to make, healthy, and delicious, these moist cream cheese brownies are sure to get you rave reviews wherever you serve them. You will be surprised at how well the ingredients go together in this chewy, fudgy keto brownie. An ideal low-carb chocolate dessert that you should make at least once.

1 teaspoon baking powder
¼ teaspoon salt
¾ cup blanched almond flour
¼ cup unsweetened cocoa powder
3 ounces (85 g) cream cheese,

softened
2 large eggs, beaten
¼ cup unsalted butter, melted
1 teaspoon vanilla extract
⅓ cup dark chocolate chips
Cooking spray

1. Preheat the oven to 325°F (160°C). Spritz a baking pan with cooking spray.
2. Mix the baking powder, salt, almond flour and cocoa powder in a large mixing bowl. Stir well to combine.
3. Fold in the cream cheese, eggs, melted butter and vanilla extract. Mix until everything comes together. Add the chocolate chips and whisk well until a smooth batter forms.
4. Transfer the batter into the greased pan and smooth the top with a spatula.
5. Bake for 38 to 40 minutes or until a sharp knife inserted in the middle comes out clean. Allow it to cool for 5 minutes before cutting into squares.

STORAGE: Store in an airtight container in the fridge for up to 4 days or in the freezer for up to 1 month.
SERVE IT WITH: To make this a complete meal, serve it with keto ice creams.
PER SERVING
calories: 102 | fat: 8.4g | total carbs: 5.0g | fiber: 0.5g | protein: 2.1g

CHIA PUDDING WITH BLUEBERRIES

Macros: Fat 73% | Protein 17% | Carbs 10%
Prep time: 10 minutes | Cook time: 0 minutes | Serves 2

This pudding recipe is perfect for you if you are looking for a low-calorie, healthy protein dessert. It smells great and tastes even better when it's properly refrigerated. It fits perfectly in the most balanced weight loss and diet plans.

1 cup unsweetened vanilla almond milk
1½ tablespoons stevia

¼ cup chia seeds
4 to 6 fresh blueberries

1. Put the milk and stevia in a blender and process for 1 minute to combine well.
2. Pour the chia seeds in a glass and add the mixture.
3. Make the pudding: Stir the mixture well and then cover the glass with plastic wrap and refrigerate for 6 to 8 hours.
4. Transfer the pudding into a glass and add the blueberries on top before serving

STORAGE: Store the pudding in a glass container with an airtight cover, or cover it with plastic wrap. The pudding can last up to 5 days in the refrigerator after preparation.
SERVE IT WITH: The pudding can be used to layer in parfaits, trifles, or as a pie filling, or you can just enjoy it as a lovely dessert.
PER SERVING
calories: 125 | fat: 10.2g | total carbs: 12.9g | fiber: 9.8g | protein: 5.2g

MACADAMIA NUT AND CHOCOLATE FAT BOMBS

Macros: Fat: 83% | Protein 4% | Carbs 13%
Prep time: 5 minutes | Cook time: 1 minute | Makes 8 fat bombs

This recipe is a sweet, salty and savoury dessert for people who have a deep appreciation for chocolate and nuts. The nutty, chocolaty taste is reminiscent of world-class chocolate treats. They are the perfect dessert for every meal.

¼ cup sugar-free dark chocolate chips
Sea salt, to taste

1 tablespoon coconut oil
24 raw macadamia nut halves

SPECIAL EQUIPMENT:
8 baking cups or truffle molds

1. Melt the chocolate chips in a microwave for 50 seconds and mix it with sea salt and oil. Stir it until well mixed.
2. Arrange 3 macadamia nut halves inside each small baking cup and completely cover the nuts in chocolate by spooning the melted chocolate over each nut. Sprinkle a pinch of sea salt over the chocolate.
3. Place the cups inside the freezer for 30 to 40 minutes or until solid.

STORAGE: Store them in Ziploc bags in a refrigerator for a maximum of about 6 months.
SERVE IT WITH: You can serve it with other nut-based snacks, or a full keto meal.
PER SERVING
calories: 161 | fat: 14.8g | total carbs: 7.5g | fiber: 2.2g | protein: 1.7g

STRAWBERRY POPSICLES

Macros: Fat: 85% | Protein: 6% | Carbs: 9%
Prep time: 5 minutes | Cook time: 0 minutes | Makes 6 popsicles

Strawberry cream pops are the perfect cheat day dessert snack. They have a rich, creamy taste, a sweet scent accompanied by an equally fantastic taste.

8 fresh strawberries, hulled and quartered
1 cup heavy whipping cream
½ cup unsweetened almond milk

2 ounces (57 g) softened cream cheese
2½ tablespoons stevia
½ teaspoon vanilla extract

SPECIAL EQUIPMENT:
6 ice pop molds

1. Blend the strawberries and cream in a blender until they form soft peaks
2. Add almond milk, cream cheese, sweetener and vanilla extract, and pulse the blender until smooth.
3. Make the Popsicles: Pour the mixture in the blender into the ice pop molds and freeze them for at least three hours.
4. To separate the ice molds and Popsicles before serving, run the molds through lukewarm or hot water.

STORAGE: Store the ice molds inside the freezer for as long as you want. Popsicle can last for up to five months.
SERVE IT WITH: Just enjoy it with your friends and burning sun.
PER SERVING
calories: 120 | fat: 11.3g | total carbs: 3.2g | fiber: 0.3g | protein: 1.7g

EASY COCONUT MOUNDS

Macros: Fat: 91% | Carbs: 4% | Protein: 5%
Prep time: 20 minutes | Cook time: 0 minutes | Makes 18 bars

Coconut mounds are essentially home-made bounty bars with fewer chemicals, preservatives and artificial sweeteners. They have a unique creamy-chocolaty taste that puts even bounty bars to shame. They are a lot less calorie-dense than regular bounty bars, and the ratio of chocolate to coconut you want is up to you.

2⅔ cups unsweetened shredded coconut
1 (14-ounce / 397-g) can unsweetened coconut milk, heated just until lukewarm
¼ cup melted coconut oil
1 tablespoon plus 1 teaspoon

erythritol
1 teaspoon vanilla extract
¼ teaspoon grounded gray sea salt
36 roasted almonds
½ cup melted and sugar-free dark chocolate chips

1. Line a baking sheet with parchment paper.
2. Pour the shredded coconut, milk, coconut oil, erythritol, vanilla, and salt in a mixing bowl. Stir to make sure every piece of coconut is coated with the mixture.
3. Scoop out 2 tablespoons of the coconut mixture and shape it up like a bar before placing on the baking sheet. Repeat with the remaining mixture.
4. Place the baking sheet in the fridge and allow it to harden for 30 minutes.
5. Place 2 almonds on each bar. Sprinkle with chocolate chips, and then place in the fridge for another 15 minutes.
6. Remove from the fridge and serve chill.

STORAGE: Store in an airtight container, and store in a refrigerator. They can be stored for 3 days or in the freezer for 1 month.
SERVE IT WITH: You can enjoy this dessert with your favorite smoothie, such as strawberry smoothie.
PER SERVING
calories: 153 | fat: 15.5g | total carb: 3.8g | fiber: 1.9g | protein: 1.4g

EASY PEANUT BUTTER COOKIES

Macros: Fat 74% | Protein 16% | Carbs 10%
Prep time: 1 hour | Cook time: 15 minutes | Serves 6

This is the recipe that is easy and quick to make with just 3 ingredients! These cookies ate irresistibly super delicious.

1 egg
½ cup peanut butter

½ cup Swerve

1. Start by preheating the oven to 350°F (180°C). Line a parchment paper on a baking pan.
2. Put egg, peanut butter and Swerve in a bowl to make the dough and mix until bubbly.
3. Using a cookie spoon to scoop the dough into balls, then arrange them in the baking pan. Press the balls with a fork.
4. Put the baking pan in the preheated oven and bake for 15 minutes.
5. Cool for 10 minutes and serve.

STORAGE: Store in an airtight container in the fridge for up to 3 days, or up to 3 months in a freezer.
SERVE IT WITH: Serve this dessert with a glass of zucchini smoothie.
PER SERVING
calories: 155 | fat: 12.7g | total carbs: 5.0g | fiber: 1.1g | protein: 6.3g

ALMOND AND CINNAMON TRUFFLES

Macros: Fat: 88% | Carbs: 6% | Protein: 6%
Prep time: 20 minutes | Cook time: 0 minutes | Makes 10 truffles

Almond truffles are scrumptious delicacies that taste even better when they are accompanied with the right mood. They are prepared exclusively for special occasions. This truffle recipe uses almonds only, but it's possible to add another coat of dark or milk chocolate if you dip them in chocolate and let them freeze.

½ cup unsweetened almond butter
¼ cup plus 2 tablespoons melted cacao butter
1 tablespoon plus 1 teaspoon ground cinnamon

1 tablespoon erythritol
½ teaspoon vanilla extract
1 pinch of gray sea salt
3 tablespoons roasted almonds, smashed to ⅛-inch thick

1. Line a rimmed baking sheet with parchment paper.
2. Make the truffle: Pour almond butter, cacao butter, cinnamon, erythritol, vanilla extract, and salt in a bowl and stir until it's smooth. Refrigerate for about 45 minutes.
3. Remove the truffle mixture from the fridge, shape 1 tablespoon of the mixture into 10 eraser sized bricks. Pour the smashed almonds in a separate bowl.
4. Pick up the little bricks, coat it with almond pieces and then set it on the baking sheet already prepared. Repeat the process until you have 10 coated truffle pieces.
5. Serve the truffle in the baking sheet under room temperature.

STORAGE: Store it in an airtight container in a fridge for up to 2 weeks. The freezer will get you about 2 extra weeks.
SERVE IT WITH: You can enjoy this dessert with your favorite smoothie, such as blueberry smoothie or zucchini smoothie.
PER SERVING
calories: 186 | fat: 18.1g | total carbs: 3.6g | fiber: 0.7g | protein: 2.8g

HEMP SEEDS AND CHOCOLATE COOKIES

Macros: Fat 82% | Protein 14% | Carbs 4%
Prep time: 20 minutes | Cook time: 0 minutes | Serves 14

This keto recipe is an easy and quick no-bake recipe. It has lots of nutrients such as fat and protein. The chocolate is sweetened with the stevia, which will leave you licking your fingers.

½ teaspoon ground cinnamon
½ teaspoon vanilla extract or powder
¼ cup melted coconut oil or cacao butter

1¼ cups hulled hemp seeds
2 drops liquid stevia
¼ cup sugar-free dark chocolate chips

1. Line parchment paper on a baking sheet.
2. In a medium bowl, combine cinnamon, vanilla, coconut oil, hemp seeds and stevia.
3. Blend the mixture in a food processor until the dough is ready. To check if it's ready, pinch it with your fingers; it is ready if it sticks together.
4. Add the chocolate chips and mix.
5. Scoop the dough with a round spoon into the baking sheet to make 14 cookies.
6. Refrigerate for at least 30 minutes and then serve.

STORAGE: Store in an airtight container in the fridge for up to 1 week, or up to 1 month in a freezer.
SERVE IT WITH: To make this a complete meal, you can serve it as an appetizer or dessert and serve with main dish and soup such as roast turkey and veggie soup.
PER SERVING
calories: 127 | fat: 11.6g | total carbs: 1.3g | fiber: 0g | protein: 4.3g

GOOEY CREAMY CAKE

Macros: Fat 76% | Protein 15% | Carbs 9%
Prep time: 55 minutes | Cook time: 22 minutes | Serves 18

This recipe is traditionally from St. Louis, Missouri. It is so sweet, filled with flavor from its delicious ingredients. You can replace coconut milk with soy milk when making this recipe.

¼ cup coconut oil, plus more for greasing the baking pan
¾ cup blanched almond flour, plus more for dusting the baking pan
1 teaspoon baking powder
½ teaspoon finely ground gray

sea salt
¾ cup erythritol, plus more for dusting
5 large whisked eggs
1½ teaspoons vanilla extract
1 cup unsweetened coconut milk, heated until lukewarm

1. Start by preheating the oven to 350℉ (180°C). Grease a baking pan with 1 tablespoon coconut oil and dust with almond flour.
2. Combine the almond flour, baking powder, and salt in a bowl.
3. Put the coconut oil in a separate bowl and whip with a hand mixer until puffed.
4. Gently mix in the erythritol, then pour the whisked egg into the mixture. Stir to combine.
5. Fold in the vanilla, then mix in the flour mixture in 3 batches.
6. Pour the mixture into the greased baking pan. Bake in the preheated oven for 20 minutes or until lightly browned. Remove the pan from the oven and let stand for 30 minutes.
7. Prick the top of the cake with a fork, then pour the lukewarm coconut milk over.
8. Wrap the pan in plastic and refrigerate for 1 day. Remove the cake from the refrigerate and let sit under room temperature for 30 minutes before serving. Sprinkle with erythritol and slice to serve.

STORAGE: Store in an airtight container in the fridge for up to 3 days.
REHEAT: Microwave, covered, until the desired temperature is reached or reheat in a frying pan or air fryer / instant pot, covered, on medium.
SERVE IT WITH: To make this a complete meal, serve the cake with plain yogurt or cherry smoothie.
PER SERVING
calories: 74 | fat: 6.3g | total carbs: 1.6g | fiber: 0g | protein: 2.8g

ALMOND SNICKERDOODLE COOKIES

Macros: Fat 69% | Protein 13% | Carbs 18%
Prep time: 13 minutes | Cook time: 12 minutes | Serves 8

Snickerdoodle cookies are a favorite among kids and are a special treat for holidays such as Christmas.

COOKIES:

½ cup unsweetened almond milk
2 teaspoons vanilla essence
1 cup almond butter
1½ cups monk fruit sweetener
2 beaten eggs
2 teaspoons tartar cream

¼ cup coconut oil
1 cup coconut flour
1 teaspoon baking soda
1¾ cups almond flour
1 teaspoon cinnamon
⅛ teaspoon sea salt

TOPPING:
3 tablespoons monk fruit sweetener
1 tablespoon cinnamon

1. Start by preheating the oven to 350°F (180°C) and line a baking sheet with parchment paper.
2. Add almond milk, vanilla essence, almond butter, monk sweetener, eggs, tartar cream, coconut oil and blend. Add coconut flour, baking soda, almond flour, cinnamon, salt and blend further.
3. Refrigerate the batter for 20 minutes.
4. Remove the batter from the fridge. Divide and form into 8 equally sized small balls.
5. In a shallow bowl, combine the monk fruit sweetener and cinnamon and add the balls to coat them with the mixture.
6. Arrange the balls on the baking sheet and bake in the preheated oven for 12 minutes.
7. Cool for about 6 minutes and serve.

STORAGE: Store in an airtight container in the fridge for up to 4 days, or up to 2 months in a freezer.
SERVE IT WITH: You can serve the cookies with vegetable juice or blueberry smoothie.
PER SERVING
calories: 553 | fat: 42.1g | total carbs: 28.9g | fiber: 3.4g | protein: 17.9g

CHOCOLATE-CRUSTED COFFEE BITES

Macros: Fat 91% | Protein 7% | Carbs 2%
Prep time: 10 minutes | Cook time: 0 minutes | Serves 8

This recipe is an ideal treat for you and your family. Biting a bitter coffee and then coupling it with yummy creamy chocolate is great at any time of the day!

BITES:
½ teaspoon sugar-free instant coffee
1 tablespoon erythritol or 1 or 2 drops liquid stevia
½ cup macadamia nuts, roasted
¼ cup plus 2 tablespoons cacao butter
2 tablespoons collagen peptides

CHOCOLATE TOPPING:
¼ cup sugar-free dark chocolate chips, melted
¼ teaspoon sea salt

1. Make the bites: In a high-powered food processor, add instant coffee, erythritol, macadamia nuts, and cacao butter. Blend for 20 seconds on high speed, or until the macadamia nuts break into pieces.
2. Add the collagen peptides and blend further to combine.
3. Scoop the mixture with a spoon into 8 silicon mold cavities and press. Refrigerate the mixture for 2 hours or freeze for 1 hour, or until the bites are ready.
4. In the meantime, line parchment paper on a baking sheet and set aside.
5. Remove the bites from the freezer or refrigerator and arrange the bites on the baking sheet. Top with the melted chocolate and season the bites with salt.
6. Refrigerate the bites for about 10 minutes and serve.

STORAGE: Store in an airtight container in the fridge for up to 2 weeks, or up to 2 months in a freezer.
SERVE IT WITH: To make this recipe complete meal, serve with monk fruit sweetened coconut milk.
PER SERVING
calories: 193 | fat: 19.5g | total carbs: 1.5g | fiber: 0.7g | protein: 3.6g

KETO MATCHA BROWNIES WITH PISTACHIOS

Macros: Fat 83% | Protein 11% | Carbs 6%
Prep time: 10 minutes | Cook time: 18 minutes | Serves 4

These are deliciously easy to make brownies that you and every member of your family will love. The brownie is moist with subtle flavors and perfectly satisfies any sweet cravings.

¼ cup butter, unsalted and melted
4 tablespoons Swerve
A pinch of salt
1 egg
1 tablespoon matcha powder
¼ cup coconut flour
½ teaspoon baking powder
½ cup pistachios, chopped

1. Preheat your oven to 350°F (180°C) and line a baking pan with parchment paper.
2. Add butter, Swerve, and a pinch of salt to a mixing bowl, and whisk until well combined.
3. Break the egg into the butter mixture and beat the mixture until well mixed.
4. Sift matcha powder coconut flour and baking powder through a fine-mesh sieve into the bowl of the egg mixture. Stir until well mixed.
5. Add the chopped pistachios and stir well to combine. Pour the mixture into the prepared baking pan and bake in the preheated oven for 18 minutes.
6. Remove from the oven and let rest for 5 minutes. Cut into brownie cubes to serve.

STORAGE: Store in an airtight container in the fridge for 5 days.
SERVE IT WITH: You can enjoy this dessert with your favorite smoothie, such as blueberry smoothie or zucchini smoothie.
PER SERVING
calories: 239 | fat: 21.9g | total carbs: 8.5g | fiber: 1.6g | protein: 6.5g

GINGERSNAP NUTMEG COOKIES

Macros: Fat 78% | Protein 12% | Carbs 10%
Prep time: 13 minutes | Cook time: 12 minutes | Serves 8

Ginger is one of the spices for cookies. Coupled with nutmeg, it makes cookies taste amazingly sweet and crunchy.

1 teaspoon vanilla essence
1 large egg
¼ cup butter, unsalted
1 cup erythritol
2 cups almond flour
½ teaspoon ground cinnamon
2 teaspoons ground ginger
¼ teaspoon ground nutmeg
¼ teaspoon ground cloves
¼ teaspoon salt

1. Start by preheating the oven to 350°F (180°C) and line a baking sheet with parchment paper.
2. With an electric mixer, add vanilla essence, egg, butter, erythritol, and mix.
3. Add almond flour, cinnamon, ginger, nutmeg, cloves and salt and stir until smooth.
4. Spoon the dough into cookies with a cookie scoop and arrange them on the baking sheet.
5. Bake for 12 minutes in the preheated oven.
6. Remove from oven and cool for 3 minutes and serve.

STORAGE: Store in an airtight container in the fridge for up to 2 weeks or up to 2 months in a freezer.
SERVE IT WITH: To make this recipe complete meal, serve with plain Greek yogurt or cherry pancake.
PER SERVING
calories: 238 | fat: 20.5g | total carbs: 6.5g | fiber: 0.2g | protein: 7.0g

MICROWAVED RHUBARB CAKES

Macros: Fat 88% | Protein 9% | Carbs 3%
Prep time: 5 minutes | Cook time: 2 minutes | Serves 2

There are easy recipes to make, but this one is among the easiest. It takes just 2 minutes to prepare! Blueberries are also a great substitute for the strawberries in this recipe.

¼ teaspoon vanilla extract or powder
1 tablespoon plus 1 teaspoon erythritol
3 tablespoons refined macadamia nut oil or avocado oil
1 large egg

¼ teaspoon baking powder
¼ teaspoon ground nutmeg
1 teaspoon ground cinnamon
¼ cup roughly ground flaxseeds
1 (2½-inch) piece rhubarb, diced
1 to 2 fresh strawberries, hulled and sliced, for garnish

1.   In a small bowl, whisk together the vanilla, erythritol, oil, and egg.
2.   In another bowl, combine the baking powder, nutmeg, cinnamon and flaxseeds. Pour into the egg mixture. Stir in the rhubarb.
3.   Divide evenly among 2 microwave-safe containers and microwave for about 2 minutes. You can check the doneness by inserting a toothpick in the center of the cake. If it comes out clean, then it is ready to serve.
4.   Top with strawberries and serve.

STORAGE: Store in an airtight container in the fridge for up to 2 days.
REHEAT: Microwave, covered, until the desired temperature is reached or reheat in a frying pan or air fryer / instant pot, covered, on medium.
SERVE IT WITH: To make this a complete meal, serve the cake with plain Greek yogurt or blueberry smoothie.
PER SERVING
calories: 335 | fat: 32.7g | total carbs: 9.5g | fiber: 7.1g | protein: 7.7g

BERRY TART

Macros: Fat 83% | Protein 9% | Carbs 8%
Prep time: 15 minutes | Cook time: 10 minutes | Serves 6

The summer is always filled with plenty of berries. The best way to make use of them is making this great and easy tart. With strawberries, blueberries and raspberries, you will love every bit of this tart.

TART CRUST:
5 tablespoons butter, melted
¼ cup erythritol, powdered

2¼ cups almond flour
¼ teaspoon sea salt

FILLING:
⅓ cup heavy cream
2 tablespoons erythritol
1 teaspoon vanilla essence

¼ teaspoon lemon zest
6 ounces (170 g) mascarpone cheese

TOPPINGS:
6 blueberries
6 raspberries

6 blackberries

1.   Start by preheating the oven to 350°F (180°C). Use melted butter to grease 6 small tart pans.
2.   Blend the erythritol, almond flour and salt in a blender until well combined.
3.   Put the mixture equally into the tart pans and press to make them firm.

4.   Bake in the preheated oven for 10 minutes.
5.   Meanwhile, mix the cream and the erythritol using an electric mixture until well combined.
6.   Add vanilla essence, lemon zest, and cheese and mix further until creamy.
7.   Divide this mixture onto the crusts and top with berries separately.
8.   Refrigerate for about 10 minutes before serving.

STORAGE: Store in an airtight container in the fridge for up to 3 days, or up to 2 months in a freezer.
PER SERVING
calories: 497 | fat: 45.6g | total carbs: 10.9g | fiber: 0.3g | protein: 11.0g

CHOCOLATE TART

Macros: Fat 78% | Protein 8% | Carbs 14%
Prep time: 12 minutes | Cook time: 28 minutes | Serves 8

You do not need to have any dough-making skills to make this creamy chocolate tart. It's simple and finger-licking good.

CRUST:
4 tablespoons melted butter, divided
1 large egg

6 tablespoons coconut flour
2 tablespoons erythritol

FILLING:
½ cup heavy whipping cream
2 ounces (57 g) unsweetened chocolate
Liquid stevia, to taste

¼ cup powdered erythritol
1 ounce (28 g) cream cheese
1 large egg

1.   Start by preheating the oven to 400°F (205°C). Grease two tart pans with 2 tablespoons melted butter.
2.   Blend the egg, the remaining melted butter, coconut flour and erythritol with a blender until mixed.
3.   Pour the mixture equally into the two tart pans, and press them to make them firm.
4.   Poke a few holes on the top of the crusts with a fork.
5.   Transfer to the preheated oven and bake for 12 minutes.
6.   In the meantime, in a saucepan over medium heat, heat the cream, add chocolate and melt it. Put the mixture into a blender and blend until soft peaks form.
7.   Add stevia, erythritol, cream cheese, egg and blend further.
8.   Divide the filling mixture among the crusts and bake again in the oven for 15 minutes. Transfer to a wire rack for about 10 minutes.
9.   Put in the fridge for at least 3 hours and then serve.

STORAGE: Store in an airtight container in the fridge for up to 4 days or up to 2 months in a freezer.
SERVE IT WITH: To make this recipe complete meal, serve with plain Greek yogurt or nutmeg cookies and peanut butter fat bombs.
PER SERVING
calories: 170 | fat: 14.8g | total carbs: 6.7g | fiber: 0.8g | protein: 3.4g

ALMOND PUMPKIN PIE

Macros: Fat 76% | Protein 17% | Carbs 7%
Prep time: 1 hour | Cook time: 10 minutes | Serves 8

The almond pumpkin pie's crust is naturally sweetened and filled with the sweet flavor of vanilla and cinnamon.

ALMOND FLOUR PIE CRUST:

4 tablespoons melted butter, divided
1 egg yolk

½ teaspoon cinnamon
1 teaspoon vanilla
2 cups almond flour

PUMPKIN SPICE FILLING:

8 ounces (227 g) cream cheese
4 eggs
1 teaspoon vanilla
⅔ cup Swerve

1 cup heavy cream
2 teaspoons pumpkin pie spice
¼ teaspoon salt

1. Start by preheating the oven to 400°F (205°C) and grease a baking pan with 2 tablespoons melted butter.
2. Mix egg yolk, cinnamon, vanilla, almond flour, and remaining butter together in a bowl. Pour the mixture into the prepared baking pan.
3. Bake for 12 minutes in the preheated oven and set aside.
4. Meanwhile, add cream cheese and egg to a bowl and whisk until foamy.
5. Add vanilla, Swerve, heavy cream, pumpkin pie spice and salt and combine well.
6. Pour the mixture onto the baked crust, and spread the mixture with a spatula to coat the bottom evenly.
7. Return to the oven and bake for 45 about minutes. Remove from the oven, transfer to a wire rack to cool for 10 minutes, then cut into pieces and serve.

STORAGE: Store in an airtight container in the fridge for up to 4 days or up to 1 month in a freezer.
SERVE IT WITH: To make this recipe complete meal, serve with tomato and zucchini smoothie or walnut cookies.
PER SERVING
calories: 556 | fat: 47.2g | total carbs: 9.1g | fiber: 0.1g | protein: 23.7g

CHILLED VANILLA ICE CREAM

Macros: Fat 91% | Protein 5% | Carbs 4%
Prep time: 30 minutes | Cook time: 0 minutes | Serves 6

There is a reason why vanilla ranks best when compared with the ice cream flavors. The flavor is like none other. This makes this ice cream special in its own way.

6 large egg yolks
1 (13½-ounce / 383-g) package unsweetened coconut milk
2 tablespoons granulated xylitol
½ cup melted coconut oil,

cooled
2 teaspoons vanilla powder or extract
¼ teaspoon kosher salt

TOPPING:
2 tablespoons roasted blanched almonds, sliced

SPECIAL EQUIPMENT:
Ice cream maker

1. Place a baking pan lined with a parchment paper or a glass bowl in a freezer.
2. In a blender, add the egg yolks, coconut milk, xylitol, coconut oil, vanilla powder, and kosher salt and pulse until smooth.

3. Put the mixture in a mason jar and chill in the refrigerator for 2 hours.
4. Put the chilled mixture into an ice cream maker and proceed as per the directions of the manufacturer.
5. Put the mixture into the chilled baking pan, or chilled glass bowl and cover. Put in a freezer for a minimum of one and a half hours.
6. Remove from the freezer and leave it to soften under room temperature for 6 to 9 minutes. Use a teaspoon of roasted almonds to garnish each serving.

STORAGE: Store in an airtight container in a freezer for up to 2 weeks.
SERVE IT WITH: You can serve it with gluten-free strawberry brownies and a chocolate smoothie.
PER SERVING (WITHOUT ALMOND TOPPING)
calories: 407 | fat: 41.3g | total carbs: 5.6g | fiber: 2.1g | protein: 5.3g

KETO CHOCOLATE CUTE MUG CAKE

Macros: Fat 77% | Protein 16% | Carbs 7%
Prep time: 5 minutes | Cook time: 1½ minutes | Serves 4

This is an ultimate dessert to serve every member of your family. It is fluffy and packed with chocolate flavor to satisfy all your chocolate cravings.

2 tablespoons coconut flour
½ cup almond flour
2 tablespoons cocoa powder
1 tablespoon granulated monk fruit sweetener
1¼ teaspoons baking powder

2 beaten eggs
½ teaspoon vanilla extract
¼ cup melted butter
½ cup sugar-free dark chocolate chips

1. Mix the coconut flour, almond flour, cocoa powder, monk fruit sweetener and baking powder in a medium mixing bowl until well incorporated.
2. Stir in eggs, vanilla extract, and butter in the dry ingredients mixture. You can use an electronic mixture for a perfectly consistent batter.
3. Stir in the chocolate chips until well distributed in the batter.
4. Divide the mixture between two mugs. Microwave for 1½ minutes or until the mug cake is just cooked.
5. Remove from the microwave and let cool for 10 minutes to serve

STORAGE: Store in an airtight container in the fridge or covered at room temperature for 1 day.
SERVE IT WITH: To make this a complete meal, serve it with a dollop of plain Greek yogurt.
PER SERVING
calories: 470 | fat: 40.0g | total carbs: 9.3g | fiber: 1.1g | protein: 19.4g

SMOOTH AND PUFFED COCONUT MOUSSE

Macros: Fat 89% | Protein 6% | Carbs 5%
Prep time: 15 minutes | Cook time: 15 minutes | Serves 4

This is a light yet rich and creamy dessert that comes together both very easily and quickly. It is packed with creamy and cold coconut flavor, making it perfect for a summer dessert.

¼ cup cold water
2 teaspoons granulated gelatin
1 cup unsweetened coconut milk
3 egg yolks

½ cup granulated monk fruit sweetener
1 cup heavy whipping cream

1. Pour the water in a mixing bowl and sprinkle granulated gelatin and stir to combine. Set aside for 10 minutes.
2. Meanwhile, add the coconut milk in a saucepan over medium-high and heat until it boils. Remove the milk from heat and set aside.
3. In a separate medium mixing bowl, whisk eggs yolks together with granulated monk fruit sweetener until well mixed.
4. Pour the boiled coconut milk into the egg yolk mixture and continue to whisk until well blended. Use a blender to expedite the mixing and for better consistency.
5. Pour the coconut milk mixture back to the saucepan and heat it while whisking for 5 minutes or until the base thickens.
6. Remove the milk mixture from heat and stir in the gelatin mixture. Set aside to cool.
7. Transfer the mixture to a bowl and refrigerate for an hour.
8. Meanwhile, place the whipping cream in a mixing bowl and whisk it until thick and fluffy.
9. Once the coconut milk mixture is cooled, fold in the whisked cream until well mixed.
10. Divide the mousse among four serving bowls and serve immediately.

STORAGE: Store in an airtight container in the fridge for up to 5 days or freeze for up to 2 months
SERVE IT WITH: To make this a complete meal, you can serve it with strawberry and blueberry smoothie.
PER SERVING
calories: 292 | fat: 29.0g | total carbs: 5.1g | fiber: 1.3g | protein: 4.0g

CARAMEL AND CREAM WITH COCONUT PANNA COTTA

Macros: Fat 78% | Protein 13% | Carbs 9%
Prep time: 5 minutes | Cook time: 60 minutes | Serves 4

⅓ cup erythritol
2 tablespoons water
4 beaten eggs
1 tablespoon vanilla extract
1 tablespoon lemon zest

½ cup erythritol
2 cups unsweetened coconut milk
2 cups heavy whipping cream
Mint leaves, for serving

SPECIAL EQUIPMENT:
4 ramekins

1. Preheat your oven to 350°F (180°C).
2. Make the caramel: Heat ⅓ cup erythritol in a shallow saucepan then add 2 tablespoons of water. Bring the mixture to a boil, then reduce heat and simmer until the caramel turns golden brown.
3. Remove from heat and divide the mixture among four ramekins. Set aside to let cool.
4. Meanwhile, add eggs, vanilla extract, lemon zest and the ½ cup erythritol to a mixing bowl. Mix well until combined. Stir in coconut milk.

5. Pour the coconut milk mixture into the ramekins while filling them with hot water. Place the ramekins in a deep baking dish.
6. Place the baking dish with ramekins in the preheated oven and bake for 45 minutes.
7. Remove the baking dish from the oven. Allow the ramekins to cool under the room temperature, then use tongs to transfer the ramekins to the fridge. Let chill for 3 hours.
8. Run a knife around the ramekins, then invert the ramekin on a platter.
9. Top with whipped cream dollops and scatter mint leaves to serve.

STORAGE: Store in an airtight container in the fridge for 5 days or freeze for up to 3 months
SERVE IT WITH: To make this a complete meal, you can serve it with a raspberry smoothie.
PER SERVING
calories: 415 | fat: 35.8g | total carbs: 9.2g | fiber: 0.2g | protein: 14.1g

CHOCOLATE AND BLUEBERRY TRUFFLES

Macros: Fat 81% | Protein 4% | Carbs 15%
Prep time: 10 minutes | Cook time: 95 seconds | Serves 8

Blueberries in chocolate! These truffles are unbelievably wonderful. They are just easy to make and mix with the flour of fruit and chocolate.

2 cups raw walnuts
2 tablespoons flaxseeds
3 tablespoons xylitol
1½ cups blueberry

10 ounces (284 g) sugar-free dark chocolate chips
3 tablespoons olive oil

1. Add walnuts and flaxseeds in a food processor. Pulse for 50 seconds or until fully crushed.
2. Add 2 tablespoons xylitol and blueberry in the food processor and pulse for 1 more minute or until everything is well combined.
3. Line your baking pan with parchment paper.
4. Use your hands to mold the mixture into 1-inch balls and arrange them on the lined baking pan.
5. Place the baking pan in a freezer and freeze for an hour or until firm to touch.
6. Add chocolate chips with olive oil and remaining xylitol in a microwave-safe bowl and melt in the microwave for 95 seconds.
7. Remove from the microwave and toss the truffles in the melted chocolate mixture and place them back on the baking pan.
8. Once you have tossed all truffles, return to the freezer and freeze for 3 more hours.
9. Let rest for 10 minutes to serve.

STORAGE: Store in an airtight container in the fridge for 4 to 5 days or freeze for up to 3 months
SERVE IT WITH: To make this a complete meal, you can serve it with keto bread or chocolate fat bombs.
PER SERVING
calories: 334 | fat: 30.1g | total carbs: 8.8g | fiber: 2.7g | protein: 3.7g

CHOCOLATE-STRAWBERRY MOUSSE

Macros: Fat 76% | Protein 10% | Carbs 14%
Prep time: 20 minutes | Cook time: 25 minutes | Serves 8

This amazing chocolate mousse with strawberries will blow away your mind. It's a real hit in a family or friends gathering and surprisingly easy and quick to make.

MOUSSE:

12 ounces (340 g) sugar-free dark chocolate	¾ cup Swerve
8 eggs, separated into whites and yolks	2 tablespoons salt
	½ cup olive oil
	3 tablespoons brewed coffee

CHERRIES:

½ cup Swerve	½ cup of water
½ stick cinnamon	1 cup strawberries, chopped
½ juiced lime	

SPECIAL EQUIPMENT:
8 medium ramekins

1. Add chocolate in a microwave-safe bowl and microwave for 90 seconds to melt the chocolate chips.
2. In a separate bowl, add the egg yolk and half of the Swerve. Whisk together until the yolk turns pale yellow.
3. Stir in salt, olive oil, and brewed coffee. Add melted chocolate and mix until the mixture is smooth.
4. In another bowl, add egg whites and use a hand mixer to mix until stiff peaks form. Use a wooden spoon to fold in the remaining sweetener.
5. Scoop 1 tablespoon of the chocolate mixture in a third bowl and fold in the egg white mixture. Add the remaining chocolate mixture and thoroughly mix until well combined.
6. Scoop the mixture into ramekins and cover the ramekins with plastic wraps. Place in the fridge and refrigerate overnight.
7. The next day, add the sweetener, cinnamon, lime juice, and water in a shallow saucepan. Simmer for 4 minutes or until the Swerve has dissolved, and a syrup is formed.
8. Add the strawberries and poach them in the water with sweetener for 20 minutes or until just soft.
9. Remove from heat and discard the cinnamon stick. Spoon the strawberries with the syrup on the mousse. Serve immediately.

STORAGE: Store in an airtight container in the fridge for 4 to 5 days or freeze for up to 2 months.
SERVE IT WITH: You can enjoy this dessert with your favorite smoothie, such as blueberry smoothie or zucchini smoothie.
PER SERVING
calories: 490 | fat: 41.3g | total carbs: 22.2g | fiber: 5.0g | protein: 12.4g

CHOCOLATE MARSHMALLOWS

Macros: Fat 64% | Protein 21% | Carbs 15%
Prep time: 21 minutes | Cook time: 9 minutes | Serves 4

These are the best marshmallows you will ever want after preparing this recipe. They are lofty, creamy, and light as air. Even better, you can customize your marshmallows as you want.

2 tablespoons coconut oil, melted	Salt to taste
1 tablespoon xanthan gum	2½ teaspoons gelatin powder
Cold water, as needed	2 tablespoons cocoa powder, unsweetened
½ cup erythritol	½ teaspoon vanilla extract

DUSTING:
1 tablespoon cocoa powder, unsweetened
1 tablespoon Swerve

1. Line a baking loaf pan with parchment paper, then grease it with coconut oil. Set it aside.
2. Add xanthan gum in a small bowl and add 1 tablespoon of water. Mix until well mixed.
3. In another medium bowl, add erythritol and mix it with 2 tablespoons of water. Mix in the xanthan gum mixture and a pinch of salt.
4. Heat the mixture in a shallow saucepan over high heat and bring the mixture to a boil. Then reduce heat and simmer at 225°F (107°C) for 8 minutes.
5. Meanwhile, add 2 more tablespoons of water and gelatin in a mixing bowl. Let the mixture rest for 5 minutes for the gelatin to dissolve.
6. Meanwhile, pour 2 tablespoons of water in a microwave-safe bowl, and heat in a microwave for 30 seconds. Remove from the microwave and mix in cocoa powder.
7. Pour the cocoa mixture in the gelatin mixture. Once the erythritol mixture has reached the desired temperature, remove it from heat and stir it into the gelatin mixture. Now beat the mixture until light and fluffy.
8. Stir the vanilla extract into the mixture until well mixed. Pour the mixture in the prepared loaf pan.
9. Place the loaf pan in the fridge for 3 hours to let the marshmallows set. Oil a knife and cut the marshmallows into cubes, then transferring them to a plate.
10. In a small bowl, mix the dusting ingredients and sift the mixture over the marshmallows before serving.

STORAGE: Store in an airtight container in the fridge for several days or freeze for up to 3 months.
SERVE IT WITH: You can enjoy this dessert with your favorite smoothie, such as strawberry smoothie.
PER SERVING
calories: 103 | fat: 7.4g | total carbs: 5.4g | fiber: 1.5g | protein: 5.3g

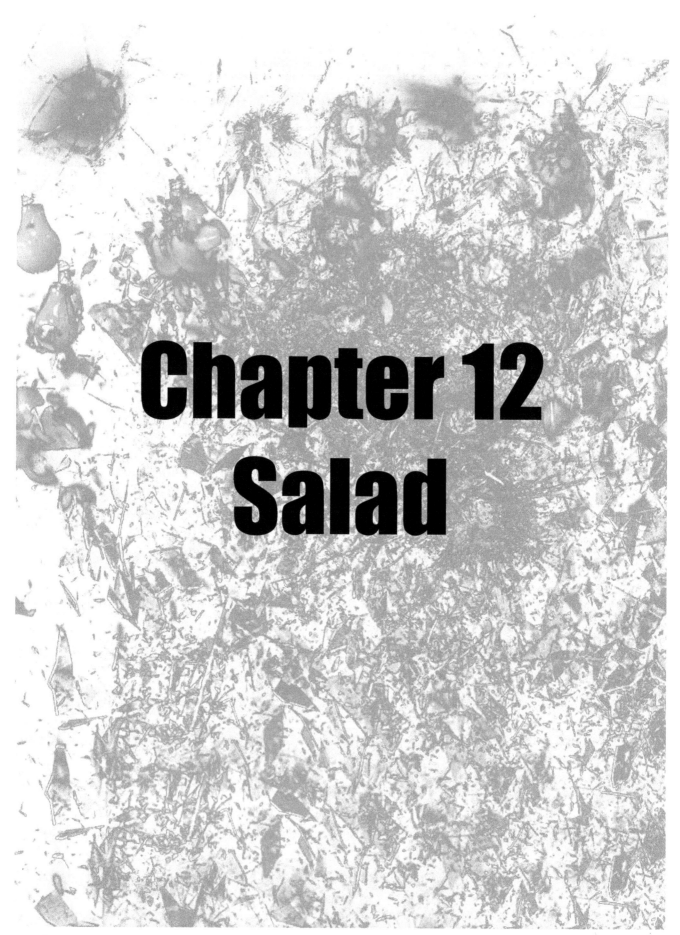

Chapter 12
Salad

WATERCRESS AND ARUGULA TURKEY SALAD

Macros: Fat 68% | Protein 27% | Carbs 5%
Prep time: 12 minutes | Cook time: 13 minutes | Serves 4

The turkey transforms this salad into a classic light dinner that is irresistibly delicious and that will leave everyone asking for more.

DRESSING:
1 tablespoon xylitol
2 tablespoons lime juice
1 tablespoon Dijon mustard
1 red onion, chopped
1¾ cups raspberries, divided

5 tablespoons olive oil, divided
¼ cup water
Salt and freshly ground black pepper, to taste

SALAD:
1 pound (454 g) boneless turkey breast, slice in half
1 cup watercress
1 cup arugula

4 ounces (113 g) goat cheese, crumbled
½ cup walnuts, halved

1. Make the dressing: Add xylitol, lime juice, Dijon mustard, onion, 1 cup of raspberries, 3 tablespoons olive oil, water, salt, and pepper in a high-powered blender. Pulse until smooth.
2. Strain the liquid from the mixture in a mixing bowl and set aside.
3. On a flat work surface, generously season the turkey breasts with salt and pepper.
4. Heat a saucepan over medium heat, then coat the bottom with 2 tablespoons olive oil. Place the turkey in the heated saucepan, skin-side down. Cook the turkey for 8 minutes, then flip the turkey and cook for 5 minutes more.
5. Meanwhile, place the watercress and arugula in a salad bowl. Add the remaining raspberries, goat cheese, and walnuts halves into the bowl.
6. Use two folks to shred the turkey into small pieces and add to the salad bowl.
7. Pour over the dressing, then stir thoroughly to mix well.
8. Let the salad rest for 10 minutes, then serve.

STORAGE: Store in an airtight container in the fridge for 3 days.
REHEAT: Microwave, covered, until the turkey pieces are just warm.
SERVE IT WITH: To make this a delicious complete meal, serve it with keto burgers.
PER SERVING
calories: 553 | fat: 42.0g | total carbs: 12.1g | fiber: 4.9g | protein: 36.5g

SPINACH SALAD WITH MUSTARD VINAIGRETTE AND BACON

Macros: Fat 81% | Protein 8% | Carbs 11%
Prep time: 15 minutes | Cook time: 10 minutes | Serves 4

This is a delicious steakhouse-style spinach salad with a vinaigrette dressing that I have ever prepared. The salad looks complex but is very easy and quick to make.

2 bacon slices, chopped
1 cup spinach
1 spring onion, sliced

½ lettuce head, shredded
1 hard-boiled egg, chopped
1 avocado, sliced

VINAIGRETTE:
¼ teaspoon garlic powder
1 teaspoon Dijon mustard
1 tablespoon white wine vinegar

3 tablespoons olive oil
Salt, to taste

1. Cook bacon in a nonstick skillet over medium heat for 8 minutes or until cooked and crispy. Remove from heat to plate lined with a paper towel to drain and cool. Set aside.
2. In a medium mixing bowl, add spinach, onion, lettuce, and chopped egg. Stir to combine well.
3. Add all the vinaigrette ingredients in a separate bowl and whisk together until well mixed.
4. Pour the vinaigrette dressing over the spinach mixture and toss thoroughly until well coated.
5. Top with cooked bacon and avocado slices. Serve immediately.

STORAGE: Store in an airtight container in the fridge for 4 to 5 days.
REHEAT: Microwave the bacon, if needed, covered, until the desired temperature is reached or reheat the bacon in a frying pan or air fryer / instant pot, covered, on medium.
SERVE IT WITH: To make this a complete meal, serve it with sliced button mushrooms and fried chicken.
PER SERVING
calories: 273 | fat: 25.2g | total carbs: 8.2g | fiber: 4.8g | protein: 6.1g

SEARED RUMP STEAK SALAD

Macros: Fat 65% | Protein 27% | Carbs 8%
Prep time: 30 minutes | Cook time: 10 minutes | Serves 4

This hearty and satisfying rump steak salad is easy to prepare and is perfect for those warm summer evenings. It highly complements keto diet and goes well with keto bread to mop up the dressing and juices.

DRESSING:
2 teaspoons yellow mustard
1 tablespoon balsamic vinegar
2 tablespoons extra-virgin olive oil

Salt and freshly ground black pepper, to taste

8 ounces (227 g) rump steak
3 green onions, sliced
1 cup green beans, steamed and sliced

3 tomatoes, sliced
2 cups mixed salad greens
1 avocado, sliced

1. Make the dressing: Add yellow mustard, vinegar, oil, salt, and pepper in a medium mixing bowl. Mix until well combined. Set aside.
2. Preheat your grill pan to high heat.
3. Meanwhile, generously season the rump steak with salt and pepper in a separate bowl.
4. Sear the rump steak in the preheated pan for 4 minutes or until browned on each side.
5. Remove the steak from heat and let cool for 5 minutes. When cooled, thinly slice the steak.
6. Add green onions, green beans, tomatoes, and mixed salad greens to a salad bowl.
7. Pour the dressing into the salad bowl and toss until well mixed.
8. Top with avocado slices, then let rest for 5 minutes before serving.

STORAGE: Store in an airtight container in the fridge for 3 days.
REHEAT: Microwave the dressing and steak separately until just warm.
SERVE IT WITH: To make this a complete meal, you can serve it with grilled chicken thighs or pork chops.
PER SERVING
calories: 280 | fat: 20.2g | total carbs: 11.8g | fiber: 5.8g | protein: 18.6g

SUN-DRIED TOMATO AND FETA CHEESE SALAD

Macros: Fat 81% | Protein 15% | Carbs 4%
Prep time: 5 minutes | Cook time: 10 minutes | Serves 4

If you are looking for a fabulous salad to impress your guests or your family members, this sun-dried tomato and feta salad with bacon has got you covered. It is packed with nutrients and flavors.

5 ounces (142 g) bacon, chopped	4 basil leaves
5 sun-dried tomatoes in oil, sliced	2 teaspoons extra-virgin olive oil
1 cup feta cheese, crumbled	1 teaspoon balsamic vinegar
	Salt, to taste

1. Cook the bacon in a saucepan over medium heat for 4 minutes on each side, or until crisp and golden brown.
2. With a slotted spoon, transfer the bacon to a paper towel-lined plate to drain excess fat. Set aside.
3. Arrange the tomato slices in a salad bowl.
4. Scatter crumbled cheese and basil leaves over the tomatoes, then put the cooked bacon on top.
5. Drizzle the olive oil and vinegar over the mixture, then season with salt to taste.
6. Let the salad rest for 5 minutes to serve.

STORAGE: Store in an airtight container in the fridge for up to 3 days or in the freezer for up to 1 week.
REHEAT: Microwave the bacon, covered, until the desired temperature is reached or reheat the bacon in a frying pan or air fryer / instant pot, covered, on medium.
SERVE IT WITH: To make this a complete meal, you can serve it with grilled chicken thighs or pork chops.
PER SERVING
calories: 272 | fat: 24.7g | total carbs: 2.9g | fiber: 0.2g | protein: 10.0g

AVOCADO, CUCUMBER AND BACON SALAD

Macros: Fat 92% | Protein 1% | Carbs 6%
Prep time: 15 minutes | Cook time: 8 minutes | Serves 8

This is an extremely easy salad to prepare. It is healthy and tasty for bacon and avocado lovers. The freshness of cucumber combined with the taste of avocado will release the potential of the salad.

1 pound (454 g) bacon, chopped	pepper, to taste
1 cup cherry tomatoes, quartered	½ cup fresh cilantro, chopped
1 cucumber, diced	4 green onions, chopped
¼ cup rice vinegar	5 avocados, peeled, pitted and diced
Salt and freshly ground black	

1. In a nonstick skillet over medium-high heat, add bacon and cook for 8 minutes until browned, flipping occasionally. Drain the bacon on a paper towel and crumble into small pieces. Set aside on a plate.
2. In a medium bowl, add tomatoes, cucumber, rice vinegar, pepper and salt. Stir well to mix.
3. Fold in the bacon, cilantro, green onions, and avocado. Toss to combine well.
4. Divide the salad among serving plates, then serve.

STORAGE: Store in an airtight container in the refrigerator for up to 4 days.
SERVE IT WITH: To make this a complete meal, serve with buttered cod.
PER SERVING
calories: 721 | fat: 74.9g | total carbs: 12.8g | fiber: 9.1g | protein: 3.1g

CHICKEN SALAD WITH PARMESAN CHEESE

Macros: Fat 75% | Protein 19% | Carbs 6%
Prep time: 20 minutes | Cook time: 10 minutes | Serves 4

If you are looking forward to serving your family with a little different dinner meal, look no further. This chicken salad with Parmesan cheese is yummy, classic and the easiest chicken salad for hot summer days.

8 ounces (227 g) chicken thighs	1 head Romaine lettuce, torn
2 garlic cloves, minced	3 Parmesan cheese crisps
¼ cup lemon juice	½ cup Parmesan cheese, grated
2 tablespoons olive oil	

DRESSING:

2 tablespoons extra virgin olive oil	Salt and freshly ground black pepper, to taste
1 tablespoon lemon juice	

1. Place the chicken thighs, garlic, lemon juice, and olive oil in a sealable bag. Zip the bag and shake thoroughly until the chicken is well coated. Refrigerate the chicken for 1 hour to marinate.
2. Preheat your grill to medium-high heat.
3. Grill the marinated chicken for 4 minutes on each side. Remove from the grill and set aside.
4. Add the dressing ingredients in a mixing bowl and stir well to combine.
5. Arrange Romaine lettuce in a separate salad bowl and place cheese crisps on top. Pour the dressing over the lettuce and cheese crisps, then toss thoroughly until well coated.
6. Top the lettuce with the grilled chicken and grated cheese.
7. Let rest for 5 minutes and serve.

STORAGE: Store in an airtight container in the fridge for up to 2 days.
REHEAT: Microwave the chicken, covered, until the desired temperature is reached or reheat in a frying pan or air fryer / instant pot, covered, on medium.
SERVE IT WITH: To make this a complete meal, you can serve it with veggie skewers.
PER SERVING
calories: 328 | fat: 27.2g | total carbs: 8.8g | fiber: 3.4g | protein: 15.5g

BEEF, PORK, AND VEGETABLE SALAD WITH YOGHURT DRESSING

Macros: Fat 63% | Protein 31% | Carbs 6%
Prep time: 15 minutes | Cook time: 15 minutes | Serves 4

A salad that is packed with vegetables and protein is all you need to energize the body. The beef, crisp vegetables with a yogurt dressing, is just perfect for a warm summer evening.

1 pound (454 g) ground beef	2 tablespoons olive oil, divided
1 tablespoon fresh parsley, chopped	1 cup arugula
1 onion, grated	1 cucumber, sliced
1 whisked egg	1 cup cherry tomatoes, halved
½ teaspoon dried oregano	1½ tablespoons lemon juice
¼ cup pork rinds, crushed	1 cup plain Greek yogurt
1 garlic clove, minced	1 tablespoon fresh mint, chopped
Salt and freshly ground black pepper, to taste	2 tablespoons unsweetened almond milk

1. Add beef, parsley, onion, egg, oregano, pork rinds, garlic, salt, and pepper in a medium mixing bowl. Stir thoroughly until well mixed.
2. Use your hands to mold small balls with the mixture and place the balls on a clean work surface.
3. Heat half of the olive oil in a skillet over medium heat and cook the meatballs for 10 minutes on both sides or until well cooked. Remove the balls from heat and set aside on a plate lined with paper towels.
4. Add arugula, cucumber, and tomatoes in a salad bowl and mix well to combine. Stir in the remaining olive oil, lemon juice, salt, and pepper in the salad until well mixed.
5. In a separate bowl, whisk together Greek yogurt, mint, and almond milk until well mixed.
6. Pour the yogurt mixture over the salad and top with the meatballs. Serve immediately.

STORAGE: Store in an airtight container in the fridge for 3 days or freeze or up to a week.
REHEAT: Microwave the meat ball, if needed, covered, until the desired temperature is reached or reheat in a frying pan or air fryer / instant pot, covered, on medium.
SERVE IT WITH: To make this a complete meal, serve it with green soup, and pork and broccoli skewers.
PER SERVING
calories: 462 | fat: 32.3g | total carbs: 8.1g | fiber: 1.1g | protein: 35.9g

ICEBERG LETTUCE SALAD WITH BACON AND GORGONZOLA CHEESE

Macros: Fat 78% | Protein 16% | Carbs 6%
Prep time: 9 minutes | Cook time: 6 minutes | Serves 4

The crunch lettuce leaves with the crisp bacon and cheese make this a sensational salad that will leave your taste buds overjoyed and asking for more.

4 ounces (113 g) bacon
1 tablespoon white wine vinegar
3 tablespoons extra virgin olive oil
Salt and freshly ground black pepper, to taste
1 head iceberg lettuce, separated into leaves
1½ cups Gorgonzola cheese, crumbled
2 tablespoons pumpkin seeds

1. Place the bacon on a cutting board and chop it into bite-sized pieces.
2. Transfer the bacon to a nonstick skillet and cook over medium heat for 6 minutes or until the bacon is crispy and evenly browned.
3. Remove from heat and transfer to plate lined with paper towels to drain the excess fat and cool
4. Add vinegar, oil, salt, and pepper to a medium-sized mixing bowl. Using a spoon to stir thoroughly until the mixture is perfectly combined. Set aside.
5. Lay the lettuce leaves on a platter and top it with cooked bacon and cheese. Drizzle the vinegar mixture over the salad and toss until well coated.
6. Top the salad with pumpkin seeds, then let rest for 10 minutes to serve.

STORAGE: Store in an airtight container in the fridge for 2 days.
REHEAT: Microwave the bacon, if needed, covered, until the desired temperature is reached or reheat the bacon in a frying pan or air fryer / instant pot, covered, on medium.
SERVE IT WITH: To make this a complete meal, serve it with green and egg drip soup or veggie skewers.
PER SERVING
calories: 432 | fat: 37.9g | total carbs: 7.6g | fiber: 2.5g | protein: 17.2g

BRUSSELS SPROUTS CITRUS BACON DRESSING

Macros: Fat 71% | Protein 16% | Carbs 13%
Prep time: 10 minutes | Cook time: 10 minutes | Serves 4

The Brussels sprouts with a bacon dressing is a nutritious delicacy that is easy to make. The lemon and apple cider vinegar gives it a unique flavor fusion.

1¼ pounds (567 g) Brussels sprouts, cut into strips
1 tablespoon olive oil
4 ounces (113 g) sliced bacon
3 tablespoons erythritol
⅓ cup apple cider vinegar
1 lemon, juiced
Salt and freshly ground black pepper, to taste
Cayenne pepper, to taste

1. In a nonstick skillet over medium heat, heat the olive oil. Add bacon and cook for 8 minutes until it buckles and curls, flipping occasionally.
2. Add the erythritol, apple cider vinegar, and lemon juice, black pepper, salt and cayenne pepper. Stir well to mix. Reduce the heat to medium-high and cook for 1 minute more.
3. Transfer the bacon mixture to a large bowl and add the Brussels sprouts. Gently toss until well combined.
4. Let it rest for 5 minutes and serve.

STORAGE: Store in an airtight container in the refrigerator for up to 4 days.
SERVE IT WITH: To make this a complete meal, serve with beef steak and berry smoothie.
PER SERVING
calories: 248 | fat: 15.0g | total carbs: 13.9g | fiber: 5.4g | protein: 8.4g

EGG SALAD WITH MUSTARD DRESSING

Macros: Fat 76% | Protein 20% | Carbs 4%
Prep time: 6 minutes | Cook time: 10 minutes | Serves 4

It is an interesting egg salad. The fresh vibe from the lemon and the Dijon mustard tang makes it a must if you love salads.

2½ cups water
6 eggs

DRESSING:
1 teaspoon Dijon mustard
¼ cup green onions, chopped
½ juiced lemon
¼ cup keto-friendly mayonnaise
½ teaspoon yellow mustard
Salt and freshly ground black pepper, to taste

1. In a saucepan, pour the water and add eggs. Bring to a boil for about 10 minutes.
2. Transfer the eggs to a bowl of cold water. Peel and chop the eggs into ½-inch chunks. Set aside.
3. Make the dressing: In a medium bowl, add the Dijon mustard, green onions, lemon juice, mayonnaise, and yellow mustard and thoroughly mix.
4. Pour the dressing over the egg chunks and sprinkle with salt, and pepper. Gently toss to combine well and serve.

STORAGE: Store in an airtight container in the refrigerator for up to 4 days.
SERVE IT WITH: To make this a complete meal, serve it with seared salmon fillets.
PER SERVING
calories: 293 | fat: 24.9g | total carbs: 2.8g | fiber: 0.3g | protein: 13.8g

LETTUCE WRAPS WITH MACKEREL

Macros: Fat 44% | Protein 53% | Carbs 3%
Prep time: 10 minutes | Cook time: 20 minutes | Serves 4

It is quick and easy to make mackerel salad. Iit is also healthy and a great low- mercury alternative to tuna salad. The lettuce cups are perfect for light dinners and packed lunches.

2 mackerel fillets, sliced	1 tomato, deseeded and chopped
1 tablespoon olive oil	2 tablespoons keto-friendly
Salt and freshly ground black	mayonnaise
pepper, to taste	½ head lettuce, separated into
2 eggs	leaves

1. Heat your heavy skillet over medium-high heat until hot.
2. Meanwhile, place the fish on a cutting board. Rub the fillets with olive oil, then season with salt and pepper.
3. Place the seasoned fish to the hot skillet and cook for 4 minutes on each side. Remove the fish from heat and set aside to cool.
4. In a pot, add 2 cups of salted water. Add the eggs and boil them for 10 minutes. Once cooked, remove the eggs from the pot to a bowl with cold water.
5. Peel the eggs and slice them into small pieces. Put the eggs in a salad bowl.
6. Add the fish, tomatoes, and mayo to the salad bowl. Use a spoon to mix thoroughly until well combined.
7. Layer a lettuce leaf as a cup on a platter and fill with 2 tablespoons of fish salad. Repeat the process with remaining lettuce leaves and fish salad.
8. Serve immediately.

STORAGE: Store in an airtight container in the fridge for 2 days.
SERVE IT WITH: To make this a complete meal, serve it with grilled beef steak or chicken roast.
PER SERVING
calories: 368 | fat: 18.1g | total carbs: 3.6g | fiber: 1.2g | protein: 45.5g

GREEN CHICKEN SALAD

Macros: Fat 71% | Protein 24% | Carbs 5%
Prep time: 10 minutes | Cook time: 15 minutes | Serves 4

This is a great way to cheer up your desire to chicken salad. The minty and chicken flavors takes the salad to the next level, making it perfect to please your crowd during a family gathering.

2 cups water	2 tablespoons olive oil
2 eggs	2 tablespoons lemon juice
1 tablespoon avocado oil	1 teaspoon Dijon mustard
1 chicken breast, cubed	Salt and freshly ground black
2 cups steamed green beans	pepper, to taste
4 cups mixed salad greens	1 tablespoon mint, chopped
1 avocado, sliced	

1. In a pot, add 2 cups of water, and sprinkle with a dash of salt, then stir to combine. Add the eggs into the pot and let boil over medium heat for 10 minutes.
2. Once the eggs are cooked, transfer to a bowl with cold water. Peel the eggs under the water and cut into medium-sized chunks.
3. Heat the avocado oil in a heavy skillet over medium heat and cook the chicken breast for 4 minutes. Remove from the heat and let cool, then slice.
4. Divide the steamed green beans and mixed salad greens between two salad bowls, then equally add the eggs, chicken, and avocado in both bowls.

5. In a separate bowl, add olive oil, lemon juice, and Dijon mustard, salt, and pepper, then whisk until well mixed.
6. Drizzle the mustard mixture over the salad in the two salad bowls.
7. Top with chopped mint, then let rest for 5 minutes to serve.

STORAGE: Store in an airtight container in the fridge for up to 3 days.
REHEAT: Microwave the chicken, if needed, covered, until the desired temperature is reached or reheat in a frying pan or air fryer / instant pot, covered, on medium.
SERVE IT WITH: To make this a complete meal, serve it with tomato and egg drip soup or veggie skewers.
PER SERVING
calories: 373 | fat: 29.6g | total carbs: 10.1g | fiber: 5.9g | protein: 22.5g

BACON, SMOKED SALMON AND POACHED EGG SALAD

Macros: Fat 81% | Protein 14% | Carbs 5%
Prep time: 10 minutes | Cook time: 15 minutes | Serves 4

Smoked salmon and poached egg make a stunning combination that can not only be served for lunch but also for a hearty filling breakfast.

DRESSING:

1 tablespoon lemon juice	1 teaspoon Tabasco sauce
½ cup mayonnaise, keto-friendly	½ teaspoon garlic purée
4 eggs	½ cup smoked salmon, sliced
4 slices bacon	Salt and freshly ground black
1 head Romaine lettuce, shredded	pepper, to taste

1. Add the dressing ingredients into a mixing bowl. Stir to combine well and set aside.
2. In a large saucepan, pour the water and sprinkle with a dash of salt, then bring to a boil. One at a time, crack the eggs into the saucepan and cook for 3 minutes. Transfer the poached eggs to a plate and set aside.
3. Cook the bacon slices in a skillet over medium heat for 8 minutes until crispy and well browned on both sides. Transfer to a separate plate lined with a paper towel and let drain and cool, then chop into bite-sized pieces.
4. Add the lettuce, salmon, cooked bacon, and dressing to a large salad bowl. Sprinkle with salt and black pepper, then toss until well combined.
5. Divide the salad among 4 plates and top each plate with one poached egg.
6. Serve immediately or refrigerate to chill.

STORAGE: Store in an airtight container in the fridge for 2 days.
REHEAT: Microwave the bacon and salmon, if needed, covered, until the desired temperature is reached or reheat the bacon in a frying pan or air fryer / instant pot, covered, on medium.
SERVE IT WITH: To make this a complete meal, serve it with keto toast slices for a filling sandwich.
PER SERVING
calories: 489 | fat: 44.3g | total carbs: 6.9g | fiber: 3.3g | protein: 17.3g

BRUSSEL SPROUTS AND SPINACH SALAD

Macros: Fat 77% | Protein 6% | Carbs 17%
Prep time: 10 minutes | Cook time: 25 minutes | Serves 4

Brussels sprouts, spinach, and hazelnuts combine to make a delicious salad that even the kids will enjoy eating. The combination of flavors and colors make this salad a perfect side dish for all summer.

1 pound (454 g) Brussels sprouts
4 tablespoons extra virgin olive oil, divided
Salt and freshly ground black pepper, to taste

½ cup hazelnuts
1 cup baby spinach
1 tablespoon Dijon mustard
1 tablespoon balsamic vinegar

1. Preheat your oven to 400°F (205°C). Line a baking pan with parchment paper and set aside.
2. Add Brussels sprouts in a mixing bowl, then drizzle with 2 tablespoons of olive oil and season with salt and pepper. Mix until the Brussels sprouts are well coated.
3. Spread the Brussels sprouts on the prepared baking pan and bake in the preheated oven for 20 minutes or until they are tender.
4. Meanwhile, toast hazelnuts in a heavy pan over medium heat for 2 minutes. Remove from heat and let cool, then chop into bite-sized pieces.
5. Once the Brussels sprouts are cooked, transfer them to a salad bowl. Add chopped hazelnuts, spinach, and Dijon mustard. Mix thoroughly until well combined.
6. In a separate bowl, add vinegar and remaining olive oil and mix thoroughly. Pour the mixture over the salad and gently toss to combine.
7. Let rest for 5 minutes and serve.

STORAGE: Store in an airtight container in the fridge for 5 days.
SERVE IT WITH: To make this a complete meal, serve it with grilled beef steak or chicken roast.
PER SERVING
calories: 258 | fat: 23.0g | total carbs: 11.7g | fiber: 4.7g | protein: 5.4g

EASY LUNCH SALAD

Macros: Fat 64% | Protein 32% | Carbs 4%
Prep time: 3 hours | Cook time: 0 minutes | Serves 4

The special lunch salad is made up of hard-boiled eggs, salmon, and vegetables. You do not have to limit the number of vegetables as long as they are keto-friendly. It is the best option as it is quick to prepare.

¾ cup avocado mayonnaise
4 hard-boiled eggs, peeled and cubed
6 ounces (170 g) cooked salmon, chopped

2 celery stalks, chopped
½ yellow onion, chopped
1 tablespoon chopped fresh dill
Salt and freshly ground black pepper, to taste

1. In a mixing bowl, put the avocado mayonnaise, boiled eggs, cooked salmon, celery stalks, dill, yellow onion, salt, and black pepper. Mix well until combined evenly.
2. Cover the bowl with plastic wrap and chill in the fridge for 3 hours.
3. Remove from the fridge and serve chilled.

STORAGE: Store in an airtight container in the fridge for up to 3 days.
SERVE IT WITH: To make this a complete meal, serve it with fresh vegetables like cherry tomatoes or cucumbers.
PER SERVING
calories: 263 | fat: 18.7g | total carbs: 5.4g | fiber: 2.6g | protein: 20.8g

CRABMEAT AND CELERY SALAD

Macros: Fat 86% | Protein 11% | Carbs 3%
Prep time: 2 hours | Cook time: 0 minutes | Serves 6

It is a healthy seafood salad delicacy. You can have the salad alone or with company. It has an amazing fusion of flavors. And the fragrance of the celery will also give you a freshness eating enjoyment.

½ cup green bell pepper, diced
½ cup red onion, diced

1 pound (454 g) flaked crab meat
½ cup celery, diced

DRESSING:
1½ cups keto-friendly mayonnaise
¼ cup sour cream
2 tablespoons lemon juice

⅔ cup Italian salad dressing
½ teaspoon oregano, dried
Salt and freshly ground black pepper, to taste

1. In a large bowl, add the diced green peppers, onions, crab meat, and celery and mix well. Set aside.
2. Make the dressing: In a separate bowl, add mayonnaise, sour cream, lemon juice, salad dressing, oregano, pepper and salt.
3. Pour the dressing into the bowl of crab mixture and gently toss to mix.
4. Cover the bowl with plastic wrap and let sit for 2 hours in the fridge.
5. Divide the salad among six plates and serve.

STORAGE: Store in an airtight container in the refrigerator for up to no more than 5 days.
SERVE IT WITH: To make this a complete meal, serve with creamy chicken.
PER SERVING
calories: 546 | fat: 53.2g | total carbs: 4.5g | fiber: 0.5g | protein: 14.3g

SUMPTUOUS EGG SALAD

Macros: Fat 80% | Protein 18% | Carbs 2%
Prep time: 6 minutes | Cook time: 20 minutes | Serves 4

The salad is easy to make and requires very few ingredients. It has a great taste and can serve your company as well. And this salad can not only be served as a salad but also served as a filling for an almond-flour-made sandwich bread.

3 cups water
8 eggs
1 teaspoon yellow mustard
¼ cup green onion, chopped

½ cup keto-friendly mayonnaise
¼ teaspoon paprika
Salt and freshly ground black pepper, to taste

1. In a saucepan, pour water and add eggs, then bring to a boil. Allow the eggs to sit in the hot water for 12 minutes.
2. Transfer the eggs to a bowl of cold water. Peel and chop the eggs into chunks.
3. In a separate bowl, add the chopped eggs. Stir in the mustard, green onion and mayonnaise, and toss to combine well.
4. Add the paprika, pepper and salt and stir well. Serve immediately.

STORAGE: Store in an airtight container in the refrigerator for up to 4 days.
SERVE IT WITH: To make this a complete meal, serve it between gluten-free almond bread or coconut crackers.
PER SERVING
calories: 449 | fat: 39.9g | total carbs: 2.9g | fiber: 0.3g | protein: 18.4g

CHICKEN, CRANBERRY, AND PECAN SALAD

Macros: Fat 71% | Protein 21% | Carbs 8%
Prep time: 1 hour 10 minutes | Cook time: 0 minutes | Serves 12

It is a special salad made uniquely with the combination of ingredients that brings out a special fusion of flavor. It is a quick fix and a favorite among many people. The pecans and cranberry will send you the taste that comes from a different field of food.

1 teaspoon paprika
1 cup keto-friendly mayonnaise
1 teaspoon seasoning salt
1 cup celery, chopped
1½ cups dried cranberries
½ cup green bell pepper, minced

1 cup chopped pecans
2 chopped green onions
4 cups cooked chicken meat, cubed
Ground black pepper, to taste

1. In a medium bowl, add paprika, mayonnaise and seasoned salt. Stir well to mix.
2. Add the celery, dried cranberries, bell pepper, pecans and onion and stir well to combine. Add chicken cubes. Sprinkle with black pepper.
3. Let it rest in the refrigerator for 1 hour before serving.

STORAGE: Store in an airtight container in the refrigerator for up to 5 days.
SERVE IT WITH: To make this a complete meal, serve with beef and pork stuffed tomatoes.
PER SERVING
calories: 274 | fat: 21.7g | total carbs: 7.5g | fiber: 2.1g | protein: 14.2g

CREAMED OMEGA-3 SALAD

Macros: Fat 53% | Protein 43% | Carbs 4%
Prep time: 10 minutes | Cook time: 10 minutes | Serves 2

Filled with nutritional value, prepare creamed Omega-3 salad especially for the babies during lunch hours. The fresh lime juice gives the salad a special flavor and unique taste.

1 tablespoon olive oil
½ pound (227 g) skinless salmon fillet, cut into 4 pieces
Salt and freshly ground black pepper, to taste
¼ zucchini, cut into small cubes

¼ tablespoon fresh lime juice
4 tablespoons sour cream
¼ teaspoon jalapeño pepper, deseeded and chopped finely
¼ tablespoon fresh dill, chopped

1. Heat the olive oil in the skillet over medium heat, then add the salmon and cook for 5 minutes per side.
2. Add the black pepper and salt, then stir well. Transfer to a serving bowl and set aside.
3. In a large bowl, mix together the zucchini cubes, lime juice, sour cream, jalapeño pepper, and dill. Pour them into the bowl of cooked salmon and toss to combine, then serve.

STORAGE: Store in an airtight container in the fridge for up to 4 days.
REHEAT: Microwave the salmon, covered, until the desired temperature is reached or reheat in a frying pan or air fryer / instant pot, covered, on medium.
PER SERVING
calories: 240 | fat: 14.3g | total carbs: 2.6g | fiber: 0.3g | protein: 24.3g

RANCH CHICKEN AND BACON SALAD

Macros: Fat 86% | Protein 13% | Carbs 1%
Prep time: 10 minutes | Cook time: 10 minutes | Serves 6

A salad made up of chicken can be taken for lunch or dinner. The combination of bacon, chicken, and vegetables equals to a tasty and nutritious meal. You can choose to garnish the salad with freshly chopped parsley or serve without the parsley.

5 slices bacon
12 ounces (340 g) cubed cooked chicken
½ chopped stalk celery
⅓ cup keto-friendly mayonnaise

3 tablespoons ranch dressing
Salt and freshly ground pepper, to taste
6 butterhead lettuce leaves, for serving

1. Fry the bacon in a skillet over medium heat for 8 minutes until crispy, then transfer to a plate lined with paper towels. When cool enough to handle, crumble the bacon into smaller pieces with a spatula.
2. In a medium bowl, put the cooked chicken. Add the celery, mayonnaise, ranch dressing, and bacon pieces. Using a fork to stir the mixture until well combined. Sprinkle the salt and pepper to season.
3. Evenly divide the salad on the lettuce leaves and serve immediately.

STORAGE: Store in separate airtight containers in the fridge for up to 3 days.
SERVE IT WITH: To make this a complete meal, you can serve it with broccoli soup.
PER SERVING
calories: 469 | fat: 45.2g | total carbs: 0.8g | fiber: 0.1g | protein: 14.4g

SIMPLE CAULIFLOWER SALAD

Macros: Fat 75% | Protein 11% | Carbs 15%
Prep time: 15 minutes | Cook time: 5 minutes | Serves 2

Enjoy the tasty cauliflower salad made with a variety of other vegetables. The grated Parmesan cheese gives the meal a unique taste that will leave you wanting more. If you love bacon, you can enjoy the salad with some bacon strips.

½ cup chopped cauliflower
⅛ cup chopped fresh basil
¾ tablespoon chopped kalamata olives
½ minced garlic clove
¾ tablespoon chopped sun-dried tomatoes

⅛ cup grated Cheddar cheese
¾ tablespoon balsamic vinegar
¾ tablespoon extra-virgin olive oil
Salt and freshly ground black pepper, to taste

1. Microwave the chopped cauliflower for 5 minutes or until just tender.
2. Meanwhile, in a mixing bowl, combine the basil, olives, garlic, tomatoes, and cheese. Add the cooked cauliflower and toss well.
3. In another bowl, whisk together the vinegar and olive oil. Pour the mixture over the cauliflower mixture. Sprinkle with salt and pepper and stir well before serving.

STORAGE: Store in separate airtight containers in the fridge for up to 3 days.
SERVE IT WITH: To make this a complete meal, serve the cauliflower salad with crispy bacon slices.
PER SERVING
calories: 101 | fat: 8.4g | total carbs: 4.0g | fiber: 1.0g | protein: 3.0g

COLORFUL CRAB CEVICHE APPETIZER

Macros: Fat 37% | Protein 47% | Carbs 16%
Prep time: 40 minutes | Cook time: 0 minutes | Serves 4

Colorful crab ceviche appetizer is the best side meal when it comes to maintaining your keto routine. What's better than a fat-free, protein full meal? You can have it on any meal in the day. Best Latino meal!

1 (8-ounce / 227-g) package crab meat flakes	2 large tomatoes, evenly chopped
1 tablespoon olive oil	1 red onion, finely chopped into slices
½ bundle cilantro, finely chopped	¼ cup lemon juice
3 Serrano peppers, finely cut into small slices	Salt and freshly ground black pepper, to taste

1. In a bowl, place the crab meat. Pour the olive oil slowly into the bowl of crab meat until well coated, then stir in the cilantro, Serrano peppers, tomato, and onion. Pour the lemon juice over the mixture and toss well.
2. Sprinkle with pepper and salt, then refrigerate for an hour before serving.

STORAGE: This appetizer can be stored in the fridge for no more than 2 days.
SERVE IT WITH: To make this a complete meal, serve it with roasted Brussels sprouts.
PER SERVING
calories: 117 | fat: 4.8g | total carbs: 9.3g | fiber: 4.5g | protein: 13.6g

VEGGIES AND CALAMARI SALAD

Macros: Fat 54% | Protein 43% | Carbs 3%
Prep time: 10 minutes | Cook time: 7 minutes | Serves 4

Vegetable and calamari salad tastes perfect for lunch. If you have a group of friends visiting, this is a good recipe to surprise them with. Flavors from the lemon zest and lemon juice make the salad more delicious.

SALAD:

12 ounces (340 g) uncooked calamari rings	and halved
1½ cups grape halved tomatoes	½ packed cup fresh parsley, chopped
½ cup kalamata olives, pitted	¼ cup sliced green onions

DRESSING:

1 tablespoon red wine vinegar	½ grated lemon zest
½ cup extra-virgin olive oil	¼ teaspoon black pepper
2 small minced garlic cloves	¼ teaspoon gray sea salt
½ juiced lemon	

1. Put the calamari in a steamer and steam for 7 minutes, then put in the freezer to cool for about 2 minutes.
2. In the meantime, start the dressing by putting all the dressing ingredients in a small bowl, then mix thoroughly and set aside.
3. Once the calamari has cooled, place it in a large bowl along with the grape tomatoes, olives, parsley, and green onions. Pour in the dressing and toss to coat well.
4. Evenly divide the salad among four serving bowls and serve.

STORAGE: Store in an airtight container in the fridge for up to 3 days.
SERVE IT WITH: To make this a complete meal, you can serve it with rich clam chowder.
PER SERVING
calories: 508 | fat: 30g | total carbs: 4.4g | fiber: 1.3g | protein: 55.1g

EASY MEDITERRANEAN SALAD

Macros: Fat 79% | Protein 10% | Carbs 11%
Prep time: 15 minutes | Cook time: 0 minutes | Serves 2

Prepare the easy Mediterranean salad for a busy afternoon. Filled with flavors from different vegetables, you will have a nutritious lunch filled with oregano flavors. You can serve the salad immediately or chill before serving.

1 shallot, sliced	Salt and freshly ground black pepper, to taste
½ cucumber, peeled and sliced	3 ounces (85 g) feta cheese, crumbled
2 ripe firm tomatoes, sliced	
½ green peppers, sliced	2 tablespoons extra-virgin olive oil
8 kalamata olives, pitted and sliced	
½ teaspoon dried oregano	

1. In a large mixing bowl, put the shallots, cucumbers, tomatoes, green peppers, and olives. Toss to mix evenly.
2. Add the oregano, black pepper, and salt. Stir well.
3. Divide the salad equally among two serving bowls, then sprinkle the crumbled cheese on top.
4. Pour 1 tablespoon of olive oil into each salad bowl and mix well, then serve.

STORAGE: Store in an airtight container in the fridge for up to 3 days.
SERVE IT WITH: To make this a complete meal, serve it with roasted beef or baked chicken breasts.

calories: 272 | fat: 24.3g | total carbs: 7.9g | fiber: 1.8g | protein: 7.1g

TASTY AVOCADO SHRIMP SALAD

Macros: Fat 86% | Protein 10% | Carbs 4%
Prep time: 8 minutes | Cook time: 0 minutes | Serves 8

Avocado and lemon shrimp salad is a perfect idea for a quick lunch. Are you that tired? Are you hungry? Prepare this quick recipe and within a few minutes, you will feel satisfied and nourished at the same time.

8 ounces (227 g) cooked shrimp, cut in half lengthwise
1 small cucumber, peeled and diced

DRESSING:

1 tablespoon freshly squeezed lemon juice	1 small and ripe avocado, roughly chopped
2 tablespoons fresh cilantro, chopped	1 tablespoon extra-virgin olive oil
2 tablespoons plain Greek yogurt	Lemon slices, for garnish

1. Divide the cooked shrimp into four serving bowls, then put the diced cucumber on top
2. Make the dressing: Blend the lemon juice, cilantro, Greek yogurt, avocado, and olive oil in a blender until smooth.
3. Pour the smooth dressing over the salads in the serving bowls, then top each with a slice of lemon for garnish.

STORAGE: Store in separate airtight containers in the fridge for up to 3 days.
PER SERVING
calories: 317 | fat: 31.0g | total carbs: 3.4g | fiber 1.9g | protein: 8.3g

GREEN SALAD WITH BAKED HALIBUT

Macros: Fat 64% | Protein 28% | Carbs 8%
Prep time: 10 minutes | Cook time: 10 minutes | Serves 12

Are you holding a meeting with friends and relatives? Here is a quick idea. Prepare baked halibut with green salad and enjoy together. To enjoy the salad, refrigerate to chill before serving.

6 cups baby spinach	1 cup chopped green onions
Black pepper, to taste	2 tablespoons hot pepper sauce
2 cucumbers, diced	1 tablespoon butter, softened
¼ teaspoon salt	3 tablespoons mayonnaise
2 cups chopped Romaine lettuce	2 tablespoons Parmesan cheese
1 tablespoon balsamic vinegar	2 pounds (907 g) skinless
2 tablespoons olive oil, divided	halibut fillet
4 tablespoons lemon juice	

1. Start the salad by mixing the spinach, pepper, cucumbers, salt, lettuce, vinegar, and 1 tablespoon olive oil in a large bowl. Toss to mix evenly, then chill until ready to serve.
2. Preheat the oven broiler and lightly grease a baking tray with remaining olive oil. Set aside.
3. In another bowl, mix the lemon juice, salt, green onions, hot pepper sauce, butter, mayonnaise, and Parmesan cheese. Stir to combine well.
4. Arrange the halibut fillet on the prepared baking tray. Broil until the fish flakes easily when tested with a fork, for about 8 minutes.
5. Remove from the oven to a plate and spread the cheese mixture on top.
6. Broil for an additional 2 minutes. Let cool for about 5 minutes and serve with the chilled salad.

STORAGE: Store in separate airtight containers in the fridge for up to 3 days.
REHEAT: Microwave, covered, until the desired temperature is reached.
PER SERVING
calories: 402 | fat: 28.8g | total carbs: 6.4g | fiber: 9.4g | protein: 28.4g

SHRIMP SALAD WITH EGG AND MAYONNAISE

Macros: Fat 56% | Protein 42% | Carbs 2%
Prep time: 15 minutes | Cook time:0 minutes | Serves 4

Is it hot outside and wants something cool and light? Here's the summer preferable salad "Shrimp Salad with Egg and Mayonnaise". A simple, fast, and protein-rich salad! Fantastic summer light meal!

1 pound (454 g) cooked shrimp, peeled and chopped	friendly
4 cooked eggs, chopped	1 teaspoon Dijon mustard
4 tablespoons mayonnaise, keto-	1 sprig fresh dill, chopped
	4 leaves lettuce

1. In a medium bowl, mix together the shrimp, eggs, mayonnaise, Dijon mustard, and fresh dill. Then, spoon the mixture over lettuce leaves and serve.

SERVE IT WITH: To add more flavors to this meal, you can serve the shrimp salad over some Romaine lettuce.
PER SERVING
calories: 346 | fat: 21.4g | total carbs: 2.1g | fiber: 0.4g | protein: 36.7g

SALMON AND ALMOND SALAD

Macros: Fat 68% | Protein 27% | Carbs 5%
Prep time: 5 minutes | Cook time: 10 minutes | Serves 2

Prepare fish and almond salad for dinner to enjoy with family. The salad has vital nutrients, including vitamins from the vegetables and fat from the fish. Encourage your children to take fish and almond salad to have a good health.

¼ cup tamari	6 halved cherry tomatoes
8 ounces (227 g) salmon	1 tablespoon olive oil
½ sliced red bell pepper	2 cups salad greens
¼ teaspoon salt	1 tablespoon avocado oil
4 sliced radishes	1 tablespoon toasted almonds,
½ tablespoon lemon juice	chopped

1. In a large bowl, pour the tamari. Add the salmon and toss to coat evenly.
2. Cover the bowl with plastic wrap, then let the fish marinate for 1 hour.
3. In another bowl, mix together the bell peppers, salt, radishes, lemon juice, tomatoes, olive oil, and salad greens. Divide the mixture between two serving plates and set aside.
4. In a large skillet, melt the avocado oil over medium-high heat. Add the salmon and cook until browned evenly, for 4 minutes per side.
5. Remove from the heat to a plate and slice into pieces.
6. Top each plate evenly with salmon pieces and almonds, then serve.

STORAGE: Store in separate airtight containers in the fridge for up to 3 days.
REHEAT: Microwave the fish, covered, until the desired temperature is reached.
SERVE IT WITH: To make this a complete meal, serve it with sautéed spinach or mushrooms.
PER SERVING
calories: 501 | fat: 38.0g | total carbs: 8.0g | fiber: 3.0g | protein: 34.0g

CAPRESE SALAD

Macros: Fat 72% | Protein 25% | Carbs 3%
Prep time: 15 minutes | Cook time: 0 minutes | Serves 6

If you are a fan of salads as a side dish for your dinner, Caprese salad will be the greatest one as you do not need much effort or time to prepare it. With help from your children, you can make this splendid meal. In simple and easy steps, we will make it together!

1 pound (454 g) Mozzarella cheese, sliced into ¼ inch thick	3 tablespoons extra virgin olive oil
4 large ripe tomatoes, cut into ¼-inch-thick slices	Sea salt and freshly ground black pepper, to taste
⅓ cup fresh basil leaves	

1. Combine the sliced Mozzarella cheese, tomato slices, and basil leaves with a pinch of olive oil, sea salt, and pepper in a large bowl.
2. Leave the bowl in the refrigerator to chill for 20 minutes before serving.

STORAGE: Store in an airtight container in the fridge for up to 3 to 5 days.
SERVE IT WITH: To make this a complete meal, serve it chilled with pecan-crusted chicken nuggets.
PER SERVING
calories: 288 | fat: 23.8g | total carbs: 2.1g | fiber: 0.1g | protein: 16.9g

BREADED CHICKEN STRIPS AND SPINACH SALAD

Macros: Fat 73% | Protein 21% | Carbs 6%
Prep time: 15 minutes | Cook time: 25 minutes | Serves 4

Made with a variety of flavors, you will enjoy the breaded chicken strips with fresh spinach salad for lunch or dinner. The meal has extra taste from coconut flavors that will leave you craving for more.

3 tablespoons refined avocado oil, for greasing the baking sheet

CHICKEN:

1 cup unsweetened shredded coconut	Cajun seasoning
1 tablespoon plus 1 teaspoon	1½ pounds (680 g) boneless, skinless chicken thighs

SALAD:

4 cups fresh spinach	½ cup roughly chopped celery
½ cup sliced green onions	1 cup ranch dressing

1. Start by preheating the oven to 375℉ (190℃). Grease a baking sheet with the avocado oil generously and set aside.
2. Put the shredded coconut in a blender and pulse until grounded coarsely, but not to a powder.
3. In a medium bowl, put the shredded coconut and Cajun seasoning, then stir to mix thoroughly.
4. Using a mallet, pound the chicken thighs until it is ¼-inch thickness. Add the chicken to the bowl of coconut and Cajun seasoning. Toss until the chicken is coated well.
5. Arrange the chicken thighs on the greased baking sheet. Bake in the preheated oven for about 25 minutes, or until cooked through.
6. Meantime, make the salad: divide the spinach equally among four serving plates.
7. Sprinkle the green onions and celery on top.
8. Transfer the chicken to plates before slicing. Serve it with ranch dressing in a small bowl or ramekin on the side.

STORAGE: Store in a separate airtight container in the fridge for up to 3 days.
REHEAT: Microwave the chicken, covered, until the desired temperature is reached or put the chicken in a casserole dish then reheat in a preheated oven at 300℉ (150℃) until warmed through for 15 minutes.
PER SERVING
calories: 705 | fat: 56.7g | total carbs: 11.2g | fiber: 6.4g | protein: 37.6g

KETO LEMON DRESSING, WALNUTS AND ZUCCHINI SALAD

Macros: Fat 87% | Protein 4% | Carbs 9%
Prep time: 15 minutes | Cook time: 10 minutes | Serves 4

The salad is nutritious and low in carbohydrates. It is very easy to make and can serve with your friends and families. The walnuts contain abundant fat and is a very nice keto-friendly recipe, and it can be also eaten as the snack during the leisure time.

DRESSING:

2 teaspoons lemon juice	¾ cup keto-friendly mayonnaise
2 tablespoons olive oil	¼ teaspoon chili powder
1 finely minced garlic clove	½ teaspoon salt

SALAD:

4 ounces (113 g) arugula lettuce	into ½-inch pieces
1 head Romaine lettuce	Salt and freshly ground black pepper, to taste
¼ cup fresh chives, finely chopped	3½ ounces (99 g) toasted walnuts, chopped
1 tablespoon olive oil	
2 zucchinis, deseeded and cut	

1. Make the dressing: In a bowl, add lemon juice, olive oil, garlic, mayonnaise, chili powder and salt. Whisk together to mix and set aside.
2. Make the salad: In a large bowl, add arugula, Romaine, and chives and mix well. Set aside.
3. In a frying pan, add olive oil and heat over medium heat. Add zucchinis, pepper and salt and sauté for 5 minutes or until the zucchinis are tender but still firm.
4. Transfer the zucchinis to the salad bowl, then add the toasted walnuts and pour over the dressing. Gently toss until fully combined. Serve immediately or refrigerate to chill.

STORAGE: Store in an airtight container in the refrigerator for up to 5 days.
SERVE IT WITH: To make this a complete meal, serve with grilled beef or shrimp skewers.
PER SERVING
calories: 587 | fat: 58.2g | total carbs: 13.9g | fiber: 6.7g | protein: 8.2g

CRISPY ALMONDS WITH BRUSSELS SPROUT SALAD

Macros: Fat 84% | Protein 9% | Carbs 7%
Prep time: 12 minutes | Cook time: 10 minutes | Serves 4

It is a simple and fresh salad that is easy to prepare. The crispy and lemon touch brought about by the almonds and lemon makes it special. It is also very nutritious.

1 tablespoon coconut oil	½ teaspoon fennel seeds
1 teaspoon chili paste	1 ounce (28 g) sunflower seeds
2 ounces (57 g) almonds	1 pinch salt
1 ounce (28 g) pumpkin seeds	

SALAD:

1 pound (454 g) Brussels sprouts, shredded	Salt and freshly ground black pepper, to taste
1 lemon, juice and zest	½ cup spicy almond and seed mix
½ cup olive oil	

1. In a frying pan, add oil and heat. Add chili, almond, pumpkin seeds, fennel seeds, and sunflower seeds into the oil and stir to mix.
2. Add salt and sauté for 2 minutes. Set aside until ready to serve.
3. Make the salad: Shred the Brussels sprouts in a food processor, then put in a bowl.
4. Combine the lemon juice and zest, olive oil, pepper and salt in a separate bowl, then pour the mixture over the Brussels sprouts. Toss to combine well and allow to marinate in the fridge for about 10 minutes.
5. On a serving plate, combine the salad and almond and seeds mixture before serving.

STORAGE: Store in an airtight container in the refrigerator for up to 4 days.
SERVE IT WITH: To make this a complete meal, serve with roasted salmon.
PER SERVING
calories: 484 | fat: 44.9g | total carbs: 16.8g | fiber: 7.9g | protein: 11.1g

FETA CHEESE AND CUCUMBER SALAD

Macros: Fat 80% | Protein 9% | Carbs 11%
Prep time: 10 minutes | Cook time: 0 minutes | Serves 5

Share this amazing feta cheese and cucumber salad with your family, especially on a sunny afternoon. To enjoy the salad, chill before serving, although you can take the salad immediately after preparation.

SALAD:

2 medium cucumbers	crumbled
½ cup thinly sliced red onions	Salt and freshly ground black
4 ounces (113 g) feta cheese,	pepper, to taste

DRESSING:

¼ cup extra-virgin olive oil	½ teaspoon dried ground
1 tablespoon Swerve	oregano
1 tablespoon red wine vinegar	

1. Peel the cucumbers to your preference. On your cutting board, cut them in half lengthwise and then slice.
2. Put the sliced cucumbers in a large bowl, then add the onions and toss fully. Sprinkle with the feta cheese and combine well. Set aside.
3. Meanwhile, start the dressing by putting all the ingredients for dressing in another bowl, then whisk thoroughly to incorporate.
4. Pour the dressing into the bowl of cucumber salad and toss well. Season as desired with salt and pepper before serving.

STORAGE: Store in a separate airtight container in the fridge for up to 3 days.
SERVE IT WITH: To make this a complete meal, you can serve it with grilled chicken or fish fillets.
PER SERVING
calories: 177 | fat: 15.8g | total carbs: 5.7g | fiber: 0.8g | protein: 3.8g

DELICIOUS STEAK SALAD

Macros: Fat 42% | Protein 25% | Carbs 33%
Prep time: 15 minutes | Cook time: 15 minutes | Serves 4

Nothing tastes better than a well-marinated steak with a tasty salad. Prepare this meal for a fulfilled lunch or dinner and enjoy with your family.

4 sirloin steaks, trimmed	black pepper
3 tablespoons extra virgin olive	2 cups cherry tomatoes
oil, divided	1 bunch arugula
2 tablespoons freshly cracked	4 cups green salad

1. Rub the steaks with 2 tablespoons olive oil. On a plate, put the black pepper, then press the steaks into the pepper until coated evenly.
2. Preheat the barbecue grill to medium-high heat, then grill the steaks until cooked through, about 5 minutes per side. Put the cooked steaks in a bowl and keep aside.
3. Meanwhile, brush the tomatoes with remaining oil, then grill them for 5 minutes until they are tender, turning occasionally.
4. Divide the arugula among four serving plates and top with grilled steaks and tomatoes. Serve them alongside the green salad.

STORAGE: Store in separate airtight containers in the fridge for up to 3 days.
REHEAT: Microwave the steak, covered, until the desired temperature is reached.
PER SERVING
calories: 238 | fat: 11.2g | total carbs: 10.8g | fiber: 8.2g | protein: 14.9g

SALMON ASPARAGUS PECAN SALAD

Macros: Fat 73% | Protein 15% | Carbs 13%
Prep time: 15 minutes | Cook time: 10 minutes | Serves 8

It's more than a salad dish! Salmon Asparagus and Smoked Salad is the best way to start your lunch meal. It also can be a complete meal on dinner in light of your keto routine. Light and tasty! Highly recommended for keto!

1 pound (454 g) fresh asparagus,	rinsed and torn
trimmed and cut into 1-inch	2 tablespoons lemon juice
pieces	¼ cup olive oil
½ cup pecans, chopped into	1 teaspoon Dijon mustard
pieces	¼ teaspoon freshly ground
4 ounces (113 g) smoked salmon,	black pepper
cut into 1-inch chunks	½ teaspoon salt
2 heads red leaf lettuce, finely	

1. Put the asparagus into a pot of salted water and bring to a boil for 5 minutes until tender.
2. Remove from the heat and drain on a paper towel. Set aside on a plate.
3. In a skillet over medium-high heat, place the pecans and cook for 5 minutes, stirring frequently, until the pecans are lightly toasted.
4. In a medium bowl, toss the salmon chunks with toasted pecans, asparagus, and red leaf lettuce.
5. In another bowl, whisk together the lemon juice, olive oil, Dijon mustard, pepper, and salt. Pour them over the salad and stir to combine, then serve.

STORAGE: Store in a sealed airtight container in the fridge for up to 2 days.
SERVE IT WITH: To make this a complete meal, serve it with shrimp skewers or scallop chowder.
PER SERVING
calories: 149 | fat: 12.5g | total carbs: 5.2g | fiber: 2.5g | protein: 6.0g

CRAB SALAD

Macros: Fat 55% | Protein 42% | Carbs 3%
Prep time: 15 minutes | Cook time: 0 minutes | Serves 4

Love seafood and love to try the different seafood dishes? The Crab Salad is your choice for a simple but magically delicious meal. If you do not love to wait like me this salad would be just perfect.

2 pounds (907 g) crab meat	4 teaspoons stevia
2½ cups celery, chopped finely	½ tablespoon freshly ground
½ cup keto-friendly mayonnaise	black pepper
2 teaspoons celery seed	1 teaspoon Old Bay Seasoning
Paprika, to taste	2 teaspoons dried parsley

1. Mix the crab meat, chopped celery, mayonnaise, celery seed, paprika, stevia, pepper, Old Bay Seasoning and parsley in a large bowl. Stir with a fork to combine well.
2. Serve immediately or refrigerate to chill until ready to serve.

STORAGE: The salad can be stored covered in the fridge for 3 to 4 days.
SERVE IT WITH: To make this a complete meal, serve it with a bed of mixed salad greens.
PER SERVING
calories: 420 | fat: 26.1g | total carbs: 3.2g | fiber: 1.4g | protein: 41.7g

KALE AND AVOCADO SALAD WITH LEMON DIJON VINAIGRETTE DRESSING

Macros: Fat 85% | Protein 3% | Carbs 11%
Prep time: 25 minutes | Cook time: 15 minutes | Serves 4

The Kale and Avocado Salad is the perfect match for keto diet, especially when it is flavored with the Lemon Dijon Vinaigrette dressing. I personally tried it and it tastes amazingly good.

DRESSING:

1½ tablespoons Dijon mustard
2 tablespoons lemon juice
¼ teaspoon ground black

pepper
Sea salt, to taste
¼ cup olive oil

SALAD:

1 bundle kale, torn into small pieces
½ avocado, sliced
½ cup cucumber, chopped
⅔ cup cherry tomatoes, quartered

2 tablespoons red onion, chopped finely
⅓ cup red bell pepper, chopped finely
1 tablespoon feta cheese

1. In a bowl, mix Dijon mustard, lemon juice, black pepper, sea salt and olive oil together until well combined. Set aside.
2. Blanch the kale in a saucepan of salted water for about 45 seconds until hot.
3. Remove from the heat to a plate. Put the avocado, cucumber, cherry tomatoes, onion, bell pepper and feta cheese on top.
4. Pour the mustard mixture over the salad and toss well, then serve.

STORAGE: The salad can be stored covered in the fridge for 3 to 5 days.
SERVE IT WITH: The Kale and Avocado Salad can be a side dish with any other main dishes.
PER SERVING
calories: 187 | fat: 18.3g | total carbs: 5.8g | fiber: 2.8g | protein: 1.9g

TASTY SHRIMP SALAD

Macros: Fat 71% | Protein 26% | Carbs 3%
Prep time: 15 minutes | Cook time: 0 minutes | Serves 6

This Tasty Shrimp Salad is one of my best ways to enjoy shrimp. It is so easy to do, and the results are amazing! The sea flavor of the shrimp and the freshness of eggs, cherry tomatoes, and celery will give you a perfect eating experience.

1 pound (454 g) cooked shrimp, peeled and deveined
¾ cup mayonnaise, keto-friendly
2 hard-boiled eggs, chopped into chunks

1 cup cherry tomatoes, quartered
Salt and freshly ground black pepper, to taste
1 cup celery, chopped
½ cup onion, chopped

1. In a bowl, mix the mayonnaise, eggs, tomatoes, salt, and pepper together.
2. Combine the mixture with the peeled shrimp. Add the celery and onion. Toss to combine well, then serve.

STORAGE: The salad can be stored covered in the fridge for 3 to 4 days.
SERVE IT WITH: The shrimp salad can be a side dish with any other main dishes and will mix very well.
PER SERVING
calories: 322 | fat: 25.8g | total carbs: 2.8g | fiber: 0.7g | protein: 20.7g

MINT AND TUNA SALAD

Macros: Fat 38% | Protein 54% | Carbs 8%
Prep time: 15 minutes | Cook time: 0 minutes | Serves 6

Did you know that mint is a rich source of vitamins A, C, B2 and valuable minerals such as calcium, copper and magnesium? Well, the Mint and Tuna Salad provide a magical combination of the fresh mint and the delicious tuna.

1 (5-ounce / 142-g) can tuna, drained
6 ounces (170 g) garlic and herb-flavored feta cheese, crumbled
3 hearts Romaine lettuce, cut into pieces
1 cucumber, peeled and chopped
4 green onions, chopped finely

¼ cup olive oil
¼ cup lemon juice
4 cloves garlic, diced finely
¼ cup fresh parsley, minced
¼ cup fresh mint leaves, minced
Salt and freshly ground black pepper, to taste

1. In a bowl, mix together the tuna, feta cheese, lettuce, cucumber and green onion.
2. In another bowl, whisk together the olive oil, lemon juice, garlic, parsley, mint leaves, salt and pepper, then pour over the salad. Gently toss until well coated, then serve.

STORAGE: The salad can be stored covered in the fridge for 3 to 4 days.
SERVE IT WITH: The Mint and Tuna Salad can be a side dish with any other main dishes and will mix very well.
PER SERVING
calories: 418 | fat: 18.0g | total carbs: 9.5g | fiber: 1.5g | protein: 57.0g

BAKED SALSA CHICKEN

Macros: Fat 65% | Protein 31% | Carbs 4%
Prep time: 5 minutes | Cook time: 40 minutes | Serves 4

Do you wonder how to cook chicken in a healthy but surprisingly delicious way?
Baked Salsa Chicken will bring you a new way of perspective on salad.

1 tablespoon olive oil
4 skinless and boneless chicken breasts, halved
4 teaspoons mix taco seasoning

1 cup salsa
1 cup Cheddar cheese, shredded
2 tablespoons sour cream

1. Preheat the oven to 375°F (190°C).
2. Lightly grease a baking dish with olive oil, then arrange the chicken breasts on it.
3. Sprinkle with the mix taco seasoning and spread the salsa on top.
4. Bake in the preheated oven for 25 to 35minutes, or until the juices run clear.
5. Sprinkle the chicken with cheese evenly and continue baking for 3 to 5minutes more, or until the cheese is melted and bubbly. Top with sour cream to serve.

STORAGE: The dish can be wrapped with aluminum foil and stored in an airtight container in the fridge for up to 4 days or in the freezer for up to 1 month.
REHEAT: Microwave, covered, until the medium temperature is reached or reheat in a frying pan or air fryer / instant pot, covered, on medium.
SERVE IT WITH: You can serve it with leafy green salad or roasted vegetables on the side.
PER SERVING
calories: 508 | fat: 37.0g | total carbs: 5.6g | fiber: 0.5g | protein: 37.0g

SHRIMP SALAD WITH AVOCADO AND TOMATOES

Macros: Fat 42% | Protein 39% | Carbs 19%
Prep time: 25 minutes | Cook time: 0 minutes | Serves 4

Shrimp salad with avocado and tomatoes is a classic dish in summer that adds so much healthy value to your table. You can serve it on any meal. Dinner, lunch, or even breakfast, this dish of salad is splendid in all cases.

1 pound (454 g) cooked shrimp, peeled and chopped	1 onion, peeled and chopped into slices
2 avocados, peeled, pitted, and minced	¼ teaspoon freshly ground black pepper
2 tomatoes, finely rinsed and cubed	¼ teaspoon salt
	2 tablespoons lemon juice

1. In a large bowl, stir together the shrimp, avocados, tomatoes, and onion.
2. Sprinkle with pepper and salt, then stir in lemon juice. Serve chilled.

STORAGE: Shrimp salad with avocado and tomatoes can be stored for no more than 2 days in the fridge.
SERVE IT WITH: You can serve it with a bed of greens, yogurt, lettuce leaves and any low-carb juice.
PER SERVING
calories: 302 | fat: 15.2g | total carbs: 15.8g | fiber: 8.2g | protein: 30.2g

GREEN ANCHOVY DRESSING

Macros: Fat 99% | Protein 1% | Carbs 0%
Prep time: 10 minutes | Cook time: 5 minutes | Serves 6

Normal salad dressing is loaded with lots of sugar and processed chemical supplement and is forbidden to eat in keto diet. Well, creating a keto-friendly salad dressing becomes imminent! The green goddess dressing of 97% fat can be enjoyed contentedly pairing with your favorite vegetables without any worry.

1 green onion, chopped finely	chopped finely
2 cups keto-friendly mayonnaise	1 tablespoon tarragon-flavored vinegar
2 teaspoons fresh chives, chopped finely	2 teaspoons fresh parsley, chopped finely
4 anchovy fillets, minced	
1 teaspoon fresh tarragon,	

1. In a bowl, mix together chopped green onion, mayonnaise, fresh chives, minced anchovy fillets, fresh tarragon, tarragon-flavored vinegar, and parsley until well combined.
2. Place the mixture in a jar and put it in the refrigerator for 20 minutes and serve chilled.

STORAGE: Stored in an airtight container in the refrigerator for about 1 week.
SERVE IT WITH: It can be served as a dip, or toss with salad greens for a dressing.
PER SERVING
calories: 555 | fat: 62.3g | total carbs: 0.5g | fiber: 0.1g | protein: 0.8g

LOBSTER SALAD

Macros: Fat 70% | Protein 30% | Carbs 0%
Prep time: 10 minutes | Cook time: 0 minutes | Serves 4

Thinking of making a tasty, simple salad that can be stored for the next few days? Dennie's Lobster Salad is an amazing option. It's rich in flavor, and heart-freshening for your special day.

1 pound (454 g) cooked lobster meat, torn into bite-sized pieces	¼ cup keto-friendly mayonnaise
¼ cup melted butter	⅛ teaspoon freshly ground black pepper

1. In a medium bowl, put the lobster pieces and dunk them in the melted butter.
2. Mix in the mayonnaise and season with black pepper. Chill in the refrigerator for 20 minutes, then serve.

STORAGE: The salad can be stored covered in the fridge for 3 to 4 days.
SERVE IT WITH: To make this a complete meal, serve it with some green leaf lettuce.
PER SERVING
calories: 306 | fat: 24.1g | total carbs: 0.1g | fiber: 0g | protein: 21.7g

KETO QUICK CAESAR DRESSING

Macros: Fat 87% | Protein 8% | Carbs 5%
Prep time: 5 minutes | Cook time: 0 minutes | Serves 4

To enjoy your meal to the utmost, try to prepare this keto quick Caesar dressing. Cool yourself down with this cheesy buttered to put it in your dinner, lunch or even supper.

1½ ounces (42 g) Parmesan cheese, grated	1 pinch ground black pepper
¼ cup olive oil	½ garlic clove, minced
1 tablespoon Dijon mustard	½ teaspoon salt
1 teaspoon red wine vinegar	½ lemon, the juice

1. Whisk the Parmesan cheese, olive oil, mustard, wine vinegar, pepper, garlic well in a bowl except for the salt, until smooth, add salt and pepper to taste. Keep stirring.
2. To reduce the density of the mixture, gradually add about a teaspoon of water or lemon juice at a time to obtain the desired consistency.

STORAGE: Store the left dressing in an airtight container in the fridge for 5 days, and it can also be kept in the freezer for 30 days. It can serve with any meal.
SERVE IT WITH: Serve it with crunchy vegetables, high-fat cheese or serve it with a dish of warm Broccoli Cheddar Soup.
PER SERVING
calories: 169 | fat: 16.6g | total carbs: 2.3g | fiber: 0.2g | protein: 3.2g

TUNA STUFFED AVOCADOS

Macros: Fat 64% | Protein 20% | Carbs 15%
Prep time: 20 minutes | Cook time: 0 minutes | Serves 4

Planning for a trip and needs something simple and freshening to take? Avocado and Tuna Tapas is the great mix you would consider for its perfect combination between avocado and tuna.

1 can (12-ounce / 340-g) solid white tuna, drained	finely
1 tablespoon keto-friendly mayonnaise	A dash of balsamic vinegar
3 cups thinly diced green onions, plus more for garnish	Garlic salt and ground black pepper, to taste
½ red bell pepper, chopped	2 ripe avocados, pitted and cut in half

1. In a medium bowl, mix together tuna, mayonnaise, green onions, red bell pepper, and balsamic vinegar. Season with pepper and garlic salt. Using a spoon, stuff the avocado halves evenly with the tuna mixture.
2. Sprinkle the green onions on top for garnish before serving.

STORAGE: Store in an airtight container in the fridge for up to 3 days.
SERVE IT WITH: To make this a complete meal, serve it with roasted vegetables on the side.
PER SERVING
calories: 287 | fat: 21.5g | total carbs: 12.3g | fiber: 7.8g | protein: 14.4g

LOW-CARB DRESSING

Macros: Fat 98% | Protein 1% | Carbs 1%
Prep time: 10 minutes | Cook time: 0 minutes | Serves 6

Looking for a dip or dressing that is keto-friendly? This low-carb dressing perfectly pairs with your keto-friendly salads.

¼ cup keto-friendly mayonnaise	2 tablespoons lemon juice
¼ cup olive oil	2 tablespoons fresh parsley, chopped finely
2 tablespoons MTC oil	
1 tablespoon Dijon mustard	Himalayan pink salt and ground black pepper, to taste
2 cloves garlic, peeled and crushed	

1. In a jar, mix together mayonnaise, olive oil, MCT oil, Dijon mustard, garlic and lemon juice.
2. Add chopped parsley, salt and pepper. Tightly cover the jar, then shake until well combined, then serve.

STORAGE: This keto dressing can be stored in an airtight container in the refrigerator for about 1 week. You can store it in the freezer for up to 1 month.
SERVE IT WITH: The keto dressing can be served as a dip, or mix with salad greens.
PER SERVING
calories: 198 | fat: 21.5g | total carbs: 1.0g | fiber: 0.2g | protein: 0.3g

CHICKEN SALAD WITH RANCH DRESSING

Macros: Fat 76% | Protein 18% | Carbs 6%
Prep time: 5 minutes | Cook time: 20 minutes | Serve 4

Are you always looking for a delicious keto-friendly recipe? This chicken salad is low-carb and keto-friendly. It's healthy, easy and fresh.

RANCH DRESSING:

3 tablespoon keto-friendly mayonnaise	2 tablespoons water
	1 tablespoon ranch seasoning
2 eggs	lettuce, chopped
3 ounces (85 g) bacon	Salt and ground black pepper
½ pound (227 g) rotisserie chicken, cut into smaller pieces	2 ounces (57 g) blue cheese, crumbled
1 avocado, sliced	1 tablespoon fresh chives, minced
1 tomato, sliced	
5 ounces (142 g) Romaine	

1. Make the ranch dressing: Combine the mayonnaise, water and ranch seasoning in a bowl. Set aside.
2. Boil the eggs in a pot of salted water for 10 minutes. Remove the eggs to a bowl of cold water. Peel and chop them into small chunks.
3. Fry bacon in a skillet over medium heat for 4 minutes per side until crispy. Remove from the heat to a paper towel-lined plate.
4. In a salad bowl, combine the bacon, chicken, sliced avocado and tomato, chopped eggs, and lettuce. Season with salt and pepper.
5. Drizzle with ranch dressing and top with blue cheese and chives before serving.

STORAGE: Store in an airtight container in the fridge for up to 3 days.
SERVE IT WITH: You can serve this dish with creamy chowder and fresh lemon juice.
PER SERVING
calories: 469 | fat: 37.9g | total carbs: 7.5g | fiber: 4.3g | protein: 26.8g

GRILLED SALMON AND GREEK SALAD

Macros: Fat 55% | Protein 32% | Carbs 13%
Prep time: 15 minutes | Cook time: 10 minutes | Serves 4

Grilled salmon when served with a chilled salad is so satisfying. The salad is perfect for the evenings where you get home tired and just want something easy to fix. Within a few minutes, you will have your complete meal.

SALAD:

2 medium heads Romaine lettuce, chopped
½ medium cucumber, chopped
¾ cup feta cheese, crumbled
¾ cup cherry tomatoes, halved

½ cup red onions, thinly sliced
½ cup Kalamata olives, pitted
1 teaspoon dried ground oregano
Salt and freshly ground black pepper, to taste

DRESSING:

2 teaspoons dried ground oregano
2 tablespoons extra-virgin olive oil
2 teaspoons onion powder

1 large clove garlic, minced
¼ cup red wine vinegar
Salt and freshly ground black pepper, to taste

SALMON:

4 (6-ounce / 170-g) skin-on salmon fillets, rinsed and drained
1 tablespoon extra-virgin olive oil

Salt and freshly ground black pepper, to taste
1 tablespoon avocado oil, for greasing the grill grates
Fresh dill, for garnish

1. Put all the ingredients for salad in a large bowl and toss to combine well.
2. Divide the salad into four serving bowls and put aside.
3. In the meantime, make the dressing by adding the oregano, olive oil, onion powder, garlic, pepper, salt, and vinegar in another bowl. Stir thoroughly, then put aside.
4. Brush the salmon with olive oil on both sides, then season with pepper and salt to taste.
5. Preheat the grill to medium-high heat, then grease the grill grates with avocado oil.
6. Grill the salmon for 3 minutes, skin facing up. Turn the salmon over and grill for about 5 minutes, or until the internal temperature reads 145℉ (63℃).
7. Let the salmon rest for about 5 minutes, then put the fillets on top of the salad in four serving bowls. Pour the dressing over the salads and sprinkle the fresh dill on top for garnish before serving.

STORAGE: Store in separate airtight containers in the fridge for up to 3 days.
REHEAT: Microwave the salmon, covered, until the desired temperature is reached.
SERVE IT WITH: To make this a complete meal, you can serve it with Chinese-flavor mushroom and chicken broth.
PER SERVING
calories: 541 | fat: 33.3g | total carbs: 19.2g | fiber: 8.6g | protein: 42.7g

CHEESY KETO CHICKEN BROCCOLI CASSEROLE

Macros: Fat 74% | Protein 23% | Carbs 3%
Prep time: 15 minutes | Cook time: 35 minutes | Serves 6

The dish is an easy-and-quick side. You just need to prepare the ingredients and toss them in the oven for baking and move to busy work or entertainment activity. When the dish is done, the oven will call for you to enjoy the yummy meal!

2 tablespoons butter
¼ cup keto-friendly mayonnaise
½ cup Gouda cheese, shredded
8 ounces (227 g) softened cream cheese
¼ cup chicken broth
2 tablespoons dry ranch dressing mix

1¾ cups chicken, diced and well cooked
2 cups cooked broccoli, cut into florets
½ teaspoon salt
A pinch of ground black pepper
1½ cups Cheddar cheese, shredded

1. Preheat the oven to 350° F (180° C).
2. In a large nonstick skillet, melt the butter over medium heat. Mix in the mayonnaise, Gouda cheese, cream cheese, chicken broth and ranch dressing. Keep on stirring over low heat for 5 minutes until fully combined.
3. Add the chicken, broccoli, salt and pepper to the mixture. Stir well and transfer the mixture to a casserole dish, then sprinkle Cheddar cheese on the top.
4. Bake in the preheated oven for about 25 minutes. When the cheese is melted and the mixture is cooked, turn the oven to broil until the cheese gets browned.
5. Allow to cool for 5 minutes before serving.

STORAGE: Store the dish in an airtight container in the fridge for 3 days.
REHEAT: Microwave, covered, until the desired temperature is reached.
SERVE IT WITH: To make this a complete meal, you can serve it with roasted chicken thighs.
PER SERVING
calories: 541 | fat: 45.1g | total carbs: 4.9g | fiber: 0.8g | protein: 29.8g

Appendix 1: Measurement Conversion Chart

VOLUME EQUIVALENTS(DRY)

US STANDARD	METRIC (APPROXIMATE)
1/8 teaspoon	0.5 mL
1/4 teaspoon	1 mL
1/2 teaspoon	2 mL
3/4 teaspoon	4 mL
1 teaspoon	5 mL
1 tablespoon	15 mL
1/4 cup	59 mL
1/2 cup	118 mL
3/4 cup	177 mL
1 cup	235 mL
2 cups	475 mL
3 cups	700 mL
4 cups	1 L

VOLUME EQUIVALENTS(LIQUID)

US STANDARD	US STANDARD (OUNCES)	METRIC (APPROXIMATE)
2 tablespoons	1 fl.oz.	30 mL
1/4 cup	2 fl.oz.	60 mL
1/2 cup	4 fl.oz.	120 mL
1 cup	8 fl.oz.	240 mL
1 1/2 cup	12 fl.oz.	355 mL
2 cups or 1 pint	16 fl.oz.	475 mL
4 cups or 1 quart	32 fl.oz.	1 L
1 gallon	128 fl.oz.	4 L

TEMPERATURES EQUIVALENTS

FAHRENHEIT(F)	CELSIUS(C) (APPROXIMATE)
225 °F	107 °C
250 °F	120 °C
275 °F	135 °C
300 °F	150 °C
325 °F	160 °C
350 °F	180 °C
375 °F	190 °C
400 °F	205 °C
425 °F	220 °C
450 °F	235 °C
475 °F	245 °C
500 °F	260 °C

WEIGHT EQUIVALENTS

US STANDARD	METRIC (APPROXIMATE)
1 ounce	28 g
2 ounces	57 g
5 ounces	142 g
10 ounces	284 g
15 ounces	425 g
16 ounces (1 pound)	455 g
1.5 pounds	680 g
2 pounds	907 g

Appendix 2: Index

A

Alfalfa Sprout
Pecan And Veggies In Collard Wraps 60

Anchovy Fillet
Green Anchovy Dressing 176

Artichoke Heart
Tasty Artichoke Dip 136
Creamy Bacon Omelet 44
Spinach, Artichoke And Cauliflower Stuffed Red Bell Peppers 60

Almond
Keto Almond Butter Fudge Slices 155
Riced Broccoli With Almonds 56
Lemony Brussels Sprout Salad With Spicy Almond And Seed Mix 57
Crispy Almonds With Brussels Sprout Salad 173
Chocolate Granola Bars 152
Cheesy Baked Jalapeño Peppers 145
Keto Pumpkin Spice Fat Bombs 150
Crusted Zucchini Sticks 54
Almond And Cinnamon Truffles 158
Chilled Vanilla Ice Cream 161
Easy Coconut Mounds 157
Cheesy Crab Stuffed Mushrooms 146
Easy Coconut Mounds 157
Cheesy Crab Stuffed Mushrooms 146

Almond Flour
Cheesy Bacon Pancake With Parsley 31
Waffle Sandwiches 43
Bacon Quiche 43
Spanish Beef Empanadas 95
Cheesy Keto Blueberry Pancake 20
Almond Fritters With Mayo Sauce 143
Creamy Chicken And Ham Meatballs 65
Pie Keto Chicken Curry 74
Cream Cheese Brownies 156
Low-Carb Chocolate Chip Cookies 156
Keto Chocolate Cute Mug Cake 161
Lemon Allspice Muffins 47
Italian Metballs Parmigiana 96
Salmon Pie 105
Low Carb Keto Sausage Balls 143
Almond Sausage Balls 141
Classic Sausage & Beef Meatloaf 99
Almond Cinnamon Cookies 149
Almond Flour Shortbread Cookies 155
Frosted Snickerdoodle Cupcakes 153
Gooey Creamy Cake 158
Almond Snickerdoodle Cookies 158
Gingersnap Nutmeg Cookies 159
Almond Pumpkin Pie 161

Almond Meal
Almond Chicken Cordon Bleu 72
Healthy Hemp Seed Porridge 39
Almond Meal Cupcakes 149
Mini Cheesecakes 151
Cheesy Keto Cupcakes 147

Arugula
Simple Arugula Salad 22
Beef, Pork, And Vegetable Salad With Yoghurt Dressing 166
Zucchini And Walnut Salad 54
Keto Lemon Dressing, Walnuts And Zucchini Salad 173
Delicious Steak Salad 174

Avocado
Cabbage Plate With Keto Salmon 110
Spicy Shrimp And Chorizo Soup With Tomatoes And Avocado 125
Spinach Salad With Mustard Vinaigrette And Bacon 165
Spiced Eggs And Bacon Breakfast 16
Deviled Eggs With Bacon And Cheese 140
Avocado, Cucumber And Bacon Salad 166
Chicken And Egg Stuffed Avocado 41
Spicy Cheesy Stuffed Avocados 67
Massaged Collard And Avocado Salad 26
Crab–Stuffed Avocado 139
Coco Avocado Truffles 154
Creamy And Cheesy Spicy Avocado Soup 132
Kale And Avocado Salad With Lemon Dijon Vinaigrette Dressing 175
Keto Egg Butter And Smoked Salmon 113
Buttered Eggs With Avocado And Salmon 31
Tasty Avocado Shrimp Salad 171
Shrimp Salad With Avocado And Tomatoes 176
Guacamole 52
Tuna Stuffed Avocados 177
Spiralized Zucchini With Avocado Sauce 56
Scrambled Eggs With Cheese And Chili 41
Egg Avocado Cups 149

Asparagus
Greedy Keto Vegetable Mix 60
Prosciutto And Asparagus Wraps 139
Salmon Asparagus Pecan Salad 174
Asparagus Seared Salmon 111
Goat Cheese And Asparagus Omelet 38
Grilled Tuna Salad With Garlic Sauce 111
Easy Grilled Asparagus 27
Easy Asparagus With Parmesan 33
Easy Asparagus f1ry 52
Easy Asparagus With Walnuts 56
Asparagus And Pork Bake 55
Asparagus Cream Soup 122

B

Blackberry
Berry Tart 160
Seeds And Nuts Parfait 61
Cheesy Keto Blueberry Pancake 20
Healthy Blueberry Fat Bombs 156
Chia Pudding With Blueberries 156
Berry Tart 160

Blueberry Preserves
Chocolate And Blueberry Truffles 162

Brazil Nut
Healthy Hemp Seed Porridge 39

Broccoli
Greedy Keto Vegetable Mix 60
Bacon And Broccoli Egg Muffins 45
Creamy Beef And Broccoli Soup 128
Cheesy Cauliflower And Broccoli Bake 56
Creamy Broccoli And Cauliflower Soup 118
Cheesy Keto Chicken Broccoli Casserole 178
Roast Chicken With Broccoli And Garlic 80
Keto Fried Chicken With Broccoli 78
Delicious Fried Chicken With Broccoli 81
Crispy Keto Wings With Rich Broccoli 67
Cheesy Broccoli With Keto Fried Salmon 112
One-Pan Sausage & Broccoli 97
Crispy Keto Creamy Fish Casserole 108
Simple Broccoli Rabe 21
Lemon Broccoli With Almond Butter 23
Easy Broccoli And Cheese 28
Simple Broccoli Casserole 143
Almond Fritters With Mayo Sauce 143
Broccoli And Mushroom Soup Casserole 53
Easy Broccoli And Dill Salad 55
Riced Broccoli With Almonds 56
Broccoli Cheddar Soup 125
Easy Green Soup 129

Brussels Sprout
Low-Carb Chicken With Tricolore Roasted Veggies 76
Beef And Buttered Brussels Sprouts 94
Amazing Brussel Sprouts Salad 29
Baked Brussels Sprouts And Pine Nut With Bacon 102
Vegetables Tricolor 57
 Lemony Brussels Sprout Salad With Spicy Almond And Seed Mix 57
Brussel Sprouts And Spinach Salad 169
Brussels Sprouts Citrus Bacon Dressing 167
Crispy Almonds With Brussels Sprout 173
Salad Easy Parmesan Roasted Bamboo Sprouts 141

Butternut Squash 62
Zoodles With Butternut Squash And Sage 124
Zucchini Soup

Beef 21
Pork Beef Italian Meatballs 141
Baked Beef, Pork And Veal Meatballs Keto 135
Baked Eggs

Keto Broiled Bell Pepper 144
Beef & Veggie Hash 43
Sausage, Beef And Chili Recipe 92
Beef Mini Meatloaves 93
Sloppy Joes 92
Keto Burgers 93
Beef And Buttered Brussels Sprouts 94
Seasoned Beef Roast 89
Spanish Beef Empanadas 95
Keto Beef Burger 97
Beef Taco Soup 122
Keto Beef Soup 122
Zesty Double Beef Stew 123
Rich Beef Stew With Dumpling 121
Creamy Beef And Broccoli Soup 128
Zucchini Lasagna 58
Beef, Pork, And Vegetable Salad With Yoghurt Dressing 166

Beef Brisket
Braised Beef Brisket 87
Simple Spicy Beef Brisket 88

Beef Chuck
Beef Chuck Roast 88

Beef Short Rib
Keto Beef Stew 126

Beef Tenderloin
Seasoned Beef Roast 89

Beef Tenderloin Steak
Beef Tenderloin Steaks Wrapped 92

Bacon
Beef Mini Meatloaves 93
Keto Beef Burger 97
Beef Tenderloin Steaks Wrapped 92
Baked Brussels Sprouts And Pine Nut With Bacon 102
Brussels Sprouts Citrus Bacon Dressing 167
Cauliflower Leek Soup 128
Ranch Chicken And Bacon Salad 170
Bacon-Wrapped Chicken Breasts Stuffed With Spinach 75
Caesar Salad 83
Chicken Breast Wrapped With Bacon And Cauliflower Purée 85
Chicken Salad With Ranch Dressing 177
New England Clam Chowder 125
Tasty Collard Greens 50
Keto Kale And Bacon With Eggs 40
Keto Cheddar And Bacon Mushrooms 137
Cheddar Cheese Jalapeño Poppers 144
Pork Tarragon Soup 118
Cheesy Pork Chops And Bacon 91
Pork Chops With Caramelized Onion 98
Bacon, Smoked Salmon And Poached Egg Salad 168
Bay Scallop And Bacon Chowder 126
Keto Bacon-Wrapped Barbecue Shrimp 137
Spanish Egg Frittata 45
Spinach Salad With Mustard Vinaigrette And Bacon 165
Creamy Bacon And Tilapia Chowder 123

Gravy Bacon And Turkey   84
Cheesy Turkey And Bacon Soup With Celery And Parsley
    133
Spiced Eggs And Bacon Breakfast   16
Cheesy Bacon Pancake With Parsley   31
Bacon-Wrapped Jalapeno Poppers   136
Hearty Bacon And Mushroom Platter   139
Deviled Eggs With Bacon And Cheese   140
Cheesy Bacon Egg Cups   37
Creamy Bacon Omelet   44
Bacon And Broccoli Egg Muffins   45
Simple Scrambled Eggs   44
Waffle Sandwiches   43
Bacon Quiche   43
Breadless Egg Sandwich   48
Cauliflower Cream Soup   117
Sun-Dried Tomato And Feta Cheese Salad   166
Iceberg Lettuce Salad With Bacon And Gorgonzola Cheese
    167
Avocado, Cucumber And Bacon Salad   166

C

Cabbage
Spicy Shrimp And Veggies Cream Soup   130
Coleslaw With Crunchy Chicken Thighs   75
Lamb Soup   126
Coconut Keto Salmon And Napa Cabbage   108
Cabbage Plate With Keto Salmon   110
Keto Taco Fishbowl   106
Easy Baked Cabbage   52
Lemony Coleslaw   55

Calamari
Garlicky Pork Soup With Cauliflower And Tomatoes   132
Veggies And Calamari Salad   171

Cauliflower
Chicken Breast Wrapped With Bacon And Cauliflower Purée
    85
Low Carb Jambalaya With Chicken   46
Spinach, Artichoke And Cauliflower Stuffed Red Bell
Peppers   60
Cauliflower Cream Soup   117
Roasted Chicken Thighs And Cauliflower   85
Garlicky Pork Soup With Cauliflower And Tomatoes   132
Scrumptious Briam   63
Cheesy Cauliflower Crackers   139
Cheesy Cauliflower Bake   140
Cauliflower Bread Sticks With Cheese   147
Cauliflower Casserole   51
Cheesy Cauliflower Bake   51
Cauliflower Hash With Poblano Peppers And Eggs   55
Riced Cauliflower And Leek Risotto   61
Cheesy Cauliflower And Broccoli Bake   56
Cheesy Cauliflower Soup   117
Creamy Broccoli And Cauliflower Soup   118
Cauliflower Curry Soup   120
Cauliflower Leek Soup   128
Green Garlic And Cauliflower Soup   126
Creamy Garlic Pork With Cauliflower Soup   131
Creamy Veggie Soup   130

Simple Cauliflower Salad   170

Calf's Liver
Hearty Calf's Liver Platter   95

Capicola
Basic Capicola Egg Cups   44

Celery
Creamy Broccoli And Cauliflower Soup   118
Crabmeat And Celery Salad   169
Low Carb Seafood Chowder   112
Cheesy Keto Tuna Casserole   114
Sweet And Sour Chicken Soup With Celery   124
Easy Lunch Salad   169

Cherry Tomato
Avocado, Cucumber And Bacon Salad   166
Vegetables Tricolor   57
Salmon And Almond Salad   172
Luscious Vegetable Quiche   62
Grilled Tuna Salad With Garlic Sauce   111
Gravy Bacon And Turkey   84
Cheesy Chicken Dish With Spinach And Tomatoes   72
Tasty Shrimp Salad   175
Delicious Steak Salad   174
Low Carb Poached Eggs With Tuna Salad   109

Coconut
Breaded Chicken Strips And Spinach Salad   173
Coconut Keto Salmon And Napa Cabbage   108

Coconut Flour
Buttery Cheesy Garlic Chicken   69
Chocolate Tart   160
Roasted Lamb Rack   87
Vanilla Mug Cake   150
Buttered Coconut Puffs   140
Keto Matcha Brownies With Pistachios   159

Cranberry
Low-Carb Kale With Pork And Eggs   25
Chicken, Cranberry, And Pecan Salad   170

Cucumber
Beef, Pork, And Vegetable Salad With Yoghurt Dressing
    166
Crab–Stuffed Avocado   139
Kale And Avocado Salad With Lemon Dijon Vinaigrette
Dressing   175
Grilled Salmon And Greek Salad   178
Tasty Avocado Shrimp Salad   171
Mint And Tuna Salad   175

Cream Of Mushroom Soup
Simple Broccoli Casserole   143
Broccoli And Mushroom Soup Casserole   53

Chia Seed
Chia Pudding With Blueberries   156
Coffee Chia Smoothie   40

Collard
Pecan And Veggies In Collard Wraps 60

Chicken
Creamy Chicken And Ham Meatballs 65
Spicy Oven-Baked Chicken 70
Cheesy Low-Carb Chicken 69
Rotisserie-Style Roast Chicken 74
Pie Keto Chicken Curry 74
Oven-Baked Chicken In Garlic 77
Chubby And Juicy Roasted Chicken 77
Chicken Turnip Soup 119
Sweet And Sour Chicken Soup With Celery 124
Chicken, Cranberry, And Pecan Salad 170
Ranch Chicken And Bacon Salad 170
Cheesy Keto Chicken Broccoli Casserole 178
Easily Baked Buffalo Chicken Dip 138
Chicken Fajitas Bake 74
Rotisserie Chicken And Keto Chili-Flavored Béarnaise Sauce 82
Chicken Salad With Ranch Dressing 177
Lemon-Rosemary Roasted Cornish Hens 80

Chicken Breast
Buttery Cheesy Garlic Chicken 69
Easy Enchilada Chicken Dip 135
Buffalo Chicken And Cheese Dip 143
Chicken And Egg Stuffed Avocado 41
Buttery Chicken And Mushrooms 65
Italian Garlic Chicken Kebab 66
Spicy Burnt-Fried Chicken 67
Spicy Cheesy Stuffed Avocados 67
Chicken In Tomatoes And Herbs 66
Buttery Cheesy Garlic Chicken 69
Pan-Fried Creamy Chicken With Tarragon 69
Sour And Spicy Chicken Breast 69
Cheesy Chicken Dish With Spinach And Tomatoes 72
Delicious Parmesan Chicken 72
Keto Chicken Casserole 68
Almond Chicken Cordon Bleu 72
Grilled Chicken Breast 73
Bacon-Wrapped Chicken Breasts Stuffed With Spinach 75
Low-Carb Chicken With Tricolore Roasted Veggies 76
Chicken Breast With Guacamole 68
Chicken And Herb Butter With Keto Zucchini Roll-Ups 71
Keto Chicken With Herb Butter 78
Lemon Herb Chicken Breasts 75
Lime Chicken Ginger 83
Chicken With Tomato Cream 79
Simple Chicken Tonnato 79
Caesar Salad 83
Chicken Breast Wrapped With Bacon And Cauliflower Purée 85
Garlicky Chicken Soup 119
Sour Chicken And Kale Soup 130
Green Chicken Salad 168
Baked Salsa Chicken 175

Chicken Drumstick
Garlic Chicken Low-Carb 73
Buffalo Drumsticks With Chili Aioli 77
Chicken Provençale 84

Chicken Leg
Sour Pepper Chicken 66
Roast Chicken With Broccoli And Garlic 80
Chicken Skins
Crispy Chicken 145

Chicken Thigh
Low Carb Jambalaya With Chicken 46
Air-Fried Garlic-Lemon Chicken 65
Grilled Spiced Chicken 70
Spicy Garlic Chicken Kebabs 71
Coleslaw With Crunchy Chicken Thighs 75
Chicken With Mushrooms And Parmesan 78
Chicken With Coconut Curry 79
Grilled Tandori Chicken Thighs 81
Chicken Nuggets With Fried Green Bean And Bbq-Mayo 73
Keto Fried Chicken With Broccoli 78
Roasted Chicken Thighs And Cauliflower 85
Delicious Fried Chicken With Broccoli 81
Baked Chicken Thighs With Lemon Butter Caper Sauce 70
Chicken And Mushroom Soup 128
Creamy Crockpot Chicken Stew 129
Chicken Salad With Parmesan Cheese 166
Breaded Chicken Strips And Spinach Salad 173

Chicken Wing
Sweet And Zesty Chicken Wings 146
Crunchy Taco Chicken Wings 67
Crispy Keto Wings With Rich Broccoli 67
Savoury And Sticky Baked Chicken Wings 76
Chicken Wings And Blue Cheese Dip 82

Chocolate
Chocolate Tart 160
Easy Coconut Mounds 157
Strawberries In Chocolate 152
Cream Cheese Brownies 156
Low-Carb Chocolate Chip Cookies 156
Macadamia Nut And Chocolate Fat Bombs 157
Hemp Seeds And Chocolate Cookies 158
Chocolate-Crusted Coffee Bites 159
Keto Chocolate Cute Mug Cake 161
Chocolate And Blueberry Truffles 162
Chocolate Vanilla Cake 151
Chocolate Peanut Fudge 151
Chocolate Granola Bars 152
Keto Lava Cake 153
Coco Avocado Truffles 154
Double Chocolate Brownies 153
Keto Mocha Ice Cream 154
Chocolate-Strawberry Mousse 163

Chorizo
Chive Deviled Eggs And Savory Chorizo 147
Spicy Shrimp And Chorizo Soup With Tomatoes And Avocado 125

Clam
New England Clam Chowder 125

Coconut
Walnut Granola 41
Easy Coconut Mounds 157

Cod
Grilled Spicy Shrimp   107

Collard Greens
Massaged Collard And Avocado Salad   26
Tasty Collard Greens   50
Shichimi Collard Greens With Red Onion   59

Crab Meat
Cheesy Crab Stuffed Mushrooms   146
Crab–Stuffed Avocado   139
Crabmeat And Celery Salad   169

Crab Flakes
Colorful Crab Ceviche Appetizer   171

Cucumber
Red Gazpacho Cream Soup   120
Feta Cheese And Cucumber Salad   174
Easy Mediterranean Salad   171

E

Eggplant
Baba Ghanoush   138
Keto Burgers   93
Scrumptious Briam   63

Endive
Sloppy Joes   92

Egg
Cheesy Keto Cupcakes   147
Simple Arugula Salad   22
Spiced Eggs And Bacon Breakfast   16
Cheesy Bacon Pancake With Parsley   31
Deviled Eggs With Bacon And Cheese   140
Cheesy Bacon Egg Cups   37
Creamy Bacon Omelet   44
Bacon And Broccoli Egg Muffins   45
Simple Scrambled Eggs   44
Waffle Sandwiches   43
Bacon Quiche   43
Breadless Egg Sandwich   48
Keto Baked Eggs   135
Beef & Veggie Hash   43
Spanish Beef Empanadas   95
Rich Beef Stew With Dumpling   121
Zucchini Lasagna   58
Cheesy Keto Blueberry Pancake   20
Basic Capicola Egg Cups   44
Cheesy Cauliflower Crackers   139
Cauliflower Bread Sticks With Cheese   147
Cauliflower Hash With Poblano Peppers And Eggs   55
Chicken And Egg Stuffed Avocado   41
Delicious Parmesan Chicken   72
Green Chicken Salad   168
Rotisserie Chicken And Keto Chili-Flavored Béarnaise Sauce   82
Chocolate Tart   160
Cream Cheese Brownies   156
Low-Carb Chocolate Chip Cookies   156

Keto Chocolate Cute Mug Cake   161
Chive Deviled Eggs And Savory Chorizo   147
Chocolate Vanilla Cake   151
Keto Lava Cake   153
Double Chocolate Brownies   153
Keto Mocha Ice Cream   154
Chocolate-Strawberry Mousse   163
Lemon Allspice Muffins   47
Keto Cinnamon Flaxseed Bun Muffins   42
Paleo Omelet Muffins   47
Fluffy Western Omelet   144
Mexican-Style Scrambled Eggs   138
Keto Kale And Bacon With Eggs   40
Lettuce Soup With Poached Egg   124
Coconut Baked Lobster   26
Lettuce Wraps With Mackerel   168
Vinaigrette And Mushroom Frittata   38
Ham And Veggie Omelet In a Bag   48
Kale Pork Platter With Fried Eggs   101
Spicy Cheesy Eggs With Avocado And Cilantro   39
Pancakes With Cream And Raspberries   36
Vanilla Mug Cake   150
Low-Carb Raspberry Cheesecake   155
Browned Salmon Cakes   104
Keto Egg Butter And Smoked Salmon   113
Easy Lunch Salad   169
Scrambled Eggs With Salmon   37
Pumpkin Bread And Salmon Sandwich   36
Creamy Bagel Omelet   37
Salmon Pie   105
Low Carb Keto Sausage Balls   143
Sausage Breakfast   40
Easy Sausage, Egg, And Cheese Casserole   38
Classic Sausage & Beef Meatloaf   99
Everything Bagel Seasoned Eggs   40
Shrimp And Chives Omelet   42
Deviled Egg With Shrimp   105
Shrimp Salad With Egg And Mayonnaise   172
Tasty Shrimp Salad   175
Goat Cheese And Asparagus Omelet   38
Buttery Eggs With Avocado Ang Spinach   37
Eggs & Spinach Florentine   41
Spanish Egg Frittata   45
Microwaved Rhubarb Cakes   160
Pan Seared Tilapia With Almond Crust   105
Spicy Eggs With Cheese   36
Creamy Spanish Scrambled Eggs   46
Flaxseed With Olive And Tomato Focaccia   61
Low Carb Poached Eggs With Tuna Salad   109
Simple Parmesan Zucchini Fries   50
Buttered Coconut Puffs   140
Scrambled Eggs With Cheese And Chili   41
Egg Broth   118
Swiss Chard Egg Soup   121
Almond Meal Cupcakes   149
Almond Cinnamon Cookies   149
Egg Avocado Cups   149
Mini Cheesecakes   151
Frosted Snickerdoodle Cupcakes   153
Gooey Creamy Cake   158
Chilled Vanilla Ice Cream   161
Easy Peanut Butter Cookies   157
Almond Snickerdoodle Cookies   158

Gingersnap Nutmeg Cookies 159
Almond Pumpkin Pie 161
Smooth And Puffed Coconut Mousse 162
Caramel And Cream With Coconut Panna Cotta 162
Keto Matcha Brownies With Pistachios 159
Sumptuous Egg Salad 169
Egg Salad With Mustard Dressing 167

F

Flaxseeds
Microwaved Rhubarb Cakes 160
Lemon Allspice Muffins 47
Keto Cinnamon Flaxseed Bun Muffins 42

Flaxseed Meal
Almond Fritters With Mayo Sauce 143
Coffee Chia Smoothie 40

Fish Steak
Spiced Fish Curry 104

Flounder Fillet
Exotic Flounder With Lemon Sauce 34

G

Green Bean
Keto Green Beans 32
Syrian-Style Green Beans 51
Green Chicken Salad 168
Chicken Nuggets With Fried Green Bean And Bbq-Mayo 73
Seared Rump Steak Salad 165
Curried Shrimp And Green Beans Soup 133
Stir-Fried Zucchini With Green Beans 58

H

Ham
Almond Chicken Cordon Bleu 72
Ham And Veggie Omelet In a Bag 48
Paleo Omelet Muffins 47
Fluffy Western Omelet 144

Hazelnut
Brussel Sprouts And Spinach Salad 169
Almond Flour Shortbread Cookies 155

Hemp Seed
Hemp Seeds And Chocolate Cookies 158
Healthy Hemp Seed Porridge 39

Halibut Fillet
Spicy Halibut In Tomato Soup 127
Green Salad With Baked Halibut 172

J

Jalapeño
Delicious Keto Ceviche 115

Marinated Steak Sirloin Kabobs 90
Creamy And Cheesy Spicy Avocado Soup 132
Mexican-Style Scrambled Eggs 138

K

Kale
Low-Carb Kale With Pork And Eggs 25
Keto Kale And Bacon With Eggs 40
Kale And Avocado Salad With Lemon Dijon Vinaigrette Dressing 175
Sour Chicken And Kale Soup 130
Kale Pork Platter With Fried Eggs 101
Grilled White Fish With Zucchini 106

L

Lettuce
Keto Burgers 93
Keto Beef Burger 97
Caesar Salad 83
Chicken Salad With Ranch Dressing 177
Green Salad With Baked Halibut 172
Bacon, Smoked Salmon And Poached Egg Salad 168
Iceberg Lettuce Salad With Bacon And Gorgonzola Cheese 167
Chicken Breast With Guacamole 68
Chicken Salad With Parmesan Cheese 166
Chicken Fajitas Bake 74
Cheesy Lamb Sliders 96
Lettuce Wraps With Mackerel 168
Grilled Salmon And Greek Salad 178
Smoked Salmon Appetizer 116
Shrimp Salad With Egg And Mayonnaise 172
Mint And Tuna Salad 175
Lettuce Soup With Poached Egg 124

Lemon
Grilled Spicy Shrimp 142
Pan Seared Tilapia With Almond Crust 105

Lemongrass
Chicken With Coconut Curry 79

Lamb
Spicy Lamb Meat 94
Tangy Lamb Patties 100
Cheesy Lamb Sliders 96
Lamb Soup 126

Lamb Chop
Kalamata Parsley Tapenade And Salted Lamp Chops 87
Mint Oil Braised Lamb Chops 99

Lamb Leg
Zesty Lamb Leg 101
Herbed Lamb Leg 100

Lamb Loin Chop
Roasted Vietnamese Lamb Chops 99

Lamb Rack
Roasted Lamb Rack   87

Lamb Shank
Wine Braised Lamb Shanks   97

Lobster Meat
Coconut Baked Lobster   26
Buttered Lobster And Cream Cheese Dip   135
Lobster Salad   176

Lobster Tail
Grilled Red Lobster Tails   112

Macadamia Nut
Macadamia Nut And Chocolate Fat Bombs   157
Chocolate-Crusted Coffee Bites   159

M

Mushroom
Vegetables Tricolor   57
Buttery Chicken And Mushrooms   65
Keto Chicken Casserole   68
Low-Carb Chicken With Tricolore Roasted Veggies   76
Luscious Vegetable Quiche   62
Spinach Mushroom Soup   119
Spinach And Cheese Stuffed Mushrooms   142
Balsamic Mushrooms   137
Stuffed Cheesy Mushrooms   142
Vinaigrette And Mushroom Frittata   38
Ham And Veggie Omelet In a Bag   48
Spinach And Mushroom Italian-Style   50
Greedy Keto Vegetable Mix   60
Milky Mushroom Soup   54
Cheesy Crab Stuffed Mushrooms   146
Sauteed Mushroom   50
Sour And Spicy Shrimp Soup With Mushrooms   120
Riced Cauliflower And Leek Risotto   61
Chicken With Tomato Cream   79
Chicken With Mushrooms And Parmesan   78

Mackerel Fillet
Lettuce Wraps With Mackerel   168

Mahi Mahi
Tasty Mahi Mahi Cakes   106

Mahi Mahi Fillet
Stewed Mahi Mahi   119

Mushroom-Flat
Chicken And Mushroom Soup   128

Mushroom-White
Simple Scrambled Eggs   44
Creamy Pork Loin And Mushrooms   91

Mushroom-Wild
Hearty Bacon And Mushroom Platter   139

Mushroom-Portobello
Grilled Portobello Mushrooms   136
Mushroom Pizzas With Tomato Slices   58

O

Onion
Chicken Turnip Soup   119
Rotisserie-Style Roast Chicken   74
Shichimi Collard Greens With Red Onion   59
Easy Sausage, Egg, And Cheese Casserole   38
Italian Sausage Satay   89

Olive
Easy Mediterranean Salad   171
Kalamata Parsley Tapenade And Salted Lamp Chops   87
Flaxseed With Olive And Tomato Focaccia   61
Veggies And Calamari Salad   171
Simple Cauliflower Salad   170
Mediterranean Baked Spinach   141

P

Pepper-Jalapeño
Cheesy Baked Jalapeño Peppers   145
Cheddar Cheese Jalapeño Poppers   144
Easy Enchilada Chicken Dip   135

Pecan
Pecan And Veggies In Collard Wraps   60
Chicken, Cranberry, And Pecan Salad   170
Salmon Asparagus Pecan Salad   174

Pork Rind
Coleslaw With Crunchy Chicken Thighs   75
Asparagus And Pork Bake   55

Pumpkin
Rich Beef Stew With Dumpling   121

Pumpkin Seed
Iceberg Lettuce Salad With Bacon And Gorgonzola Cheese
                                                                167
Crispy Almonds With Brussels Sprout Salad   173

Peanut
Chocolate Peanut Fudge   151

Pepper-Bell
Crabmeat And Celery Salad   169
Colorful Sausage & Bell Peppers Combo   102
Keto Broiled Bell Pepper   144

Pepper-Red
Red Pepper Roasted Dip   137

Pepper-Poblano
Cauliflower Hash With Poblano Peppers And Eggs   55

Pine Nut
Seeds And Nuts Parfait   61
Baked Brussels Sprouts And Pine Nut With Bacon   102

Pork

Baked Beef, Pork And Veal Meatballs	141
Creamy Garlic Pork With Cauliflower Soup	131
Pork Beef Italian Meatballs	21
Divine Stuffed Pork Chops	33
Baked Pork Gyros	94
Italian Metballs Parmigiana	96
Pork Tarragon Soup	118
Stewed Meat And Pumpkin	129
Spicy Pork And Spinach Stew	131

Pork Chop

Cheese Stuffed Pork Chops	90
Seasoned Pork Chops	89
Basil-Rubbed Pork Chops	91
Cheesy Pork Chops And Bacon	91
Pork Chops With Dijon Mustard	93
Coconut Pork Chops	95
Pork Chops With Caramelized Onion	98

Pork Loin

Pecan Crusted Pork Chops	28
Saucy Pernil Pork	88
Creamy Pork Loin And Mushrooms	91
Lemony Pork Loin Roast	98
Thai Pork Meal	99

Pork Loin Chop

Pork Chops Stuffed With Cheese-Bacon Mix	98

Pork Rib

Garlicky Pork Soup With Cauliflower And Tomatoes	132

Pork Belly-Smoked

Low-Carb Kale With Pork And Eggs	25
Kale Pork Platter With Fried Eggs	101

Prosciutto

Creamy Pork Tenderloin	88

Pumpkin Puree

Stewed Meat And Pumpkin	129
Pumpkin Bread And Salmon Sandwich	36

Pork Shoulder

Lemony Pork Bake	91

Pork Tenderloin

Sweet And Spicy Pork	101
Creamy Pork Tenderloin	88
Garlicky Pork Roast	89
Spiced Pork Tenderloin	90
Bbq Party Pork Kabobs	96

Prosciutto

Prosciutto And Asparagus Wraps	139

Pumpkin Purée

Keto Pumpkin Spice Fat Bombs	150

Q

Queso Fresco

Spicy Cheesy Eggs With Avocado And Cilantro	39

R

Rainbow Trout Fillet

Trout Fillets With Lemony Yogurt Sauce	115

Raspberry

Pancakes With Cream And Raspberries	36
Vanilla Mug Cake	150
Low-Carb Raspberry Cheesecake	155
Raspberry And Chocolate Fat Bombs	152
Berry Tart	160
Watercress And Arugula Turkey Salad	165

Rump Steak

Seared Rump Steak Salad	165

Radish

Creamy Crockpot Chicken Stew	129
Bay Scallop And Bacon Chowder	126
Shrimp Mushroom Chowder	117
Creamy Bacon And Tilapia Chowder	123
Keto Beef Stew	126
Salmon And Almond Salad	172

Rutabaga

Sausage And Spinach Hash Bowl	47
Walnut Granola	41

S

Spinach

Keto Chicken Casserole	68
Bacon-Wrapped Chicken Breasts Stuffed With Spinach	75
Easy Green Soup	129
Brussel Sprouts And Spinach Salad	169
Creamy Veggie Soup	130
Cheesy Chicken Dish With Spinach And Tomatoes	72
Creamy Crockpot Chicken Stew	129
Breaded Chicken Strips And Spinach Salad	173
Spinach And Cheese Stuffed Mushrooms	142
Spinach And Mushroom Italian-Style	50
Divine Stuffed Pork Chops	33
Spicy Pork And Spinach Stew	131
Keto Chili-Covered Salmon With Spinach	113
Simple Baked Salmon Salad	34
Cheesy Sausage Soup With Tomatoes And Spinach	132
Cheesy Keto Tuna Casserole	114
Cheesy Chicken Dish With Spinach And Tomatoes	72
Coconut Cream Spinach	18
Mediterranean Baked Spinach	141
Goat Cheese And Asparagus Omelet	38
Buttery Eggs With Avocado Ang Spinach	37
Eggs & Spinach Florentine	41
Sausage And Spinach Hash Bowl	47
Spanish Egg Frittata	45
Spinach Casserole	51

Luscious Vegetable Quiche	62
Spinach, Artichoke And Cauliflower Stuffed Red Bell Peppers	60
Spinach Mushroom Soup	119
Creamy Spinach Soup	131
Creamy Minty Spinach Soup	123
Spinach Salad With Mustard Vinaigrette And Bacon	165
Green Salad With Baked Halibut	172

Shrimp

Spicy Shrimp And Veggies Cream Soup	130
Low Carb Seafood Chowder	112
Sauteed Sausage And Shrimp	22
Keto Bacon-Wrapped Barbecue Shrimp	137
Grilled Spicy Shrimp	142
Shrimp And Chives Omelet	42
Deviled Egg With Shrimp	105
Grilled Spicy Shrimp	107
Keto Maui Wowie Shrimp	110
Cheesy Verde Shrimp	113
Best Marinated Grilled Shrimp	114
Classic Shrimp Scampi	109
Shrimp Mushroom Chowder	117
Curried Shrimp And Green Beans Soup	133
Easy Brazilian Shrimp Stew (Moqueca De Camaroes)	127
Spicy Shrimp And Chorizo Soup With Tomatoes And Avocado	125
Sour And Spicy Shrimp Soup With Mushrooms	120
Tasty Avocado Shrimp Salad	171
Shrimp Salad With Avocado And Tomatoes	176
Shrimp Salad With Egg And Mayonnaise	172
Tasty Shrimp Salad	175

Sausage

Low Carb Keto Sausage Balls	143
Almond Sausage Balls	141
Sausage Breakfast	40
Easy Sausage, Egg, And Cheese Casserole	38
Italian Sausage Satay	89
One-Pan Sausage & Broccoli	97
Colorful Sausage & Bell Peppers Combo	102
Classic Sausage & Beef Meatloaf	99
Cheesy Sausage Soup With Tomatoes And Spinach	132
Sausage, Beef And Chili Recipe	92
Low Carb Jambalaya With Chicken	46
Sauteed Sausage And Shrimp	22
Sausage And Spinach Hash Bowl	47

Strawberry

Seeds And Nuts Parfait	61
Chocolate-Strawberry Mousse	163
Strawberry Smoothie Bowl	45
Cheesecake Strawberries	150
Strawberries In Chocolate	152
Strawberry Popsicles	157
Microwaved Rhubarb Cakes	160
Seeds And Nuts Parfait	61

Scallop

Bay Scallop And Bacon Chowder	126

Sesame Seed

Everything Bagel Seasoned Eggs	40

Sirloin Steak

Marinated Steak Sirloin Kabobs	90
Delicious Steak Salad	174

Snow Crab

Snow Crab Clusters With Garlic Butter	104

Sirloin Beef Steak

Low-Carb Buttered Sirloin Steak	32
Garlicky Beef Steak	94

Swordfish Steak

Stuffed Mediterranean Swordfish	109

Spaghetti Squash

Sausage Breakfast	40

Salmon

Browned Salmon Cakes	104
Cheesy Broccoli With Keto Fried Salmon	112
Keto Chili-Covered Salmon With Spinach	113
Keto Egg Butter And Smoked Salmon	113
Keto Baked Salmon With Butter	113
Coconut Keto Salmon And Napa Cabbage	108
Cabbage Plate With Keto Salmon	110
Buttery Salmon And Leek Soup	124
Bacon, Smoked Salmon And Poached Egg Salad	168
Easy Lunch Salad	169
Salmon And Almond Salad	172
Salmon Asparagus Pecan Salad	174
Scrambled Eggs With Salmon	37
Buttered Eggs With Avocado And Salmon	31
Keto Smoked Salmon Fat Bombs	138
Pumpkin Bread And Salmon Sandwich	36
Creamy Bagel Omelet	37
Salmon Pie	105
Smoked Salmon Appetizer	116
Creamy Salmon Sauce Zoodles	114

Salmon Fillet

Easy Stewed Salmon	27
Simple Baked Salmon Salad	34
Salmon Blackened Fillets	108
Salmon Fillets With Dill And Lemon	107
Easy Salmon Steaks With Dill	107
Salmon With Tomato And Basil	107
Keto Baked Salmon With Butter	113
Low Carb Seafood Chowder	112
Salmon Fillets Baked With Dijon	115
Salmon With Garlic Dijon Mustard	111
Asparagus Seared Salmon	111
Grilled Salmon And Greek Salad	178
Creamed Omega-3 Salad	170

T

Tomato

Sausage, Beef And Chili Recipe	92
Spicy Cheesy Stuffed Avocados	67
Cheesy Chicken Dish With Spinach And Tomatoes	72
Chicken With Tomato Cream	79
Easy Mediterranean Salad	171

Cheesy Lamb Sliders	96
Garlicky Pork Soup With Cauliflower And Tomatoes	132
Seared Rump Steak Salad	165
Shrimp Salad With Avocado And Tomatoes	176
Keto Taco Fishbowl	106
Sun-Dried Tomato And Feta Cheese Salad	166
Beef Taco Soup	122
Veggies And Calamari Salad	171
Simple Cauliflower Salad	170
Chicken In Tomatoes And Herbs	66
Colorful Crab Ceviche Appetizer	171
Red Gazpacho Cream Soup	120
Spiced Fish Curry	104
Spicy Halibut In Tomato Soup	127
Mexican-Style Scrambled Eggs	138
Mushroom Pizzas With Tomato Slices	58
Spicy Cheesy Eggs With Avocado And Cilantro	39
Salmon With Tomato And Basil	107
Buttery Eggs With Avocado Ang Spinach	37
Ritzy Ratatouille	53
Creamy Tomato Soup	123
Tomatoes And Jalapeño Salsa	136
Spicy Eggs With Cheese	36
Creamy Spanish Scrambled Eggs	46
Guacamole	52
Flaxseed With Olive And Tomato Focaccia	61
Caprese Salad	172

Turnip
Pork Tarragon Soup	118
Chicken Turnip Soup	119

Tomatillo
Tomatoes And Jalapeño Salsa	136

Tuna
Simple Chicken Tonnato	79
Low Carb Poached Eggs With Tuna Salad	109
Grilled Tuna Salad With Garlic Sauce	111
Cheesy Keto Tuna Casserole	114
Mint And Tuna Salad	175
Tuna Stuffed Avocados	177

Tuna Steak
Ahi Tuna Steaks	111

Tilapia
Creamy Bacon And Tilapia Chowder	123

Tilapia Fillet
Pan Seared Tilapia With Almond Crust	105

Trout Fillet
Blackened Trout	115
Michigander-Style Turkey	76
Gravy Bacon And Turkey	84
Cheesy Turkey And Bacon Soup With Celery And Parsley	133

Turkey Breast
Watercress And Arugula Turkey Salad	165

V

Veal
Baked Beef, Pork And Veal Meatballs	141

W

Walnut
Chocolate Granola Bars	152
Zucchini And Walnut Salad	54
Keto Lemon Dressing, Walnuts And Zucchini Salad	173
Easy Asparagus With Walnuts	56
Chocolate And Blueberry Truffles	162
Walnut Granola	41
Strawberry Smoothie Bowl	45
Cardamom Orange Bark	155

White Fish
Keto Taco Fishbowl	106
Crispy Keto Creamy Fish Casserole	108
Grilled White Fish With Zucchini	106
Delicious Keto Ceviche	115

Watercress
Watercress And Arugula Turkey Salad	165
Creamy Veggie Soup	130

Z

Zucchini
Sour And Spicy Shrimp Soup With Mushrooms	120
Beef & Veggie Hash	43
Zucchini Lasagna	58
Chicken And Herb Butter With Keto Zucchini Roll-Ups	71
Creamed Omega-3 Salad	170
Creamy Salmon Sauce Zoodles	114
Shrimp Mushroom Chowder	117
Grilled White Fish With Zucchini	106
Simple Parmesan Zucchini Fries	50
Oven-Baked Keto Zucchini	52
Crusted Zucchini Sticks	54
Zucchini And Walnut Salad	54
Spiralized Zucchini With Avocado Sauce	56
Ritzy Ratatouille	53
Zoodles With Butternut Squash And Sage	62
Zucchini Manicotti	59
Scrumptious Briam	63
Stir-Fried Zucchini With Green Beans	58
Zucchini Cream Soup	121
Sour Garlic Zucchini Soup	127
Cheesy Zucchini Soup	122
Keto Lemon Dressing, Walnuts And Zucchini Salad	173

Dear Readers and Friends:

This is an invitation to step closer to us by voicing your opinion about our book.

We are a group of dietitians and nutritionists who are so keen about diets, nutrition, and lifestyle that we have devoted our past 6 years researching, developing, testing, and writing recipes and cookbooks. This is the profession we take so much pride in, and we strive to write high-quality recipes and produce value-packed cookbooks.

If you like our books, please do us a favor and leave an objective, honest and detailed review on our amazon page, the more specific, the better! It may take only a couple of minutes, but would mean the world to us.

We will never stop devoting our careers and minds to producing more high-quality cookbooks to serve you better.

CPSIA information can be obtained
at www.ICGtesting.com
Printed in the USA
BVHW050156130820
586212BV00007B/150